T0205845

Statistics in the Health Sciences

Statistics in the Health Sciences
Theory, Applications, and Computing

By
Albert Vexler
The State University of New York at Buffalo, USA
Alan D. Hutson
Roswell Park Cancer Institute, USA

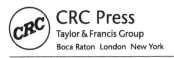

CRC Press
Taylor & Francis Group
Boca Raton London New York

CRC Press is an imprint of the
Taylor & Francis Group, an **Informa** business

CRC Press
Taylor & Francis Group
6000 Broken Sound Parkway NW, Suite 300
Boca Raton, FL 33487-2742

First issued in paperback 2022

© 2018 by Taylor & Francis Group, LLC
CRC Press is an imprint of Taylor & Francis Group, an Informa business

No claim to original U.S. Government works

ISBN 13: 978-1-03-240200-0 (pbk)
ISBN 13: 978-1-138-19689-6 (hbk)

DOI: 10.1201/b21899

Library of Congress Cataloging-in-Publication Data

Names: Vexler, Albert, author. | Hutson, Alan D., author.
Title: Statistics in the health sciences : theory, applications, and computing / Albert Vexler and Alan D. Hutson.
Description: Boca Raton, Florida : CRC Press, [2018] | Includes bibliographical references and index.
Identifiers: LCCN 2017031841| ISBN 9781138196896 (hardback) | ISBN 9781315293776 (e-book) | ISBN 9781315293769 (e-book) | ISBN 9781315293752 (e-book) | ISBN 9781315293745 (e-book)
Subjects: LCSH: Medical statistics. | Medicine–Research–Statistical methods. | Epidemiology–Statistical methods. | Statistical hypothesis testing.
Classification: LCC R853.S7 V48 2018 | DDC 610.2/1–dc23
LC record available at https://lccn.loc.gov/2017031841

Visit the Taylor & Francis Web site at
http://www.taylorandfrancis.com

and the CRC Press Web site at
http://www.crcpress.com

To my parents, Octyabrina and Alexander, and my son, David

Albert Vexler

To my wife, Brenda, and three kids, Nick, Chance, and Trey

Alan D. Hutson

Table of Contents

Preface—Please Read!

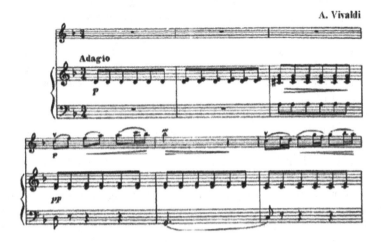

A. Vivaldi

In all likelihood, the Universe of Statistical Science is "relatively" or "privately" infinite and expanding in a similar manner to our Universe, satisfying the property of a science that is alive. Hence, it would be absolute impossibility to include everything in one book written by humans. One of our major goals is to provide the readers a small but efficient "probe" that could assist in Statistical Space discoveries.

The primary objective of the this book is to provide a compendium of statistical techniques ranging from classical methods through bootstrap strategies to modern recently developed statistical techniques. These methodologies may be applied to various problems encountered in health-related studies.

Historically, initial developments in statistical science were induced by real-life problems, when appropriate statistical instruments employed empirical arguments. Perhaps, since the eighteenth century, the heavy convolution between mathematics, probability theory, and statistical methods has provided the fundamental structures for correct statistical and biostatistical techniques. However, we cannot ignore a recent trend toward redundant simplifications of statistical considerations via so called "intuitive" and "applied" claims in complex statistical applications. It is our experience that applied statisticians or users often neglect the underlying postulates when implementing formal statistical procedures and with respect to the interpretation of their results. A very important motivation towards writing this book was to better refocus the scientist towards understanding the underpinnings of appropriate statistical inference in a well-rounded fashion. Maybe now is the time to draw more attention of theoretical and applied researchers to methodological standards in statistics and biostatistics? In contrast with many biostatistical books, we focus on rigorous formal proof schemes and their extensions regarding different statistical principles. We also show the basic ingredients and methods for constructing and examining correct and powerful statistical processes.

The material in the book should be appropriate for use both as a text and as a reference. In our book readers can find classical and new theoretical methods, open problems, and new procedures across a variety of topics for their scholarly investigations. We present results that are novel to the current set of books on the market and results that are even new with respect to the modern scientific literature. Our aim is to draw the attention of theoretical statisticians and practitioners in epidemiology and/or clinical research to the necessity of new developments, extensions and investigations related to statistical methods and their applications. In this context, for example, we would like to emphasize for whom is interested in advanced topics the following aspects. Chapter 1 lays out a variety of notations, techniques and foundations basic to the material that is treated in this book. Chapter 2 introduces the powerful analytical instruments that, e.g., consist of principles of Tauberian theorems, including new results, with applications to convolution problems, evaluations of sequential procedures, renewal functions, and risk-efficient estimations. In this chapter we also consider problems of reconstructing the general distribution based on the distribution of some observed statistics. Chapter 3 shows certain nontrivial conclusions regarding the parametric likelihood ratios. Chapter 4 is developed to demonstrate a strong theoretical instrument based on martingales and their statistical applications, which include the martingale principle for testing statistical hypotheses and comparisons between the cumulative sum technique and the Shiryayev–Roberts approach employed in change point detection policies. A part of material shown in Chapter 4 can be found only in this book. Chapter 5 can assist the statistician in developing and analyzing various Bayesian procedures. Chapter 8 provides the fundamental components for constructing unconventional statistical decision-making procedures with power one. Chapter 9 proposes novel approaches to examine, compare, and visualize properties of various statistical tests using correct p-value-based mechanisms. Chapter 10 introduces the empirical likelihood methodology. The theoretical propositions shown in Chapter 10 can lead to a quite mechanical and simple way to investigate properties of nonparametric likelihood–based statistical schemes. Several of these results can be found only in this book. In Chapter 14 one can discover interesting open problems. This book also provides software code based on both the R and SAS statistical software packages to exemplify the statistical methodological topics and their applied aspects.

Indeed, we focused essentially on developing a very informative textbook that introduces classical and novel statistical methods with respect to various biostatistical applications. Towards this end we employ our experience and relevant material obtained via our research and teaching activity across

10–15 years of biostatistical practice and training Master and PhD level students in the department of biostatistics. This book is intended for graduate students majoring in statistics, biostatistics, epidemiology, health-related sciences, and/or in a field where a statistics concentration is desirable, particularly for those who are interested in formal statistical mechanisms and their evaluations. In this context Chapters 1–10 and 12–14 provides teaching sources for a high level statistical theory course that can be taught in a statistical/biostatistical department. The presented material evolved in conjunction with teaching such a one-semester course at The New York State University at Buffalo. This course, entitled "Theory of Statistical Inference," has belonged to a set of the four core courses required for our biostatistics PhD program.

This textbook delivers a "ready-to-go" well-structured product to be employed in developing advanced biostatistical courses. We offer lectures, homework questions, and their solutions, examples of midterm, final, and Ph.D. qualifying exams as well as examples of students' projects.

One of the ideas regarding this book's development is that we combine presentations of traditional applied and theoretical statistical methods with computationally extensive bootstrap type procedures that are relatively novel data-driven statistical tools. Chapter 11 is proposed to help instructors acquire a statistical course that introduces the Jackknife and Bootstrap methods. The focus is on the statistical functional as the key component of the theoretical developments with applied examples provided to illustrate the corresponding theory.

We strongly suggest to begin lectures by asking students to smile!

It is recommended to start each lecture class by answering students' inquiries regarding the previously assigned homework problems. In this course, we assume that students are encouraged to present their work in class regarding individually tailored research projects (e.g., Chapter 14). In this manner, the material of the course can be significantly extended.

Our intent is not that this book competes with classical fundamental guides such as, e.g., Bickel and Doksum (2007), Borovkov (1998), and Serfling (2002). In our course, we encourage scholars to read the essential works of the world-renown authors. We aim to present different theoretical approaches that are commonly used in modern statistics and biostatistics to (1) analyze properties of statistical mechanisms; (2) compare statistical procedures; and (3) develop efficient (optimal) statistical schemes. Our target is to provide scholars research seeds to spark new ideas. Towards this end, we demonstrate open problems, basic ingredients in learning complex statistical notations and tools as well as advanced nonconventional methods, even in simple cases of statistical operations, providing "**Warning**" remarks to show potential difficulties related to the issues that were discussed.

Finally, we would like to note that this book attempts to represent a part of our life that definitely consists of mistakes, stereotypes, puzzles, and so on, that we all love. Thus our book cannot be perfect. We truly thank the reader

for his/her participation in our life! We hope that the presented material can
play a role as prior information for various research outputs.

Albert Vexler
Alan D. Hutson

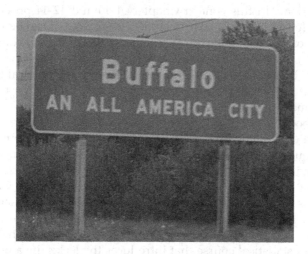

Authors

Albert Vexler, PhD, obtained his PhD degree in Statistics and Probability Theory from the Hebrew University of Jerusalem in 2003. His PhD advisor was Moshe Pollak, a fellow of the American Statistical Association and Marcy Bogen Professor of Statistics at Hebrew University. Dr. Vexler was a postdoctoral research fellow in the Biometry and Mathematical Statistics Branch at the National Institute of Child Health and Human Development (National Institutes of Health). Currently, Dr. Vexler is a tenured Full Professor at the State University of New York at Buffalo, Department of Biostatistics. Dr. Vexler has authored and co-authored various publications that contribute to both the theoretical and applied aspects of statistics in medical research. Many of his papers and statistical software developments have appeared in statistical/biostatistical journals, which have top-rated impact factors and are historically recognized as the leading scientific journals, and include: *Biometrics, Biometrika, Journal of Statistical Software, The American Statistician, The Annals of Applied Statistics, Statistical Methods in Medical Research, Biostatistics, Journal of Computational Biology, Statistics in Medicine, Statistics and Computing, Computational Statistics and Data Analysis, Scandinavian Journal of Statistics, Biometrical Journal, Statistics in Biopharmaceutical Research, Stochastic Processes and Their Applications, Journal of Statistical Planning and Inference, Annals of the Institute of Statistical Mathematics, The Canadian Journal of Statistics, Metrika, Statistics, Journal of Applied Statistics, Journal of Nonparametric Statistics, Communications in Statistics, Sequential Analysis, The STATA Journal; American Journal of Epidemiology, Epidemiology, Paediatric and Perinatal Epidemiology, Academic Radiology, The Journal of Clinical Endocrinology & Metabolism, Journal of Addiction Medicine, and Reproductive Toxicology and Human Reproduction.*

Dr. Vexler was awarded National Institutes of Health (NIH) grants to develop novel nonparametric data analysis and statistical methodology. His research interests are related to the following subjects: receiver operating characteristic curves analysis; measurement error; optimal designs; regression models; censored data; change point problems; sequential analysis; statistical epidemiology; Bayesian decision-making mechanisms; asymptotic methods of statistics; forecasting; sampling; optimal testing; nonparametric tests; empirical likelihoods, renewal theory; Tauberian theorems; time series; categorical analysis; multivariate analysis; multivariate testing of complex hypotheses; factor and principal component analysis; statistical biomarker evaluations; and best combinations of biomarkers. Dr. Vexler is Associate Editor for *Biometrics* and *Journal of Applied Statistics*. These journals belong to the first cohort of academic literature related to the methodology of biostatistical and epidemiological research and clinical trials.

Alan D. Hutson, PhD, received his BA (1988) and MA (1990) in Statistics from the State University of New York (SUNY) at Buffalo. He then worked for Otsuka America Pharmaceuticals for two years as a biostatistician. Dr. Hutson then received his MA (1993) and PhD (1996) in Statistics from the University of Rochester. His PhD advisor was Professor Govind Mudholkar, a world-renown researcher in Statistics and Biostatistics. He was hired as a biostatistician at the University of Florida in 1996 as a Research Assistant Professor and worked his way to a tenured Associate Professor. He had several roles at the University of Florida including Interim Director of the Division of Biostatistics and Director of the General Clinical Research Informatics Core. Dr. Hutson moved to the University at Buffalo in 2002 as an Associate Professor and Chief of the Division of Biostatistics. He was the founding chair of the new Department of Biostatistics in 2003 and became a full professor in 2007. His accomplishments as Chair included the implementation of several new undergraduate and graduate degree programs and a substantial growth in the size and quality of the department faculty and students. In 2005, Dr. Hutson also became Chair of Biostatistics (now Biostatistics and Bioinformatics) at Roswell Park Cancer Institute (RPCI), was appointed Professor of Oncology, and became the Director of the Core Cancer Center Biostatistics Core. Dr. Hutson helped implement the new Bioinformatics Core at RPCI. He recently became the Deputy Group Statistician for the NCI national NRG cancer cooperative group. Dr. Hutson is Fellow of the American Statistical Association. He is Associate Editor of *Communications in Statistics,* Associate Editor of the *Sri Lankan Journal of Applied Statistics,* and is a New York State NYSTAR Distinguished Professor. He has membership on several data safety and monitoring boards and has served on several high level scientific review panels. He has over 200 peer-reviewed publications. In 2013, Dr. Hutson was inducted into the Delta Omega Public Health Honor Society, Gamma Lambda Chapter. His methodological work focuses on nonparametric methods for biostatistical applications as it pertains to statistical functionals. He has several years of experience in the design and analysis of clinical trials.

1

Prelude: Preliminary Tools and Foundations

1.1 Introduction

The purpose of this opening chapter is to supplement the reader's knowledge of elementary mathematical analysis, probability theory, and statistics, which the reader is assumed to have at his or her disposal. This chapter is intended to outline the foundational components and definitions as treated in subsequent chapters. The introductory literature, including various foundational textbooks in the fields, can be easily found to complete this chapter material in details. In this chapter we also present several important comments regarding the implementation of mathematical constructs in the proofs of the statistical theorems that will provide the reader with a rigorous understanding of certain fundamental concepts. In addition to the literature cited in this chapter we suggest the reader consult the book of Petrov (1995) as a fundamental source. The book of Vexler et al. (2016 a) will provide the readers an entree into the following cross-cutting topics: *Data, Statistical Hypotheses, Errors Related to the Statistical Testing Mechanism (Type I and II Errors), P-values, Parametric and Nonparametric Approaches, Bootstrap, Permutation Testing, Measurement Errors.*

In this book we primarily deal with certain methodological and practical tools of biostatistics. Before introducing powerful statistical and biostatistical methods it is necessary to outline some important fundamental concepts such as mathematical limits, random variables, distribution functions, integration, convergence, complex variables and examples of statistical software in the following sections.

1.2 Limits

The statistical discipline deals particularly with real-world objects but its asymptotic theory oftentimes consists of concepts that employ the symbols "$\rightarrow$" (convergence) and "∞" (infinity). These concepts are not related directly to a fantasy, they just represent formal notations associated with asymptotic techniques relative to how a theoretical approximation may actually behave in real-world applications with finite objects. For example, we will use the formal limit notation $f(x) \to a$ as $x \to \infty$ (or $\lim_{x \to \infty} f(x) = a$), where a is a constant. In this case we do not pretend that there is a real number such that $x = \infty$ or x has a value that is close to infinity. We formulate that for all $\varepsilon > 0$ (in the math language: $\forall \varepsilon > 0$) there exists a constant A ($\exists A > 0$) such that the inequality $\|f(x) - a\| < \varepsilon$ holds for all $x > A$. By the notation $\|.\|$ we mean generally a measure, an operation that satisfies certain properties. In the example mentioned above $\|f(x) - a\|$ can be considered as the absolute value of the distance $f(x) - a$, that is, $\|f(x) - a\| = |f(x) - a|$. In this context, one can say for any real value $\varepsilon > 0$ we can find a number A to such that $-\varepsilon < f(x) - a < \varepsilon$ for all $x > A$. In this framework it is not difficult to denote different asymptotic notational devices. For example, the form $f(x) \to \infty$ as $x \to \infty$ (or $\lim_{x \to \infty} f(x) = \infty$) means $\forall \varepsilon > 0$: $\exists A > 0$ $|f(x)| > \varepsilon$, for $\forall x > A$. The function f can denote a series or a sequence of variables, when f is a function of the natural number $n = 1, 2, 3, \ldots$ In this case we use the notation f_n and can consider, e.g., the formal definition of $\lim_{n \to \infty} f_n$ in a similar manner to that of $\lim_{x \to \infty} f(x)$.

Oftentimes asymptotic propositions treat their results using the symbols $O(\cdot)$, $o(\cdot)$, and $\sim$, which are called *"big Oh," "little oh,"* and *"tilde/twiddle,"* respectively. These symbols provide comparisons between the magnitude of two functions, say $u(x)$ and $v(x)$. The notation $u(x) = O(v(x))$ means that $|u(x)/v(x)|$ remains bounded if the argument x is sufficiently near to some given limit L, which is not necessarily finite. In particular, $O(1)$ stands for a bounded function. The notation $u(x) = o(v(x))$, as $x \to L$, denotes that $\lim_{x \to L} \{u(x)/v(x)\} = 0$. In this case, $o(1)$ means a function which tends to zero. By $u(x) \sim v(x)$, as $x \to L$, we define the relationship $\lim_{x \to L} \{u(x)/v(x)\} = 1$.

Examples

1. A function $G(x)$ with $x > 0$ is called *slowly varying* (at infinity) if for all $a > 0$ we have $G(ax) \sim G(x)$, as $x \to \infty$, e.g., $\log(x)$ is a slowly varying function.
2. It is clear that we can obtain the different representations of the function $\sin(x)$, including $\sin(x) = O(|x|)$ as $x \to 0$, $\sin(x) = o(x^2)$ as $x \to \infty$, and $\sin(x) = O(1)$.
3. $x^2 = o(x^3)$ as $x \to \infty$.
4. $f_n = 1 - (1 - 1/n)^2 = o(1)$ as $n \to \infty$.

1.3 Random Variables

In order to describe statistical experiments in a mathematical framework we first introduce a space of elementary events, say $\omega_1, \omega_2, \ldots$, that are independent. For example, we observe a patient who can have red eyes that are caused by allergy and then we can represent these traits as $\omega_1 = $ "*has*", $\omega_2 = $ "*does not have*". In general, the space $\Omega = \{\omega_1, \omega_2, ...\}$ can consist of a continuous number of points. This scenario can be associated, e.g., with experiments when we measure a temperature or plot randomly distributed dots in an interval. We refer the reader to various probability theory textbooks that introduce definitions of underlying probability spaces, random variables, and probability functions in detail (e.g., Chung, 2000; Proschan and Shaw, 2016). In this section we shortly recall a random variable $\xi(\omega)$: $\Omega \to E$ to be a measurable transformation of Ω elements, possible outcomes, into some set E. Oftentimes, $E = R$, the real line, or R^d, the d-dimensional real space. The technical axiomatic definition requires both Ω and E to be measurable spaces. In particular, we deal with random variables that work in a "one-to-one mapping" manner, transforming each random event ω_i to a specific real number, $\xi(\omega_i) \neq \xi(\omega_j), i \neq j$.

1.4 Probability Distributions

In clinical studies, researchers collect and analyze data with the goal of soliciting useful information and making inferences. Oftentimes recorded data represents values (realizations) of random variables. However, in general, experimental data cannot identically and fully characterize relevant random variables. Full information associated with a random variable ξ can be derived from its distribution function, denoted in the form $F_\xi(x) = \Pr(\xi \leq x)$. In this example, we consider a right continuous distribution function of the one-dimensional real-valued random variable. The reader should be familiar with the ideas of left continuous distribution functions and the corresponding definitions related to random vectors.

Assume we have a function $F(x)$. In order for it to be a distribution function for a random variable there are certain conditions that need to be satisfied. For the sake of brevity we introduce the following notation: $F(+\infty) = \lim_{x \to \infty} F(x)$, $F(-\infty) = \lim_{x \to -\infty} F(x)$, $F(x+0) = \lim_{h \downarrow 0} F(x+h)$, and $F(x-0) = \lim_{h \downarrow 0} F(x-h)$, where the notation $h \downarrow 0$ means that $h > 0$ tends to zero from above. Then we call a function $F(x)$ a **distribution function** if $F(x)$ satisfies the following conditions: (1) $F(x)$ is nondecreasing, that is, $F(x+h) \geq F(x)$, for all $h > 0$; (2) $F(x)$ is right-continuous, that is, $F(x+0) = F(x)$; and (3) $F(+\infty) = 1$ and $F(-\infty) = 0$. This definition insures that distribution functions are bounded, monotone, and can have only discontinues of the first kind, i.e., x_0-type arguments at which $F(x_0 - 0) \neq F(x_0 + 0)$.

Note that the definition mentioned above regarding a distribution function $F(x)$ does not provide for the existence of $dF(x)/dx$ in general cases. In a scenario with an absolutely continuous distribution function $F(x)$, one can define

$$F(x) = \int_{-\infty}^{x} f(t)dt \quad \text{with} \quad f(x) = dF(x)/dx,$$

where $f(x)$ is the **density function** and the integral is assumed to be defined according to the chapter material presented below. In order to recognize a density function, one can use the definition of a distribution function to say that every function $g(x)$ is the density function of an absolutely continuous distribution function if $g(x)$ satisfies the conditions: (1) $g(x) \geq 0$, for all x, and (2) $F(+\infty) = \int_{-\infty}^{\infty} g(t)dt = 1$. The ability to describe random variables using density functions is restricted by opportunities to prove corresponding density functions exist. The ideas presented above pertain to univariate distribution functions and extend to higher dimensions termed multivariate distribution functions. An excellent review book on continuous multivariate distributions is presented by Kotz et al. (2000).

Note that in parallel with the role of density functions for continuous random variables one can define **probability mass functions** in the context associated with **discrete random variables**. Denote a set of a finite or countably infinity number of values $u_1, u_2, u_3, \ldots$. Then a random variable ξ is discrete if $\sum_j \Pr(\xi = u_j) = 1$. The function $f(u) = \Pr(\xi = u)$ is the probability mass function. In this case the right-continuous distribution function of ξ has the form $F(x) = \Pr(\xi \leq x) = \sum_{u_j \leq x} f(u_j)$.

Oftentimes, statistical propositions consider **independent and identically distributed (iid)** random variables, say $\xi_1, \xi_2, \xi_3, \ldots$. In these cases, a sequence or other collection of random variables is iid if each random variable has the same probability distribution as the others and all random variables are mutually independent. That is to say

$$\Pr(\xi_1 \leq t_1, \xi_2 \leq t_2, \xi_3 \leq t_3, \ldots) = \Pr(\xi_1 \leq t_1)\Pr(\xi_2 \leq t_2)\Pr(\xi_3 \leq t_3)\ldots$$
$$= F(t_1)F(t_2)F(t_3)\ldots,$$

where the distribution function $F(t) = \Pr(\xi_1 \leq t)$.

In order to summarize experimental data our desired goal can be to estimate distribution functions, either nonparametrically, semi-parametrically, or parametrically. In each setting the goal is to develop accurate, robust, and efficient tools for estimation. In general, estimation of the mean (if it exists) and/or the standard deviation (if it exists) of a random variable only partially describe the underlying data distribution.

1.5 Commonly Used Parametric Distribution Functions

There are a multitude of distribution functions employed in biostatistical studies such as the normal or Gaussian, log-normal, t, χ^2, gamma, F, binomial, uniform, Wishart, and Poisson distributions. In reality there have been thousands of functional forms of distributions that have been published, studied, and available for use via software packages. Parametric distribution functions can be defined up to finite set of parameters (Lindsey, 1996). For example, in the one-dimensional case, the normal (Gaussian) distribution has the notation $N(\mu, \sigma^2)$, which corresponds to density function defined as $f(x) = (\sigma\sqrt{2\pi})^{-1} \exp(-(x-\mu)^2/(2\sigma^2))$, where the parameters μ and σ^2 represent the mean and variance of the population and the support for x is over the entire real line. The shape of the density has been described famously as the bell-shaped curve. The values of the parameters μ and σ^2 may be assumed to be unknown. If the random variable X has a normal distribution, then $Y = \exp(X)$ has a log-normal distribution. Other examples include the gamma distribution, denoted Gamma(α, β), with shape parameter α and rate parameter β. The density function for the gamma distribution is given as $(\beta^\alpha/\Gamma(\alpha))x^{\alpha-1}\exp(-\beta x)$, $x > 0$, where $\Gamma(\alpha)$ is a complete gamma function. The exponential distribution, denoted exp(λ), has rate parameter λ with the corresponding density function given as $\lambda\exp(-\lambda x)$, $x > 0$. Note that the exponential distribution is a special case of the gamma distribution with $\alpha = 1$. It is often the case that simpler well-known models are nested within more complex models with additional parameters. While the more complex models may fit the data better there is a trade-off in terms of efficiency when a simpler model also fits the data well.

Figure 1.1 depicts the density functions of the N(0,1), Gamma(2,1) and exp(1) distributions, for example.

Note that oftentimes measurements related to biological processes follow a log-normal distribution (Koch, 1966). For example, exponential growth is combined with further symmetrical variation: with a mean concentration of, say, 10^6 bacteria, one cell division more or less will result in 2×10^6 or 5×10^5 cells. Therefore, the range will be multiplied or divided by 2 around the mean, that is, the density is asymmetrical. Such skewed distributions of these types of biological processes have long been known to fit the log-normal distribution function (Powers, 1936; Sinnott, 1937). Skewed distributions that often closely fit the log-normal distribution are particularly common when mean values are low, variances are large, and values of random variables cannot be negative, as is the case, for instance, with species abundance and lengths of latent periods of infectious diseases (Lee and Wang, 2013; Balakrishnan et al., 1994). Limpert et al. (2001) discussed various applications of log-normal distributions in different

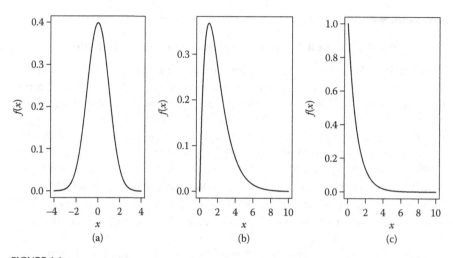

FIGURE 1.1
The density plots where the panels (a)–(c) display the density functions of the standard normal distribution, of the Gamma(2,1) distribution, and of the exp(1) distribution, respectively.

fields of science, including geology, human medicine, environment, atmospheric sciences, microbiology, plant physiology and the social sciences.

1.6 Expectation and Integration

Certain important properties of random variables may be represented sufficiently in the context of mathematical expectations, or simply expectations. For example, the terms: standard deviation, covariance, mean are examples of expectations, which are frequently found in the statistical literature. The expectation of a random variable ξ is denoted in the form $E(\xi)$ and is defined as the integral of ξ with respect to its distribution function, that is, $E(\xi) = \int u \, d\mathrm{Pr}(\xi \leq u)$. In general, for a function ψ about the random variable ξ we can define

$$E\{\psi(\xi)\} = \int \psi(u) d\mathrm{Pr}(\xi \leq u), \text{ e.g., } Var(\xi) = \int \{u - E(\xi)\}^2 d\mathrm{Pr}(\xi \leq u).$$

When we have the density function $f(x) = dF(x)/dx$, $F(x) = \mathrm{Pr}(\xi \leq x)$ the definition of expectation is clear. In this case, expectation is presented as the traditional ***Riemann–Stieltjes integral***, e.g., accurately approaching $E(\xi)$ by the sums

$$\sum_i \min\{f(u_{i-1}), f(u_i)\}(u_i - u_{i-1}) \leq E(\xi) = \int f(u) du \leq \sum_i \max\{f(u_{i-1}), f(u_i)\}(u_i - u_{i-1}),$$

where $u_i < u_j$, for $i < j$, partition the integral support.

In many scenarios, formally speaking, the derivative $dF(x)/dx$ does not exist, for example, when a corresponding random variable is categorical (discrete). Thus, what does the component $d\Pr(\xi \le u)$ in the $E(\xi)$ definition mean? In general, the definition of expectation consists of a **Lebesgue–Stieltjes integral**. To outline this concept we define the operations **infimum** and **supremum**. Assume that $A \subset R$ is a set of real numbers. If $M \in R$ is an upper (a lower) bound of A satisfying $M \le M'$ ($M \ge M'$) for every upper (lower) bound M' of A, then M is the supremum (infimum) of A, that is, $M = \sup(A)$ ($M = \inf(A)$). These notations are similar to the maximum and minimum, but are more useful in analysis, since they can characterize special cases which may have *no minimum or maximum*. For instance, let A be the set $\{x \in R : a \le x \le b\}$ for fixed variables $a < b$. Then $\sup(A) = \max(A) = b$ and $\inf(A) = \min(A) = a$. Defining $A = \{x \in R : 0 < x < b\}$, we have $\sup(A) = b$ and $\inf(A) = 0$, whereas this set A does not have a maximum and minimum, because, e.g., any given element of A could simply be divided in half resulting in a smaller number that is still in A, but there is exactly one infimum $\inf(A) = 0 \notin A$, which is smaller than all the positive real numbers and greater than any other number which could be used as a lower bound.

Lebesgue revealed the revolutionary idea to define the integration $\int_D^U \psi(u)du$. He did not follow Newton, Leibniz, Cauchy, and Riemann who partitioned the x-axis between D and U, the integral bounds. Instead, $l = \inf_{u \in [D,U]} (\psi(u))$ and $L = \sup_{u \in [D,U]} (\psi(u))$ were proposed to be defined in order to partition the y-axis between l and L. That is, instead of cutting the area under ψ using a finite number of vertical cuts, we use a finite number of horizontal cuts. The panels (a) and (b) of Figure 1.2 show an attempting to integrate the "problematic" function $\psi(u) = u^2 I(u < 1) + (u^2 + 1) I(u \ge 1)$, where $I(.) = 0, 1$ denotes the **indicator function**, using a Riemann-type approach via the sums $\sum_i \psi(u_{i-1})(u_i - u_{i-1})$ and $\sum_i \psi(u_i)(u_i - u_{i-1})$. Alternatively the hatched area in the panel (c) visualizes Lebesgue integration.

Thus, the main difference between the Lebesgue and Riemann integrals is that the Lebesgue principle attends to the values of the function, subdividing its range instead of just subdividing the interval on which the function is defined. This fact makes a difference when the function is "problematic," e.g., when it has large oscillations or discontinuities. For an excellent review of Lebesgue's methodology we refer the reader to Bressoud (2008).

We may note, for example, observing n independent and identically distributed data points $\xi_1, ..., \xi_n$, one can estimate their distribution function via the **empirical distribution function** $F_n(t) = \sum_{i=1}^{n} I(\xi_i \le t)$. Then the average

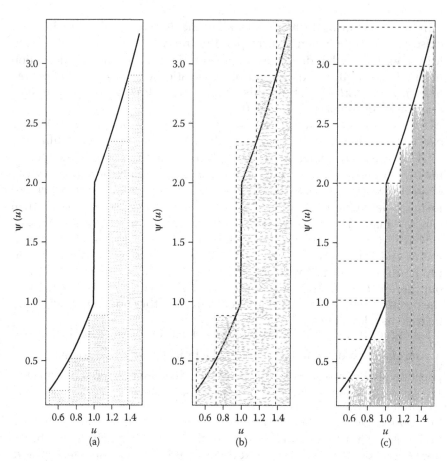

FIGURE 1.2
Riemann-type integration (a, b) and Lebesgue integration (c).

$\bar{\xi} = n^{-1} \sum_{i=1}^{n} \xi_i$, an estimator of $E(\xi)$, can be presented in the integral form $\int t \, dF_n(t)$ using Lebesgue's integration.

1.7 Basic Modes of Convergence of a Sequence of Random Variables

In the context of limit definitions, the measure of a distance between functions and their limit values denoted as $\|\cdot\|$ was mentioned in Section 1.2. Regarding limits of sequences of random variables, this measure can be defined differently, depending on the characterizations of random variables in which we are interested. Thus, statistical asymptotic propositions can employ the following forms of convergence.

1.7.1 Convergence in Probability

Let $\xi_1, ..., \xi_n$ be a sequence of random variables. We write $\xi_n \overset{p}{\to} \zeta$ as $n \to \infty$, if $\lim_{n \to \infty} \Pr\left(|\xi_n - \zeta| < \varepsilon\right) = 1$ for $\forall \varepsilon > 0$, where ζ can be a random variable. Equivalently we can formalize this statement in the following form: for $\forall \varepsilon > 0$ and $\forall \delta > 0$, $\exists N : \forall n > N$ we have $\Pr\left(|\xi_n - \zeta| \geq \varepsilon\right) \leq \delta$. The formalism $\xi_n \overset{p}{\to} \zeta$ is named *convergence in probability*.

In this framework, frequently applied in the asymptotic analysis result, is the **Continuous Mapping Theorem** that states that for every continuous function $h(\cdot)$, if $\xi_n \overset{p}{\to} \zeta$ then we also have $h(\xi_n) \overset{p}{\to} h(\zeta)$ (e.g., Serfling, 2002).

1.7.2 Almost Sure Convergence

Let $\xi_1, ..., \xi_n$ be a sequence of random variables and let ζ be a random variable. Define a sequence $|\xi_n - \zeta|$. Then $\xi_1, ..., \xi_n$ is said to converge to ζ *almost surely* (or almost everywhere, with probability one, strongly, etc.) if $\Pr(\lim_{n \to \infty} \xi_n = \zeta) = 1$. This can be written in the form $\xi_n \overset{a.s.}{\to} \zeta$ as $n \to \infty$.

The almost sure convergence is a stronger mode of convergence than that of the convergence in probability. In fact, an equivalent condition for convergence almost surely is that $\lim_{n \to \infty} \Pr(|\xi_m - \zeta| < \varepsilon, \text{ for all } m \geq n) = 1$, for each $\varepsilon > 0$.

The almost sure convergence is essentially the pointwise convergence of a sequence of functions. In particular, random variables $\xi_1, ..., \xi_n$ and ζ can be regarded as functions of an element ω from the sample space S, that is, $\xi_i \equiv \xi_i(\omega), i = 1, ..., n$, and $\zeta \equiv \zeta(\omega)$. Then $\xi_n \overset{a.s.}{\to} \zeta$ as $n \to \infty$, if the function $\xi_n(\omega)$ converges to $\zeta(\omega)$ for all $\omega \in S$, except for those $\omega \in W, W \subset S$ and $\Pr(W) = 0$. Hence this convergence is named *almost surely*.

1.7.3 Convergence in Distribution

Let $\xi_1, ..., \xi_n$ and ζ be real-valued random variables. We say that ξ_n *converges in distribution* (converge in law or converge weakly) to ζ, writing $\xi_n \overset{L}{\to} \zeta$ ($\xi_n \overset{d}{\to} \zeta$), if $\Pr(\xi_n \leq x) \to P(\zeta \leq x)$ as $n \to \infty$ at every point x that is a continuity point of the distribution function of ζ.

Convergence in distribution is one of the many ways of describing how ξ_n converges to the limiting random variable ζ. In particular, we are usually interested in the case that ζ is a constant and the ξ_i's are sample means; this situation is formally stated as the (weak) *law of large numbers*.

1.7.4 Convergence in *r*th Mean

For $r > 0$, we obtain that $\xi_1, ..., \xi_n$, a sequence of random variables, converges in the *r*th mean to ζ, if $\lim_{n \to \infty} E|\xi_n - \zeta|^r = 0$.

1.7.5 O(.) and o(.) Revised under Stochastic Regimes

For two sequences of random variables $\{U_n\}$ and $\{V_n\}$, we formulate that the notation $U_n = O_p(V_n)$ denotes that $|U_n/V_n| = O_p(1)$, where the subscript p means O(.) in probability. Similarly, the notation $U_n = o_p(V_n)$, denotes that $U_n/V_n \xrightarrow{p} 0$.

1.7.6 Basic Associations between the Modes of Convergence

The following results are frequently useful in theoretical calculations:

1. Convergence in probability implies convergence in distribution.
2. In the opposite direction, convergence in distribution implies convergence in probability only when the limiting random variable ζ is a constant.
3. Convergence in probability does not imply almost sure convergence.
4. Almost sure convergence implies convergence in probability, and hence implies convergence in distribution. It is the notion of convergence used in the strong law of large numbers.

The fundamental book of Serfling (2002) covers a broad range of useful materials regarding asymptotic behavior of random variables and their characteristics.

1.8 Indicator Functions and Their Bounds as Applied to Simple Proofs of Propositions

In Section 1.6 we employed the indicator function $I(.)$. For any event G, the *indicator function* $I(G) = 1$, if G is true and $I(G) = 0$, if G is false.

Consider four simple results that can be essentially helpful for various statistical explanations. (1) $I(G) = 1 - I(\text{not } G)$. (2) $I(G_1, G_2) \leq I(G_k), k = 1, 2$. (3) The indicator function $I(G)$ denotes a random variable with two values 0 and 1. Therefore, $EI(G) = 1 \times \Pr\{I(G) = 1\} + 0 \times \Pr\{I(G) = 0\} = \Pr\{G \text{ is true}\}$. For example, for a random variable ξ, its distribution function $F(x) = \Pr(\xi \leq x)$ satisfies $F(x) = E\{I(\xi \leq x)\}$. (4) It is clear that if a and b are positive then $I(a \geq b) \leq a/b$.

Examples

1. *Chebyshev's inequality* plays one of the main roles in theoretical statistical inference. In this frame, we suppose that a function $\varphi(x) > 0$ increases to show that

$$\Pr(\xi \geq x) = \Pr\{\varphi(\xi) \geq \varphi(x)\} = E\left[I\{\varphi(\xi) \geq \varphi(x)\}\right] \leq E\left\{\frac{\varphi(\xi)}{\varphi(x)}\right\},$$

where it is assumed that $E\{\varphi(\xi)\} < \infty$. Defining $x > 0$, $\varphi(x) = x$, and $\xi = |\zeta - E(\zeta)|^r, r > 0$, we have *Chebyshev's inequality*.

2. Let $\xi_1, \ldots, \xi_n$ be a sequence of iid positive random variables and $S_n = \sum_{i=1}^{n} \xi_i$. Then, for $x > 0$, we have

$$\Pr(S_n \leq x) = \Pr\{\exp(-S_n / x) \geq \exp(-1)\} \leq eE\{\exp(-S_n / x)\} = eq^n,$$

where $q = E\{\exp(-\xi_1/x)\} \leq 1$ and $e = \exp(1)$.

3. A frequently used method for theoretical statistical evaluations is similar to the following strategy. For example, one may be interested in the approximation of the expectation $E\{\psi(A_n)\}$, where ψ is an increasing function and A_n is a statistic with the property $A_n / n \xrightarrow{p} 1$ as $n \to \infty$. To get some intuition about the asymptotic behavior of $E\{\psi(A_n)\}$, we have, for $0 < \varepsilon < 1$,

$$E\{\psi(A_n)\} = E\{\psi(A_n)I(A_n \leq n + n^\varepsilon)\} + E\{\psi(A_n)I(A_n > n + n^\varepsilon)\}$$

$$\leq E\{\psi(n + n^\varepsilon)I(A_n \leq n + n^\varepsilon)\} + E\{\psi(A_n)I(A_n > n + n^\varepsilon)\}$$

$$\leq \psi(n + n^\varepsilon) + \left[E\{\psi(A_n)\}^2 \{\Pr(A_n > n + n^\varepsilon)\}\right]^{1/2},$$

$$E\{\psi(A_n)\} \geq E\{\psi(A_n)I(A_n \geq n - n^\varepsilon)\} \geq E\{\psi(n - n^\varepsilon)I(A_n \geq n - n^\varepsilon)\}$$

$$\geq \psi(n - n^\varepsilon) - E\{\psi(A_n)I(A_n < n - n^\varepsilon)\}$$

$$\geq \psi(n - n^\varepsilon) - \left[E\{\psi(A_n)\}^2 \{\Pr(A_n < n - n^\varepsilon)\}\right]^{1/2},$$

where the *Cauchy–Schwarz inequality*, $\{E(\xi\zeta)\}^2 \leq E(\xi^2)E(\zeta^2)$ for random variables ξ and ζ, was applied. Now, in order to show the remainder terms $\left[E\{\psi(A_n)\}^2 \{\Pr(A_n > n + n^\varepsilon)\}\right]^{1/2}$ and $\left[E\{\psi(A_n)\}^2 \{\Pr(A_n < n - n^\varepsilon)\}\right]^{1/2}$ potentially vanish to zero, a rough bound for $E\{\psi(A_n)\}^2$ might be shown to be in effect. If this is the case then a Chebyshev-type inequality could be applied to $\Pr(A_n > n + n^\varepsilon)$ and $\Pr(A_n < n - n^\varepsilon)$. Note that, since $A_n \sim n$, we choose the "vanished" events $\{A_n > n + n^\varepsilon\}$ and $\{A_n < n - n^\varepsilon\}$ to be present in the remainder terms. In the case where ψ is a decreasing function, in a similar manner to that shown above, one can start with

$$E\{\psi(A_n)\} = E\{\psi(A_n)I(A_n \geq n - n^\varepsilon)\} + E\{\psi(A_n)I(A_n < n - n^\varepsilon)\}$$

$$\leq E\{\psi(n - n^\varepsilon)I(A_n \geq n - n^\varepsilon)\} + E\{\psi(A_n)I(A_n < n - n^\varepsilon)\},$$

$$E\{\psi(A_n)\} \geq E\{\psi(A_n)I(A_n \leq n + n^\varepsilon)\} \geq E\{\psi(n + n^\varepsilon)I(A_n \leq n + n^\varepsilon)\}$$

$$\geq \psi(n + n^\varepsilon) - E\{\psi(A_n)I(A_n > n + n^\varepsilon)\}.$$

1.9 Taylor's Theorem

An essential toolkit for statisticians to prove various theoretical propositions includes methods for expanding functions in powers of their arguments by a formula similar to that provided by Taylor's theorem–type results. In mathematics, a Taylor series is a representation of a function as an infinite sum of terms that are calculated from the values of the function's derivatives at a single point. The basic Taylor's theorem states:

(i) When a function $g(x)$ has derivatives of all orders at $x = a$, the infinite Taylor series expanded about $x = a$ is $g(x) = \sum_{j=0}^{\infty} g^{(j)}(a)(x-a)^j / j!$, where, for an integer k, $k! = \prod_{i=1}^{k} i$ and $g^{(k)}(a) = d^k g(x) / \prod_{i=1}^{k} dx \Big|_{x=a}$.

(ii) Assume that a function $g(x)$ has $k + 1$ derivatives on an open interval containing a. Then, for each x in the interval, we have

$$g(x) = \sum_{j=0}^{k} \frac{g^{(j)}(a)}{j!}(x-a)^j + R_{k+1}(x),$$

where the **remainder term** $R_{k+1}(x)$ satisfies $R_{k+1}(x) = \frac{g^{(k+1)}(c)}{(k+1)!}(x-a)^{k+1}$ for some c between a and x, $c = a + \theta(x-a), 0 \leq \theta \leq 1$.

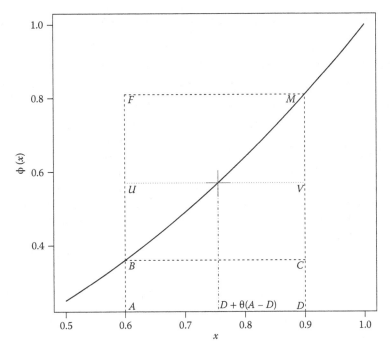

FIGURE 1.3
Illustration of Taylor's theorem.

To display some intuition regarding the proof of Taylor's theorem, we depict Figure 1.3.

Assume we would like to find the area under a function $\phi(x)$ with $x \in [A, D]$, using a rectangle. It is clear the rectangle $ABCD$ is too small and the rectangle $AFMD$ is too large to represent $\int_A^D \phi(x)\,dx$. The area of $AUVD$ is $(U-A)$ $(D-A)$ and is appropriate to calculate the integral. The segment UV should cross the curve of $\phi(x)$, when $x \in [A, D]$, at the point $D + \theta(D-A), \theta \in (0,1)$. Then $\int_A^D \phi(x)\,dx = (D-A)\phi(c)$, where $c = D + \theta(A-D)$. Define $\phi(x) = dg(x)/dx$ to obtain the Taylor theorem with $k = 0$. Now, following the mathematical induction principle and using integration by parts, one can obtain the Taylor result.

We remark that Taylor's theorem can be generalized for multivariate functions; for details see Mikusinski and Taylor (2002) and Serfling (2002).

Warning: It is very critical to note that while applying the Taylor expansion one should carefully evaluate the corresponding remainder terms. Unfortunately, if not implemented carefully Taylor's theorem is easily misapplied. Examples of errors are numerous in the statistical literature. A typical example of a misstep using Taylor's theorem can be found in several publications and is as follows: Let $\xi_1, \ldots, \xi_n$ be a sequence of iid random variables with $E\xi_1 = \mu \neq 0$ and $S_n = \sum_{i=1}^{n} \xi_i$. Suppose one is interested in evaluating the expectation $E(1/S_n)$. Taking into account that $ES_n = \mu n$ and then "using" the Taylor theorem applied to the function $1/x$, we "have" $E(1/S_n) \approx 1/(\mu n) - E\{(S_n - \mu n)/(\mu n)^2\}$ that, e.g., "results in" $nE(1/S_n) = O(1)$. In this case, the expectation $E(1/S_n)$ may not exist, e.g., when ξ_1 is from a normal distribution. This scenario belongs to cases that do not carefully consider the corresponding remainder terms. Prototypes of the example above can be found in the statistical literature that deals with estimators of regression models. In many cases, complications related to evaluations of remainder terms can be comparable with those of the corresponding initial problem statement. This may be a consequence of the universal law of conservation of energy or mere sloppiness.

In the context of the example mentioned above, it is interesting to show that it turns out that even when $E(1/S_n)$ does not exist, we obtain $E(S_m/S_n) = m/n$, for $m \leq n$, since we have $1 = E(S_m/S_n) = \sum_{i=1}^{n} E(\xi_i/S_n) = nE(\xi_i/S_n)$ and then $E(\xi_1/S_n) = 1/n$ implies $E(S_m/S_n) = \sum_{i=1}^{m} E(\xi_i/S_n) = mE(\xi_i/S_n) = m/n.$

Example

In several applications, for a function φ, we need to compare $E\{\varphi(\xi)\}$ with $\varphi(E(\xi))$, where ξ is a random variable. Applying Taylor's theorem to $\varphi(\xi)$, we can obtain that

$$\varphi(\xi) = \varphi(E(\xi)) + \{\xi - E(\xi)\}\varphi'(E(\xi)) + \{\xi - E(\xi)\}^2 \varphi''(E(\xi) + \theta\{\xi - E(\xi)\})/2, \theta \in (0,1).$$

Then, provided that φ'' is positive or negative, we can easily obtain $E\{\varphi(\xi)\} \geq \varphi(E(\xi))$ or $E\{\varphi(\xi)\} \leq \varphi(E(\xi))$, respectively. For example, $E(1/\xi) \geq 1/E(\xi)$. This is a simple way for checking **Jensen's inequality**, which states that if ξ is a random variable and φ is a convex or concave function, then $E\{\varphi(\xi)\} \geq \varphi(E(\xi))$ or $E\{\varphi(\xi)\} \leq \varphi(E(\xi))$, respectively.

1.10 Complex Variables

It is just as easy to define a *complex variable* $z = a + ib$ with $i = \sqrt{-1}$ as it is to define real variables a and b. Complex variables consist of an imaginary unit i that satisfies $i^2 = -1$. Mathematicians love to be consistent, if we can solve the elementary equation $x^2 - 1 = 0$ then we should know how to solve the equation $x^2 + 1 = 0$. This principle provides a possibility to denote k roots of the general equation $\sum_{i=0}^{k} a_i x^k = 0$ with an integer k and given coefficients $a_1, \ldots, a_k$. Complex variables are involved in this process, adding a dimension to mathematical analysis. Intuitively, we can consider a complex number $z = a + \mathrm{i}b$ as a vector with components a and b.

Formally, for $z = a + \mathrm{i}b$, $z \in C$, the real number a is called the real part of the complex variable z and the real number b is called the imaginary part of z, expressing $\mathrm{Re}(z) = a$ and $\mathrm{Im}(z) = b$. It can be noted that complex variables are naturally thought of as existing on a two-dimensional plane, there is no natural linear ordering on the set of complex numbers. We cannot say that a complex variable z_1 is greater or less than a complex variable z_2. However many mathematical operations require one to consider distances between variables and their comparisons, e.g., in the context of asymptotic mechanisms or in different aspects of integrations. Toward this end, the absolute value of a complex variable is defined. The **absolute value** (or *modulus or magnitude*) of a complex number $z = a + \mathrm{i}b$ is $r = |z| = \sqrt{a^2 + b^2}$.

The **complex conjugate** of the complex variable $z = a + \mathrm{i}b$ is defined to be $z = a - \mathrm{i}b$ and denoted as $\bar{z}$.

The definitions mentioned above are simple, but in order to show completeness of complex analysis, e.g., in the context of analytic functions, we need to attend to the complicated question: do functions of complex variables belong to C, having the form $a + \mathrm{i}b$? If yes, then how does one quantify their absolute values using only the definitions mentioned above? For example, it is required to obtain a method for proving that $\log(z) = \mathrm{Re}\{\log(z)\} + \mathrm{i}\,\mathrm{Im}\{\log(z)\}$, $\exp(z) = \mathrm{Re}\{\exp(z)\} + \mathrm{i}\,\mathrm{Im}\{\exp(z)\}$, and so on. In this case **Euler's formula** can be assigned to play a vital role.

In complex analysis, the following formula establishes the fundamental relationship between trigonometric functions and the complex exponential function. Euler's formula states that, for any real number x, $e^{\mathrm{i}x} = \cos(x) + \mathrm{i}\sin(x)$, where e is the base of the natural logarithm.

Proof. Note that $\mathrm{i}^2 = -1$, $\mathrm{i}^3 = -\mathrm{i}$, $\mathrm{i}^4 = 1$, and so on. Using the Taylor expansion, we have

$$e^x = \sum_{j=0}^{\infty} \frac{x^j}{j!}, \quad \sin(x) = \sum_{j=0}^{\infty} (-1)^{2j+1} \frac{x^{2j+1}}{(2j+1)!}, \quad \text{and} \quad \cos(x) = \sum_{j=0}^{\infty} (-1)^{2j} \frac{x^{2j}}{(2j)!}.$$

This result implies that

$$e^{\mathrm{i}x} = 1 + \frac{\mathrm{i}x}{1!} - \frac{x^2}{2!} + \ldots = \cos(x) + \mathrm{i}\sin(x),$$

yielding Euler's formula.

Euler's formula shows that $\left|e^{\mathrm{i}xt}\right| = 1$, for all $x, t \in R$. Then, for example, for all random variables, $E\left(e^{\mathrm{i}t\xi}\right)$ exists, since $\left|E\left(e^{\mathrm{i}t\xi}\right)\right| \le E\left|e^{\mathrm{i}t\xi}\right| = 1$.

Thus, one can show that complex variables can be presented as $r \exp(\mathrm{i}w)$, where r, w are real-valued variables. This assists to show that analytic functions of complex variables are "$a + ib$" type complex variables and then to define their absolute values.

Euler's formula has inspired mathematical passions and minds. For example, using $x = \pi/2$, we have $i = e^{i\pi/2}$, which leads to $i^i = e^{-\pi/2}$. Is this a "door" from the "unreal" realm to the "real" realm? In this case, we remind the reader that $\exp(x) = \lim_{n \to \infty}(1 + x/n)^n$ and then interpretations of $i^i = e^{-\pi/2}$ are left to the reader's imagination.

Warning: In general, definitions and evaluations of a function of a complex variable require very careful attention. For example, we have $e^{ix} = \cos x + \sin x$, but we also can write $e^{ix} = \cos(x + 2\pi j) + i\sin(x + 2\pi k)$, $j = 1, 2, \ldots; k = 1, 2, \ldots$, taking into account the period of the trigonometric functions. Thus it is not a simple task to define unique functions that are similar to $\log\{\varphi(z)\}$ and $\{\varphi(z)\}^{1/p}$, where p is an integer. In this context, we refer the reader to Finkelestein et al. (1997) and Chung (1974) for examples of the relevant problems and their solutions. In statistical terms, the issue mentioned above can make estimation of functions of complex variables complicated since, e.g., a problem of unique reconstruction of $\{\varphi(z)\}^{1/p}$ based on $\varphi(z)$ is in effect (see for example Chapter 2).

1.11 Statistical Software: R and SAS

In this section, we outline the elementary components of the R (R Development Core Team, 2014) and SAS (Delwiche and Slaughter, 2012) statistical software packages. Both packages allow the user to implement powerful built-in routines and user community developed code or employ programming features for customization. For example, Desquilbet and Mariotti (2010) presented the use of an SAS macro (customized SAS code) using data from the third National Health and Nutrition Examination Survey to investigate adjusted dose–response associations (with different models) between calcium intake and bone mineral density (linear regression), folate intake and hyperhomocysteinemia (logistic regression), and serum high-density lipoprotein cholesterol and cardiovascular mortality (Cox model). Examples of R and SAS programs are employed throughout the book.

1.11.1 R Software

R is an open-source, case-sensitive, command line-driven software for statistical computing and graphics. The R program is installed using the directions found at *www.r-project.org*.

Once R has been loaded, the main input window appears, showing a short introductory message (Gardener, 2012). There may be slight differences in appearance depending upon the operating system. For example, Figure 1.4 shows the main input window in the Windows operating system, which has

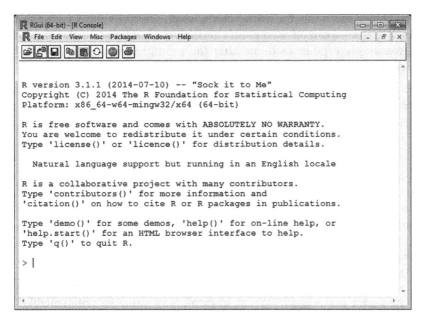

FIGURE 1.4
The main input window of R in Windows.

menu options available at the top of the page. Below the header is a screen prompt symbol > in the left-hand margin indicating the command line.

Rules for names of variables and R data sets:
A syntactically valid R name consists of letters, numbers and the dot or underline characters and starts with either a letter or the dot not followed by a number. Reserved words are not syntactic names.

Comments in R:
Comments can be inserted starting with a pound (#) throughout the R code without disrupting the program flow.

Inputting data in R:
R operates on named data structures. The simplest form is the numeric vector, which is a single entity consisting of an ordered collection of numbers. One way to input data is through the use of the function c(), which takes an arbitrary number of vector arguments and whose value is a vector got by concatenating its arguments end to end. For example, to set up a vector x, consisting of four numbers, namely, 3, 5, 10, and 7, the assignment can be done with

```
> x<-c(3,5,10,7)
```

Notice that the assignment operator (<–), which consists of the two characters, less than (<) and minus (–), occurring strictly side-by-side and "points" to the object receiving the value of the expression. In most contexts the equal operator (=) can be used as an alternative. In order to display the value of x, we simply type in its name after the prompt symbol > and press the Return key.

```
> x
```

As a result, R provides the following output:

```
[1]   3   5 10   7
```

Assignment can also be made using the function assign(). An equivalent way of making the same assignment as above is with:

```
> assign("x", c(3,5,10,7))
```

The usual assignment operator (<−) can be thought of as a syntactic short-cut to this.

In some cases the elements of a vector may not be completely known and the vector is *incomplete*. When an element or value is "not available" or a "missing value" in the statistical sense, a place within a vector may be reserved for it by assigning it the special value NA. In general, without further suboption specification, any operation on an NA becomes an NA.

Note that there is a second kind of "missing" values, which are produced by numerical computation, the so-called Not a Number, NaN, values. The following examples give NaN since the result cannot be defined sensibly:

```
> 0/0
> Inf - Inf
```

The function is.na(x) gives a logical vector of the same size as x with value TRUE if and only if the corresponding element in x is NA or NaN. The function is.nan(x) is only TRUE when the corresponding element in x is NaNs.

Missing values are sometimes printed as <NA> when character vectors are printed without quotes.

Manipulating data in R

In R, vectors can be used in arithmetic expressions, in which case the operations are performed element by element. The elementary arithmetic operators are the usual + (addition), − (subtraction), * (multiplication), / (division), and ^ (exponentiation). The following example illustrates the assignment of y, which equals $x^2 + 3$:

```
> y <- x^2 + 3
```

R can be programmed to perform simple statistical calculations as well as complex computations. Table 1.1 shows some simple commands that produce

TABLE 1.1

Selected R Commands That Produce the Descriptive Statistics of a Numerical Vector x

Syntax	Definition
mean(x, na.rm = FALSE)	Gives the arithmetic mean
sd(x, na.rm = FALSE)	Gives the standard deviation
var(x, na.rm = FALSE)	Gives the variance
sum(x, na.rm = FALSE)	Gives the sum of the vector elements

descriptive statistics of a vector x given a sample of measurements $x_1, ..., x_n$. The setting "na.rm = FALSE" is set to indicate a missing statistic value is returned if there are missing values in the data vector.

Instead of using the built-in functions contained in R, such as those shown in Table 1.1, customized functions can be created to carry out additional specific tasks. For this purpose the function() command can be used. The following example shows a simple function "mymean" that determines the running mean of the first i, $i = 1, ..., n$ elements of a vector x, where n is the number of elements in x. Results are shown for x, our toy dataset from above, by applying the customized function mymean.

```
> # to define the function
> mymean <- function(x) {
+    tmp <- c()
+    for(i in 1:length(x)) tmp[i] <- mean(x[1:i])
+    return(tmp)
+ }
> # execute the function using the data defined above
> mymean(x)
[1] 3.00 4.00 6.00 6.25
```

Note that the symbol plus (+) is shown at the left-hand side of the screen instead of the symbol greater than (>) to indicate the function commands are being input. The built-in R functions "length," "return," and "mean" are used within the new function mymean. For more details about R functions and data structures, we refer the reader to Crawley (2012).

In addition to vectors, R allows manipulation of *logical* quantities. The elements of a logical vector can be values TRUE (abbreviated as T), FALSE (abbreviated as F), and NA (in the case of "not available"). Note however that T and F are just variables that are set to TRUE and FALSE by default, but are not reserved words and hence can be overwritten by the user. Therefore, it would be better to use TRUE and FALSE.

Logical vectors are generated by conditions. For example,

```
> cond <- x > y
```

TABLE 1.2

Selected R Comparison Operators

Symbolic	Meaning
==	Equals
!=	not equal
>	greater than
<	less than
>=	greater than or equal
<=	less than or equal
%in%	determines whether specific elements are in a longer vector

sets cond as a vector of the same length as x and y, with values FALSE corresponding to elements of x and y if the condition is not met and TRUE where it is. Table 1.2 shows some basic comparison operators in R.

A group of logical expression, say cond1 and cond2, can be combined with the symbol & (and) or | (or), where cond1 & cond2 is their intersection and cond1 | cond2 is their union (or). !cond1 is the negation of cond1.

Often, the user may want to make choices and take action dependent on a certain value. In this case, an if statement can be very useful, which takes the following form:

```
if (cond) {statements}
```

Three components are contained in the if statement: if, the keyword; (cond), a single logical value between parentheses (or an expression that leads to a single logical value); and {statements}, a block of codes between braces ({}) that has to be executed when the logical value is TRUE. When there is only one statement, the braces can be omitted. For example, the following statement set the variable y equal to 10 if the variable Gender equals "F":

```
if (Gender == "F") y <- 10
```

To execute repetitive code statements for a particular number of times, a "for" loop in R can be used. For loops are controlled by a looping vector. In each iteration of the loop, one value in the looping vector is assigned to a variable that can be used in the statements of the body of the loop. Usually, the number of loop iterations is defined by the number of values stored in the looping vector; they are processed in the same order as they are stored in the looping vector. Generally, for loop construction takes the following form:

```
for (variable in seq) {
        statements
}
```

If the goal is to create a new vector, a vector to store member variables should be set up before creating a loop. For example,

```
x <- NULL
for (j in 1:50) {
      x[j] <- j^2
}
```

The program creates a vector of 50 observations $x = j^2$, where j ranges from 1 to 50.

Printing data in R

In order to display the data or the variable, we can simply type in its name after the prompt symbol >, and press the Return key.

There are many routines in R developed by researchers around the world that can be downloaded and installed from CRAN-like repositories or local files using the command install.packages("packagename"), where packagename is the name of the package to be installed and must be in quotes; single or double quotes are both fine as long as they are not mixed. Once the package is installed, it can be loaded by issuing the command library(packagename) after which commands specific to the package can be accessed. Through an extensive help system built into R, a help entry for a specified command can be brought up via the help(commandname) command. As a simple example, we introduce the command "EL.means" in the EL library.

```
> install.packages("EL")
Installing package into 'C:/Users/xiwei/Documents/R/win-library/3.1'
(as 'lib' is unspecified)
trying URL 'http://cran.rstudio.com/bin/windows/contrib/3.1/
EL_1.0.zip'
Content type 'application/zip' length 53774 bytes (52 Kb)
opened URL
downloaded 52 Kb

package 'EL' successfully unpacked and MD5 sums checked

The downloaded binary packages are in
        C:\Users\xiwei\AppData\Local\Temp\Rtmp4uRCPS\downloaded_packages
> library(EL)
> help(EL.means)
```

The EL.means function provides the software tool for implementing the empirical likelihood tests we will introduce in detail in this book.

As another concrete example, we show the "mvrnorm" command in the MASS library.

```
> install.packages("MASS")
Installing package into 'C:/Users/xiwei/Documents/R/win-library/3.1'
(as 'lib' is unspecified)
```

```
trying URL 'http://cran.rstudio.com/bin/windows/contrib/3.1/MASS_7.3-34.zip'
Content type 'application/zip' length 1083003 bytes (1.0 Mb)
opened URL
downloaded 1.0 Mb

package 'MASS' successfully unpacked and MD5 sums checked

The downloaded binary packages are in
        C:\Users\xiwei\AppData\Local\Temp\Rtmp4uRCPS\downloaded_packages
> library(MASS)
> help(mvrnorm)
```

The mvrnorm command is very useful for simulating data from a multivariate normal distribution. To illustrate, we simulate bivariate normal data with mean $(0,0)^T$ and an identity covariance matrix with a sample size of 5.

```
> n <- 5  # define the sample size
> mu <- c(0,0)  # define the mean vector
> Sigma <- matrix(c(1,0,0,1), byrow=TRUE, ncol=2) # define covariance matrix
> set.seed(123)  # define the seed to fix the sample
> X <- mvrnorm (n, mu=mu, Sigma=Sigma) # generate data
> X
              [,1]          [,2]
[1,]  -1.7150650  -0.56047565
[2,]  -0.4609162  -0.23017749
[3,]   1.2650612   1.55870831
[4,]   0.6868529   0.07050839
[5,]   0.4456620   0.12928774
```

For more details about the implementation of R, we refer the reader to, e.g., Gardener (2012) and Crawley (2012).

1.11.2 SAS Software

SAS software is widely used to analyze data from various clinical trials and manage large datasets. SAS runs on a wide range of operating systems. More information about SAS can be found at the website: http://www.sas.com/.

SAS can be run in both an interactive and batch mode. To run SAS interactively type SAS at your system prompt (UNIX/LINUX), or click the SAS icon (PC). Figure 1.5 shows the SAS interface in Microsoft Windows.

In the interactive SAS environment, one can write, edit, and submit programs for processing, as well as view and print the results.

A SAS program is a sequence of statements executed in order. A statement provides instructions for SAS to execute and must be appropriately placed in the program. Statements can consist of SAS keywords, SAS names, special characters, and operators. SAS is a free format language in that SAS statements:

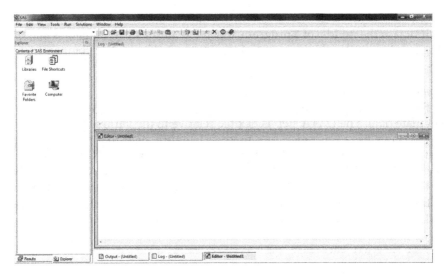

FIGURE 1.5
The interface of SAS.

- Are not case-sensitive, except those inside of quoted strings
- Can start in any column
- Can continue on the next line or be on the same line as other statements.

The most important rule is that every SAS statement ends with a semicolon (;).

Rules for names of variables and SAS data sets
When making up names for variables and data sets (data set names follow similar rules as variables, but they have a different name space), the following rules should be followed:

- Names must be 32 characters or less in length, containing only letters, digits, or the underscore character (_).
- Names must start with a letter or an underscore; however, it is a good idea to avoid starting variable names with an underscore, because special system variables are named that way.

In SAS, there are virtually no reserved words; it differentiates user-defined names with keywords or special system variables names by context.

Comments in SAS
Note that there are two styles of comments in SAS: one starts with an asterisk (*) and ends with a semicolon (;) as is shown in the example. The other style starts with a backslash asterisk (/*) and ends with an asterisk backslash (*/).

In the case of unmatched comments, SAS can't read the entire program and will stop in the middle of a program, much like unmatched quotation marks. The solution, in batch mode, is to insert the missing part of comment and resubmit the program.

Inputting data in SAS

In SAS, DATA steps are used to read and modify data, and can also be used to simulate data. The DATA step is flexible relative to the various data formats. DATA steps have an underlying matrix structure such that programming statements will be executed for each row of the data matrix. There are multiple ways to import data into SAS. Either way, you must type raw data directly in the SAS program, link SAS to a database, or direct SAS to the data file.

The following SAS program illustrates how to type raw data and use the INPUT and DATALINES statement:

```
* Read internal data into SAS data set Namelists;
DATA Namelists;
     INPUT Name $ Gender $ Age;
     DATALINES;
Lincoln M 46
Sara F 32
Catherine F 18
Mike M 35
   ;
RUN;
```

The keywords, e.g., DATA, INPUT, DATALINES, and RUN, identify the type of statement and instruct the execution in SAS. For example, the INPUT statement, a part of the DATA step, indicates to SAS the variable names and their formats. To write an INPUT statement using list input, simply list the variable names after the INPUT keyword in the order they appear in the data file. If the variable is a character, then leave a space and place a dollar sign ($) after the corresponding variable name.

Separating the data from the program avoids the possibility that data will accidentally be altered when editing the SAS program. For data contained in external files, the INFILE statement can be used to direct SAS to the data from ASCII files. The INFILE statement follows the DATA statement and must precede the INPUT statement. After the INFILE keyword, the file path and the file name are enclosed in quotation marks.

By default, the DATA step starts reading with the first data line and, if SAS runs out of data on a line, it automatically goes to the next line to read values for the rest of the variables. Most of the time this works fine, but sometimes data files cannot be read using the default settings. In the INFILE statement, the options placed after the filename can change the way SAS reads raw data files. For instance, the FIRSTOBS= option tells SAS at what line to begin reading data; the OBS= option can be used anytime you want to read only a part of your data file; the MISSOVER option tells

SAS that if it runs out of data, do not go to the next data line but assign missing values to any remaining variables instead; and the DELIMITER=, or DLM=, option allows SAS to read data files with other delimiters (the default is a blank space).

Moreover, SAS assumes that the number of characters including spaces in a data line (termed a record length) of external files is no more than 256 in some operating environments, e.g., the Windows operating system. If the data contains records that are longer than 256 characters, use the LRECL= option in the INFILE statement to specify a record length at least as long as the longest record in the data file. For more details about the INFILE options, we refer the reader to Delwiche and Slaughter (2012). More complex data import and export features are available in SAS, but go beyond the scope of our applications.

To illustrate, the following program reads data from a tab-separated external file into an SAS data set using the INFILE statement:

```
* Read internal data into SAS data set Namelists;
DATA Namelists;
    INFILE 'c:\MyRawData\Namelists.dat' DLM = '09'X;
    INPUT Name $ Gender $ Age;
RUN;
```

With SAS, there is commonly more than one way to accomplish the same result, including the input of data. For more details about other ways of inputting data, e.g., the IMPORT procedure, we refer the reader to Delwiche and Slaughter (2012).

When a variable exists in SAS but does not have a value, the value is said to be *missing*. SAS assigns a period (.) for numeric data and a blank for character data. By the MISSING statement, the user may specify other characters instead of a period or a blank to be treated as missing data. To illustrate how the missing data coding works, the following example declares that the character u is to be treated as a missing value for the character variable Gender whenever it is encountered in a record:

```
DATA two;
    MISSING u;
    INPUT $ Gender;
CARDS;
RUN;
```

Missing values have a value of false when used with logical operators such as AND or OR.

Manipulating data in SAS

In SAS, the users can create and redefine variables with assignment statements using the following basic form:

```
variable = expression;
```

On the left side of the equal sign is a variable name, either new or old. On the right side of the equal sign can be a constant, another variable, or a mathematical expression. The basic types of assignment statements may use operators such as + (addition), - (subtraction), * (multiplication), / (division), and ** (exponentiation). The following example illustrates the assignment of Newvar, which equals the square of OldVar plus 3:

```
NewVar = OldVar ** 2 + 3;
```

In the case where a simple expression using only arithmetic operators is not enough, SAS provides a set of numerous useful and built-in functions. Table 1.3 shows selected SAS numeric functions; see Delwiche and Slaughter (2012) for more numeric functions and character functions.

There are a variety of *control statements* that control the flow of execution of statements in the data step.

If the user wants to conditionally execute a SAS statement based on certain conditional logic, that is, to conduct computations under certain conditions, the IF-THEN statement can be used, which takes the following general form:

```
IF condition THEN action;
```

The condition is an expression comparing arguments, and the action is what SAS will execute when the expression is true, often an assignment statement. For example,

```
IF Gender = 'F' THEN y=10;
```

This statement tells SAS to set the variable y equal to 10 whenever the variable Gender equals F. The terms on either side of the comparison, separated by a comparison operator, may be constants, variables, or expressions. The comparison operator may be either symbolic or mnemonic, depending on the user's preference. Table 1.4 shows some basic comparison operators.

A single IF-THEN statement can only have one action. To specify multiple conditions, we can combine the condition with the keywords AND (&) or OR (|). For example,

TABLE 1.3

Selected SAS Numeric Functions

Syntax	Definition
MEAN(arg-1,arg-2,...arg-n)	Arithmetic mean of nonmissing values
STD(arg-1,arg-2,...arg-n)	Standard deviation of nonmissing values
VAR(arg-1,arg-2,...arg-n)	Variance of nonmissing values
SUM(arg-1,arg-2,...arg-n)	Sum of nonmissing values

TABLE 1.4

Selected SAS Comparison Operators

Symbolic	Mnemonic	Meaning
=	EQ	equals
¬ =, ^ =, or ~ =	NE	not equal
>	GT	greater than
<	LT	less than
>=	GE	greater than or equal
<=	LE	less than or equal
	IN	determine whether a variable's value is among a list of values

```
IF condition AND condition THEN action;
```

A group of actions can be executed by adding the keywords DO and END:

```
IF condition THEN DO;
    action;
    action;
END;
```

The DO statement designates a group of statements to be executed as a unit until a matching END statement appears. The DO statement, the matching END statement, and all the statements between them define a DO loop. There are several variations of the DO-END statement. The following example presents an iterative DO statement that executes a group of SAS statements repetitively between the DO and END statements:

```
DO index = start TO stop BY increment;
    statements;
END;
```

The number of times statements are executed is determined as follows. Initially the variable index is set to the value of start and statements are executed. Next the value of increment is added to the index and the new value is compared to the value of stop. The statements are executed again only if the new value of index is less than or equal to stop. If no increment is specified, the default is 1. The process continues iteratively until the value of index is greater than the value of stop. We illustrate with a simple example:

```
DATA one;
    DO j = 1 TO 50;
    x = j**2;
    OUTPUT one;
END;
DROP j;
CARDS;
RUN;
```

The program creates a SAS data set one with 50 observations and a variable $x = j^2$, where the index variable j ranges from 1 to 50. The DROP statement help get rid of the index variable j. The OUTPUT statement tells SAS to write the current observation to the output data set before returning to the beginning of the DATA step to process the next observation.

Printing data in SAS

The PROC PRINT procedure lists data in a SAS data set as a table of observations by variables. The following statements can be used with PROC PRINT:

```
PROC PRINT DATA = SASdataset;
    VAR variables;
    ID variable;
    BY variables;
    TITLE 'Print SAS Data Set';
RUN;
```

where SASdataset is the name of the data set printed. If none is specified, then the last SAS data set created will be printed. If no VAR statement is included, then all variables in the data set are printed; otherwise only those listed, and in the order in which they are listed, are printed. When an ID statement is used, SAS prints each observation with the values of the ID variables first instead of the observation number, the default setting. The BY statement specifies the variable that the procedure uses to form BY groups; the observations in the data set must either be sorted by all the variables specified (e.g., use the PROC SORT procedure), or they must be indexed appropriately, unless the NOTSORTED option in the BY statement is used. For more details, we refer the read to Delwiche and Slaughter (2012).

Summarizing data in SAS

After reading the data and making sure it is correct, one may summarize and analyze the data using built-in SAS procedures or PROCs. For example, PROC MEANS provides a set of descriptive statistics for numeric variables. Vitually all SAS PROCs have additional options or features, which can be accessed with subcommands, e.g., one can use PROC MEANS to carry out a one-sample t-test.

As another example, the following program sorts the SAS data set Namelists by gender using PROC SORT, and then summarizes the Age by Gender using PROC MEANS with a BY statement (the MAXDEC option is set to zero, so no decimal places will be printed.):

```
* Sort the data by Gender;
PROC SORT DATA = Namelists;
    BY Gender;
* Calculate means by Gender for Age;
PROC MEANS DATA = Namelists MAXDEC = 0;
```

```
    BY Gender;
    VAR Age;
    TITLE 'Summary of Age by Gender';
RUN;
```

Here are the results of the PROC MEANS by gender:

Summary of Age by Gender

For more details about the data summarization by descriptive statistics and/or graphs, we refer the reader to Delwiche and Slaughter (2012).

For a majority of the examples in later chapters, the reader is expected to understand the basics commands of the DATA step, such as DO loops and the OUTPUT statement, and be familiar with the various statistical PROCs that he or she might use generally given parametric assumptions. Some knowledge of the basic SAS macro language and PROC IML (a separate way to program in SAS) will also be helpful. It is our goal that most of the code provided in this book will be easily modified to handle a variety of problems found in practice. It should be noted that R routines can be implemented within SAS PROC IML.

The MEANS Procedure
Gender = F

Analysis Variable: Age

N	Mean	Std Dev	Minimum	Maximum
2	25	10	18	32

Gender = M

Analysis Variable: Age

N	Mean	Std Dev	Minimum	Maximum
2	41	8	35	46

2

Characteristic Function–Based Inference

2.1 Introduction

In this chapter we present powerful characteristic function–based tools as an approach for investigating the properties of distribution functions and their associated quantities. As it turns out the information contained within the characteristic function structure has a one-to-one correspondence with the distribution function framework. In this context characteristic functions can be extremely helpful in both theoretical and applied biostatistical work. In particular, characteristic functions can be used to simplify many analytical proofs in statistics. In certain situations, the form of a characteristic function can easily define a family of distribution functions, thus generalizing known conjugate families. This is very important, for example, in parametric statistics and the construction of *Bayesian priors*. Oftentimes a relatively simple characteristic function can mathematically represent a random variable in terms of its given properties even when the distribution function does not have an explicit analytical form.

In a similar manner to the analysis based on characteristic functions we also introduce Laplace transformations of distribution functions in this chapter. In the statistical context, oftentimes we need to estimate distribution functions based on observations subject to different noise effects or that are based on using data that are directly presented as sums or maximums. These scenarios and various tasks of statistical sequential procedures, as well as in the context of renewal theory, are examples of situations where characteristic functions and Laplace transformations can play a main role in analytical analyses.

We suggest that the reader who is interested in more details regarding characteristic functions beyond those presented in this book consult the book of Lukacs (1970) as a fundamental guide.

In Section 2.2 we consider the elementary properties of characteristic functions as well as convolution statements in which characteristic functions can be involved. The one-to-one mapping propositions related to characteristic and distribution functions are presented in Section 2.3. In Section 2.4 we outline various applications of characteristic functions to biostatistical topics, e.g., those related to renewal functions, sequential procedures, **Tauberian theorems**, risk-efficient estimation, the law of large numbers, the central limit theorem, issues of reconstructing the general distribution based on the distribution of some statistics, extensions and estimations of families of distribution functions. In this chapter we also attend to measurement error problems, cost-efficient designs, and several principles pertaining to Monte Carlo simulation.

2.2 Elementary Properties of Characteristic Functions

We define the *characteristic function* $\varphi_\xi(t), t \in R$, of a distribution function $F(x) = \Pr\{\xi \leq x\}$, where ξ is a random variable, by the following expression:

$$\varphi_\xi(t) = \int_{-\infty}^{\infty} e^{itx}\, dF(x) = E\left(e^{it\xi}\right), \hat{\text{i}} = \sqrt{-1}.$$

Thanks to Euler's formula, the characteristic function can be presented as $\varphi_\xi(t) = E\{\cos(t\xi) + \hat{\text{i}}\sin(t\xi)\}$, which leads immediately to the following properties:

Proposition 2.2.1. Let $F(x)$ denote a distribution function with characteristic function $\varphi_\xi(t)$. Then

1. $\varphi_\xi(0) = 1$;

2. $|\varphi_\xi(t)| \leq 1$, for all t;

3. $\varphi_{-\xi}(t) = \overline{\varphi_\xi(t)}$, where the horizontal bar atop of $\varphi_\xi(t)$ defines the complex conjugate of $\varphi_\xi(t)$.

For example, in order to obtain property (2) above we use the elementary inequality

$$\left|E\left(e^{it\xi}\right)\right| \leq E\left|e^{it\xi}\right| = E\left\{\cos^2(t\xi) + \sin^2(t\xi)\right\}^{1/2} = 1.$$

An attractive property of characteristic functions is related to the following set of results. Consider independent random variables ξ_1 and ξ_2. The distribution function of the sum

$$F_{\xi_1+\xi_2}(x) = \Pr\left(\xi_1 + \xi_2 \leq x\right) = E\left\{I\left(\xi_1 + \xi_2 \leq x\right)\right\}$$

has the form

$$F_{\xi_1+\xi_2}(x) = \iint I(u_1 + u_2 \leq x)d\Pr(\xi_1 \leq u_1, \xi_2 \leq u_2)$$

$$= \iint I(u_1 + u_2 \leq x)dF_{\xi_1}(u_1)dF_{\xi_2}(u_2),$$

since ξ_1 and ξ_2 are independent. Then

$$F_{\xi_1+\xi_2}(x) = \iint I(u_1 \leq x - u_2)dF_{\xi_1}(u_1)dF_{\xi_2}(u_2) = \int_{-\infty}^{\infty} \left\{ \int_{-\infty}^{x-u_2} dF_{\xi_1}(u_1) \right\} dF_{\xi_2}(u_2)$$

$$= \int_{-\infty}^{\infty} F_{\xi_1}(x - u_2)dF_{\xi_2}(u_2),$$

since it is clear that $F(u) = \int_{-\infty}^{u} dF(u)$ with $F(-\infty) = 0$. In the case with dependent random variables ξ_1 and ξ_2, using the definition of conditional probability one can show that the distribution of the sum is given as

$$F_{\xi_1+\xi_2}(x) = \int_{-\infty}^{\infty} \Pr(\xi_1 \leq x - u_2 \mid \xi_2 = u_2)dF_{\xi_2}(u_2). \tag{2.1}$$

Intuitively, this equation means that in the right-hand side of the formula above the random variable ξ_2 is fixed. However, we allow ξ_2 to vary according to its probability distribution. Thus, Equation (2.1) holds.

The integral form (2.1) of $F_{\xi_1+\xi_2}(x)$ shown above is called a *convolution*. When we have $n > 1$ independent $\xi_1, ..., \xi_n$ random variables, it is clear that

$$F_{\xi_1+\xi_2+...+\xi_n}(x) = \underbrace{\iiint \cdots}_{(n-1)\ \text{times}} F_{\xi_1}\left(x - \sum_{i=2}^{n} u_i\right) \prod_{i=2}^{n} dF_{\xi_i}(u_i).$$

Thus, the evaluation of distribution functions of sums of random variables using their components' distribution functions is not a simple task, even when the random variables are iid.

In parallel to this issue, the characteristic function of a sum of independent $\xi_1, ..., \xi_n$ random variables satisfies the simple equation

$$\varphi_{\xi_1+\xi_2+...+\xi_n}(t) = E\left\{e^{it(\xi_1+\xi_2+...+\xi_n)}\right\} = \prod_{i=1}^{n} E\left\{e^{it(\xi_i)}\right\}.$$

that is, $\varphi_{\xi_1+\xi_2+...+\xi_n}(t) = q^n$ with $q = E\left(e^{it\xi_1}\right)$, when $\xi_1, ..., \xi_n$ are iid, since the random variables $e^{it\xi_i}, i = 1, ..., n$, are independent, that is, $E\left(e^{it\xi_k + it\xi_l}\right) = E\left(e^{it\xi_k}\right)E\left(e^{it\xi_l}\right)$, $1 \leq k \neq l \leq n$. Thus characteristic functions can be used to derive the distribution of a sum of random variables. Hence, we can bypass using the direct convolution method for determining the distribution of the sum $\xi_1 + \ldots + \xi_n$, thus simplifying the analysis.

Note that we can completely enjoy the benefits of employing characteristic functions if we show that characteristic functions and distribution functions are equivalent in the context of explaining the properties of random variables.

2.3 One-to-One Mapping

The major reason for our interest in characteristic functions is that they uniquely describe the corresponding distribution functions. In order to show a one-to-one mapping between distribution functions and their corresponding characteristic functions, we should begin by reporting that the conclusion of part (2) of Proposition 2.2.1 states that characteristic functions exist for all random variables. This is important to note, since distribution functions do exist for all random variables by the definition. It is clear that the definition $\varphi_\xi(t) = \int e^{itx}\, dF(x)$ provides the characteristic function if the distribution function is specified. The second stage is to prove that probabilities of intervals can be recovered from the characteristic functions using the following inversion theorem.

Theorem 2.3.1. (Inversion Theorem)

Suppose x and y are arguments of the distribution function $F(u) = \Pr(\xi \leq u)$ that is continuous at x and y. Then

$$F(y) - F(x) = \lim_{\sigma \to 0} \frac{1}{2\pi} \int_{-\infty}^{\infty} \frac{e^{-itx} - e^{-ity}}{\mathring{\imath}t}\, \varphi(t) e^{-t^2\sigma^2/2}\, dt, \tag{2.2}$$

where $\varphi(t) = E\left(e^{it\xi}\right)$ is the characteristic function.

Comments:

   (i). The statement "the function F is continuous at x and y" does not mean F is a continuous function. We assume there are no saltus (jumps) of F specifically at x and y.

   (ii). The integral at (2.2) may have at first glance seemed to be problematic around the point $t = 0$. However, even when $\sigma = 0$, by virtue of Taylor's theorem applied to $e^{-itx} - e^{-ity}$ around $t = 0$, we have

$$\int_{-\delta}^{\delta} \frac{e^{-itx} - e^{-ity}}{\mathring{\imath}t}\, \varphi(t)\, dt = \int_{-\delta}^{\delta} (y - x)\varphi(t)\, dt + O(\delta)$$

with $|\varphi(t)| \le 1$, for all t and fixed $\delta > 0$. Thus, while restricting F (or φ) to hold

$$\int_{\delta}^{\infty} |\varphi(t)/t| \, dt < \infty \quad \text{and} \quad \int_{-\infty}^{-\delta} |\varphi(t)/t| \, dt < \infty, \tag{2.3}$$

for some $\delta > 0$, we could put $\lim_{\sigma \to 0}$ into the integral at (2.2), yielding

$$F(y) - F(x) = \frac{1}{2\pi} \int_{-\infty}^{\infty} \frac{e^{-itx} - e^{-ity}}{\mathring{\imath}t} \varphi(t) dt. \tag{2.4}$$

It turns out that in the case when the density function $f(u) = dF(u)/du$ exists we can write $\varphi(t) = \int e^{itu} f(u) \, du = \left\{ \int f(u) de^{itu} \right\} / (\mathring{\imath}t)$ and then the reader can use the method of integration by parts to obtain conditions on F in order to satisfy (2.3). For example, $\varphi(t) = 1/(1 + t^2)$ (a *Laplace distribution*), $\varphi(t) = e^{-|t|}$ (a *Cauchy distribution*) satisfy (2.3). Thus, we conclude that a class of distribution functions in the form (2.4) is not empty.

(iii). Oftentimes, in the mathematical literature, the Inversion Theorem is presented in the form

$$F(y) - F(x) = \lim_{T \to \infty} \frac{1}{2\pi} \int_{-T}^{T} \frac{e^{-itx} - e^{-ity}}{\mathring{\imath}t} \varphi(t) dt,$$

which is equivalent to (2.2).

2.3.1 Proof of the Inversion Theorem

We outline the proof of Theorem 2.3.1 via the following steps:

Step 1: Assume the random variable ξ is well-behaved so as to have a characteristic function that satisfies constraint (2.3) and is integrable. Then, comment *(ii)* above yields

$$\lim_{\sigma \to 0} \frac{1}{2\pi} \int_{-\infty}^{\infty} \frac{e^{-itx} - e^{-ity}}{\mathring{\imath}t} \varphi(t) e^{-t^2\sigma^2/2} dt = \frac{1}{2\pi} \int_{-\infty}^{\infty} \frac{e^{-itx} - e^{-ity}}{\mathring{\imath}t} \varphi(t) dt$$

$$= \frac{1}{2\pi} E\left(\int_{-\infty}^{\infty} \frac{e^{-itx} - e^{-ity}}{\mathring{\imath}t} e^{it\xi} dt \right) = \frac{1}{2\pi} E\left\{ \int_{-\infty}^{\infty} \frac{e^{-it(x-\xi)} - e^{-it(y-\xi)}}{\mathring{\imath}t} dt \right\}.$$

Since Euler's formula provides

$$e^{-it(x-\xi)} - e^{-it(y-\xi)} = \cos\left(t(x-\xi)\right) - i\sin\left(t(x-\xi)\right) - \cos\left(t(y-\xi)\right) + i\sin\left(t(y-\xi)\right),$$

we consider $\int_{-\infty}^{\infty} \{\cos(t)/t\} dt$. The fact that $\cos(t)/t = -\{\cos(-t)/(-t)\}$ implies

$$\int_{-\infty}^{\infty} \{\cos(t)/t\} dt = \int_{-\infty}^{0} \{\cos(t)/t\} dt + \int_{0}^{\infty} \{\cos(t)/t\} dt = 0.$$

Thus

$$\frac{1}{2\pi} E\left\{ \int_{-\infty}^{\infty} \frac{e^{-it(x-\xi)} - e^{-it(y-\xi)}}{it} dt \right\} = \frac{1}{2\pi} E\left\{ \int_{-\infty}^{\infty} \frac{\sin\left(t(y-\xi)\right) - \sin\left(t(x-\xi)\right)}{t} dt \right\} \quad (2.5)$$

and we need to attend to $\int_{-\infty}^{\infty} \{\sin(t)/t\} dt$. Note that this integral is interesting in itself. Taking into account that $\sin(t) = O(1)$ and $\int_{\delta}^{\infty} (1/t) dt = \infty$, for $\delta > 0$, then one concern is with respect to the finiteness of $\int_{-\infty}^{\infty} \{\sin(t)/t\} dt$. Toward this end, using the property $\sin(-t) = -\sin(t)$, we represent

$$\int_{-\infty}^{\infty} \frac{\sin(t)}{t} dt = 2 \int_{0}^{\infty} \frac{\sin(t)}{t} dt = 2 \int_{0}^{\infty} \sin(t) \int_{0}^{\infty} e^{-ut} du dt = 2 \int_{0}^{\infty}\int_{0}^{\infty} e^{-ut} \sin(t) dt du,$$

where integration by parts implies

$$\int_{0}^{\infty} e^{-ut} \sin(t) dt = -\frac{1}{u} \int_{0}^{\infty} \sin(t) de^{-ut} = -\frac{1}{u} \left\{ e^{-ut} \sin(t) \Big|_{0}^{\infty} - \int_{0}^{\infty} e^{-ut} d\sin(t) \right\}$$

$$= \frac{1}{u} \int_{0}^{\infty} e^{-ut} \cos(t) dt$$

$$= -\frac{1}{u^2} \int_{0}^{\infty} \cos(t) de^{-ut} = -\frac{1}{u^2} \left\{ e^{-ut} \cos(t) \Big|_{0}^{\infty} - \int_{0}^{\infty} e^{-ut} d\cos(t) \right\}$$

$$= \frac{1}{u^2} - \frac{1}{u^2} \int_{0}^{\infty} e^{-ut} \sin(t) dt,$$

that is, $\int_0^\infty e^{-ut}\sin(t)dt = \left(1+u^2\right)^{-1}$. Thus we obtain

$$\int_{-\infty}^\infty \frac{\sin(t)}{t}dt = 2\int_0^\infty \frac{\sin(t)}{t}dt = 2\int_0^\infty \sin(t)\int_0^\infty e^{-ut}\,du\,dt = 2\int_0^\infty \frac{1}{1+u^2}du.$$

This result resolves the problem regarding the existence of $\int_{-\infty}^\infty \{\sin(t)/t\}\,dt$. It is well known that $\int_0^\infty \left(1+u^2\right)^{-1}du = \pi$ (e.g., Titchmarsh, 1976) so that

$$\int_{-\infty}^\infty \frac{\sin(t)}{t}dt = 2\arctan(t)\Big|_0^\infty = \pi.$$

This is the **Dirichlet integral**, which can be easily applied to conclude that

$$\int_{-\infty}^\infty \frac{\sin(\gamma t)}{t}dt = \begin{cases} \pi, & \text{if } \gamma > 0 \\ -\pi, & \text{if } \gamma < 0 \\ 0, & \text{if } \gamma = 0 \end{cases} = \pi I(\gamma \geq 0) - \pi I(\gamma < 0).$$

Then, reconsidering Equation (2.5), we have

$$\frac{1}{2\pi}E\left\{\int_{-\infty}^\infty \frac{e^{-it(x-\xi)}-e^{-it(y-\xi)}}{it}dt\right\}$$

$$= \frac{1}{2\pi}E\left[\pi I\{(y-\xi)\geq 0\} - \pi I\{(y-\xi)<0\} - \pi I\{(x-\xi)\geq 0\} + \pi I\{(x-\xi)<0\}\right]$$

$$= \frac{1}{2}E\left[I\{\xi \leq y\} - \{1-I\{\xi \leq y\}\} - I\{\xi \leq x\} + \{1-I\{\xi \leq x\}\}\right]$$

$$= \Pr(\xi \leq y) - \Pr(\xi \leq x)$$

$$= F(y) - F(x),$$

which completes the proof of Theorem 2.3.1 in the case ξ is well-behaved.

Step 2: Assume the random variable ξ is not as well-behaved as required in Step 1 above. In this case we will use a random variable in the neighborhood of ξ that does satisfy the requirements as seen in Step 1 above. The idea is that instead of considering ξ we can focus on $\zeta = \xi + \eta$, where the random variable η is continuous and independent of ξ. In this setting the convolution principle can lead to

$$F_\zeta(u) = \Pr(\eta + \xi \leq u) = \int \Pr(\eta \leq u - x)d\Pr(\xi \leq x)$$

and then, for example, the density function $f_\zeta(u) = dF_\zeta(u)/du = \int f_\eta(u-x)dF(x)$ with $f_\eta(u) = dF_\eta(u)/du$ exists. Even when $\xi = 1,2,\dots$ is discrete, we have

$$F_\zeta(u) = \sum_{j=1}^{\infty} F_\eta(u-j)\Pr(\xi = j), \quad f_\zeta(u) = \sum_{j=1}^{\infty} f_\eta(u-j)\Pr(\xi = j).$$

In this case, in accordance to Step 1, it is clear that

$$F_\zeta(y) - F_\zeta(x) = \frac{1}{2\pi}\int_{-\infty}^{\infty} \frac{e^{-itx} - e^{-ity}}{it} E\left(e^{it\zeta}\right)dt = \frac{1}{2\pi}\int_{-\infty}^{\infty} \frac{e^{-itx} - e^{-ity}}{it} \varphi(t)E\left(e^{it\eta}\right)dt. \quad (2.6)$$

Then "Der η hat seine Arbeit getan, der η kann gehen" (German: Schiller, 2013) and we let η go. To formalize this result we start by proving the following lemma.

Lemma 2.3.1.

Let a random variable η be ***normally*** $N(\mu,\sigma^2)$ -distributed. Then the characteristic function for η is given by $\varphi_\eta(t) = E\left(e^{it\eta}\right) = \exp\left(i\mu t - \sigma^2 t^2/2\right)$.

Proof. If we define the random variable $\eta_1 \sim N(0,1)$ then its characteristic function is given as $\varphi_{\eta_1}(t) = (2\pi)^{-1}\int_{-\infty}^{\infty} e^{itu} e^{-u^2/2}\, du$, since the density function of η_1 is $(2\pi)^{-1} e^{-u^2/2}$. Thus

$$d\varphi_{\eta_1}(t)/dt = (2\pi)^{-1}\int_{-\infty}^{\infty} iu e^{itu - u^2/2}\, du = -(2\pi)^{-1} i\int_{-\infty}^{\infty} e^{itu}\, de^{-u^2/2}.$$

Integrating the above expression by parts, we arrive at
$d\varphi_{\eta_1}(t)/dt = -(2\pi)^{-1} t\int_{-\infty}^{\infty} e^{itu - u^2/2}\, du = -t\varphi_{\eta_1}(t)$, that is, $\{d\varphi_{\eta_1}(t)/dt\}/\varphi_{\eta_1}(t) = -t$ or $d\{\ln(\varphi_{\eta_1}(t))\}/dt = -t$. This differential equation has the solution $\varphi_{\eta_1}(t) = \exp(-t^2/2) + C$, for all constants C. Taking into account that $\varphi_{\eta_1}(0) = 1$, we can admit only $C = 0$. Then $\varphi_{\eta_1}(t) = \exp(-t^2/2)$. The random variable $\eta = \mu + \sigma\eta_1 \sim N(\mu,\sigma^2)$ and hence has the characteristic function $\varphi_\eta(t) = e^{i\mu t}E\left(e^{i\sigma t\eta_1}\right) = e^{i\mu t}\varphi_{\eta_1}(\sigma t)$.
Now the proof of Lemma 2.3.1 is complete.

Set $\eta \sim N(0, \sigma^2)$. Lemma 2.3.1 applied to Equation (2.6) yields

$$F_\zeta(y) - F_\zeta(x) = \frac{1}{2\pi} \int_{-\infty}^{\infty} \frac{e^{-itx} - e^{-ity}}{it} \varphi(t) e^{-\frac{\sigma^2 t^2}{2}} dt, \quad \zeta = \xi + \eta.$$

Since the distribution function F of ξ is continuous at x and y, we have that

$$\lim_{\sigma \to 0} \{F_\zeta(y) - F_\zeta(x)\} = \frac{1}{2\pi} \lim_{\sigma \to 0} \int_{-\infty}^{\infty} \frac{e^{-itx} - e^{-ity}}{it} \varphi(t) e^{-\frac{\sigma^2 t^2}{2}} dt,$$

which leads to

$$F(y) - F(x) = \frac{1}{2\pi} \lim_{\sigma \to 0} \int_{-\infty}^{\infty} \frac{e^{-itx} - e^{-ity}}{it} \varphi(t) e^{-\frac{\sigma^2 t^2}{2}} dt,$$

since $\Pr(|\eta| > \delta) \to 0$, for all $\delta > 0$, as $\sigma \to 0$ (here presenting $\eta_k \sim N(0, \sigma_k^2)$ it is then clear that we have $\xi + \eta_k \xrightarrow{p} \xi$ and $F_{\xi+\eta_k} \to F$ as $\sigma_k \to 0$, $k \to \infty$). This completes the proof of Theorem 2.3.1.

Note that the difference $F(y) - F(x)$ uniquely denotes the distribution function F. Thus, we conclude that characteristic functions uniquely define their distribution functions and vice versa.

Assume the density $f(x)$ of ξ exists. In view of Theoerm 2.3.1, we can write

$$\{F(x + h) - F(x)\} / h = \frac{1}{2\pi} \int_{-\infty}^{\infty} \frac{e^{-it(x)} - e^{-it(x+h)}}{iht} \varphi(t) dt,$$

using $y = x + h$. From this with $h \to 0$ and the definitions $f(x) = \lim_{h \to 0} \{F(x+h) - F(x)\}/h$, $d\{e^{-it(x)}\}/dx = -\lim_{h \to 0}\left[\{e^{-it(x)} - e^{-it(x+h)}\}/h\right]$ we have the following result.

Theorem 2.3.2.

Let the characteristic function $\varphi(t)$ be integrable. Then

$$f(x) = \frac{1}{2\pi} \int_{-\infty}^{\infty} e^{-itx} \varphi(t) dt.$$

2.4 Applications

The common scheme to apply mechanisms based on characteristic functions consists of the following algorithm:

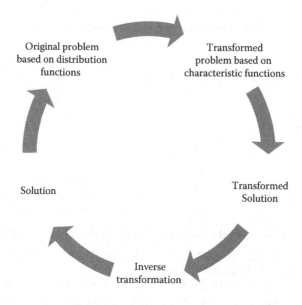

We apply this algorithm within the set of examples given below.

2.4.1 Expected Lengths of Random Stopping Times and Renewal Functions in Light of Tauberian Theorems

Assume, for example, that H denotes the hours that a physician can serve patients during a specific time span. The patients are surveyed sequentially and each patient, i, requires X_i hours to be observed. Suppose $X_i > 0, i = 1, 2, ...,$ are iid random variables. Then the physician will observe a random number of patients denoted as

$$N(H) = \min\left\{ n \geq 1 : \sum_{i=1}^{n} X_i \geq H \right\}.$$

In this case, the physician will end his/her shift when $\sum_{i=1}^{n} X_i$ overshoots the threshold $H > 0$.

In statistical applications, constructions similar to $N(H)$ above fall in the realm of **Renewal Theory** (e.g., Cox, 1962). The integer random variable $N(H)$ is a **stopping time** and its expectation $E\{N(H)\}$ is called as a **renewal function**.

In general $X_i, i = 1, 2...$ can be negative. In this case the stopping time has the form $N(H) = \inf\left\{n \geq 1 : \sum_{i=1}^{n} X_i \geq H\right\}$ and we need to require that $\Pr\{N(H) < \infty\} = 1$ in order to stop at all.

In this section we analyze the expectation $E\{N(H)\}$, when $X_i > 0, i = 1, 2,...$ are **continuous** random variables. Toward this end we begin with the simple expression

$$E\{N(H)\} = \sum_{j=1}^{\infty} j \Pr\{N(H) = j\} = \sum_{j=1}^{\infty} j \Pr\left\{\sum_{i=1}^{j-1} X_i < H, \sum_{i=1}^{j} X_i \geq H\right\},$$

where we define $\sum_{i=1}^{0} X_i = 0$ and use the rule that the process stops the **first time** at j when the event $\left\{\sum_{i=1}^{j-1} X_i < H, \sum_{i=1}^{j} X_i \geq H\right\}$ occurs. (Note that if not all $X_i > 0, i = 1, 2...$, then we should consider $\{N(H) = j\} = \left\{\max_{1 \leq k \leq j-1}\left(\sum_{i=1}^{k-1} X_i\right) < H, \max_{1 \leq k \leq j}\left(\sum_{i=1}^{k} X_i\right) \geq H\right\}$, see Figure 2.1 for details.) Thus

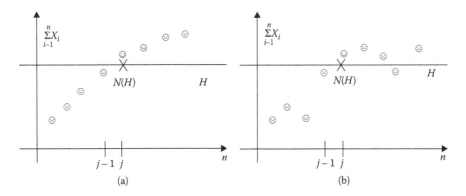

FIGURE 2.1

The sum $\sum_{i=1}^{n} X_i$ crosses the threshold H at j when (a) all $X_i > 0, i = 1, 2...$ and (b) we have several negative observations.

$$
\begin{aligned}
E\{N(H)\} &= \sum_{j=1}^{\infty} j\left[\Pr\left\{\sum_{i=1}^{j-1} X_i < H\right\} - \Pr\left\{\sum_{i=1}^{j-1} X_i < H, \sum_{i=1}^{j} X_i < H\right\}\right] \\
&= \sum_{j=1}^{\infty} j\left[\Pr\left\{\sum_{i=1}^{j-1} X_i < H\right\} - \Pr\left\{\sum_{i=1}^{j} X_i < H\right\}\right] \\
&= \sum_{j=1}^{\infty} j\Pr\left\{\sum_{i=1}^{j-1} X_i < H\right\} - \sum_{j=1}^{\infty} j\Pr\left\{\sum_{i=1}^{j} X_i < H\right\} \qquad (2.7) \\
&= 1 + \sum_{j=1}^{\infty} (j+1)\Pr\left\{\sum_{i=1}^{j} X_i < H\right\} - \sum_{j=1}^{\infty} j\Pr\left\{\sum_{i=1}^{j} X_i < H\right\} \\
&= 1 + \sum_{j=1}^{\infty} \Pr\left\{\sum_{i=1}^{j} X_i < H\right\}.
\end{aligned}
$$

This result leads to *the non-asymptotic upper bound of the renewal function*, since by (2.7) we have

$$
\begin{aligned}
E\{N(H)\} - 1 &= \sum_{j=1}^{\infty} \Pr\left\{\exp\left(-\frac{1}{H}\sum_{i=1}^{j} X_i\right) > e^{-1}\right\} \\
&= \sum_{j=1}^{\infty} E\left[I\left\{\exp\left(-\frac{1}{H}\sum_{i=1}^{j} X_i\right) > e^{-1}\right\}\right] \\
&\leq e\sum_{j=1}^{\infty} E\left\{\exp\left(-\frac{1}{H}\sum_{i=1}^{j} X_i\right)\right\} = e\sum_{j=1}^{\infty} \prod_{i=1}^{j} E\left(e^{-\frac{1}{H}X_i}\right) \\
&= e\sum_{j=1}^{\infty} \left\{E\left(e^{-\frac{1}{H}X_1}\right)\right\}^{j}, \quad e = \exp(1),
\end{aligned}
$$

where the fact that $I(a > b) \leq a/b$, for all positive a and b, was used. Noting that $E\left(e^{-X_1/H}\right) \leq 1$ and using the sum formula for a geometric progression, we obtain

$$
E\{N(H)\} \leq 1 + e\,E\left(e^{-\frac{1}{H}X_1}\right)\left\{1 - E\left(e^{-\frac{1}{H}X_1}\right)\right\}^{-1}.
$$

One can apply Taylor's theorem to $E\left(e^{-X_1/H}\right)$ by considering $1/H$ around 0 as $H \to \infty$ to easily show that the upper bound for $E\{N(H)\}$ is asymptotically linear with respect to H, when $E\left(X_1^2\right) < \infty$.

Now let us study the asymptotic behavior of $E\{N(H)\}$ as $H \to \infty$. Toward this end we consider the following nonformal arguments: (1) Characteristic functions correspond to distribution functions that increase and are bounded by 1. Certainly, the properties of a characteristic function will be satisfied if we assume the corresponding "distribution functions" are bounded by 2 or, more generally, by linear-type functions. In this context the function $E\{N(H)\}$ increases monotonically and is bounded. Thus we can focus on the transformation $\psi(t) = \int_0^\infty e^{itu} d\left[E\{N(u)\}\right]$ of $E\{N(u)\} > 0$ in a similar manner to that of characteristic functions. (2) Intuitively, relatively small values of t can provide $\psi(t)$ to represent a behavior of $E\{N(H)\}$, when H is large, because schematically it may be displayed that

$$\psi(t \to 0) \sim \int_0^\infty e^{iu(t \to 0)} d\left[E\{N(u)\}\right] \sim E\{N(u \to \infty)\}.$$

In a rigorous manner, these arguments can be found in the context of **Tauberian theorems** (e.g., Korevaar, 2004; Subkhankulov, 1976; Yakimiv, 2005) that can associate formally $\psi(t)$, as $t \to 0$, with $E\{N(H)\}$, as $H \to \infty$.

In this chapter we will prove a simple Tauberian theorem to complete the asymptotic evaluation of $E\{N(H)\}$ (see Proposition 2.4.1 below).

By virtue of (2.7), the function $\psi(t)$ can be presented as

$$\psi(t) = \int_0^\infty e^{itu} d\left[1 + \sum_{j=1}^\infty \Pr\left\{\sum_{i=1}^j X_i < u\right\}\right] = \sum_{j=1}^\infty \int_0^\infty e^{itu} d\Pr\left\{\sum_{i=1}^j X_i < u\right\}$$

$$= \sum_{j=1}^\infty E\left\{\exp\left(it\sum_{i=1}^j X_i\right)\right\} = \sum_{j=1}^\infty q^j$$

with $q = E\left(e^{itX_1}\right)$ and $|q| < 1$. The sum formula for a geometric progression provides

$$\psi(t) = \frac{q}{1-q}.$$

Applying Taylor's theorem to $q = E\left(e^{itX_1}\right)$ with respect to t around 0, we have $q = 1 + E\left(itX_1\right) + o(t)$, when we assume $E\left(X_1^2\right) < \infty$, and then

$\psi(t) \sim -1/\{t\mathring{\imath}E(X_1)\} = \mathring{\imath}/\{tE(X_1)\}$ as $t \to 0$. The transformation $\mathring{\imath}/\{tE(X_1)\}$ corresponds to the function $A(u) = u/\{E(X_1)\}, u > 0$, since (see Theorem 2.3.2)

$$\frac{dA(u)}{du} = \frac{1}{2\pi}\int_{-\infty}^{\infty} e^{-\mathring{\imath}tu}\frac{\mathring{\imath}}{tE(X_1)}dt = \frac{\mathring{\imath}}{2\pi E(X_1)}\int_{-\infty}^{\infty}\frac{\cos(tu) - \mathring{\imath}\sin(tu)}{t}dt = \frac{1}{E(X_1)}$$

(see the proof of Theorem 2.3.1 to obtain values of the integrals $\int_{-\infty}^{\infty}\{\cos(ut)/t\}dt$ and $\int_{-\infty}^{\infty}\{\sin(ut)/t\}dt$). Thus $E\{N(H)\} \sim H/E(X_1)$ as $H \to \infty$.

Let us derive the asymptotic result about $E\{N(H)\}$ given above in a formal way. By the definition of $N(H)$ we obtain

$$\sum_{i=1}^{N(H)} X_i \geq H \text{ and then } E\left\{\sum_{i=1}^{N(H)} X_i\right\} \geq H.$$

Using **Wald's lemma** (this result will be proven elsewhere in this book, see Chapter 4), we note that

$$E\left\{\sum_{i=1}^{N(H)} X_i\right\} = E(X_1)E\{N(H)\} \text{ and then } E\{N(H)\} \geq H/E(X_1). \qquad (2.8)$$

Consider the following scenario where we define $g(u) > 0$ to be an increasing function. Then the real-valued *Laplace transformation* of $g(u)$ has the form $G(s) = \int_0^{\infty} e^{-su}dg(u), s > 0$. The form of the Laplace transformation belongs to a family of transformations that includes the characteristic functions considered above. In this case, we have the Tauberian-type result given as follows:

Proposition 2.4.1. Assume $a > 0$ is a constant and the increasing function $g(u)$ satisfies the conditions *(i)* $g(u) \geq au$ and *(ii)* $g(u) = o(e^u)$ as $u \to \infty$. If $G(s) < \infty$, for all $s > 0$, then

$$g(u) \leq \frac{G(1/u) - au}{(w-1)}e^w + auwe^{w-1},$$

for all $u > 0$ and $w > 1$.

Proof. By virtue of condition *(ii)*, integrating by parts, we obtain

$$G(s) = s\int_0^{\infty} e^{-su}g(y)dy.$$

Since $g(u)$ increases and $g(u) \geq au$, for $s \in R$, we have

$$G(s) = s \int_0^u e^{-sy} g(y) dy + s \int_u^{wu} e^{-sy} g(y) dy + s \int_{wu}^\infty e^{-sy} g(y) dy$$

$$\geq sa \int_0^u e^{-sy} y \, dy + sg(u) \int_u^{wu} e^{-sy} \, dy + sa \int_{wu}^\infty e^{-sy} y \, dy.$$

Thus

$$G(s) \geq \frac{a}{s} \left\{ 1 - e^{-su}(1+su) \right\} + g(u)\left(e^{-su} - e^{-swu} \right) + \frac{a}{s}\left\{ e^{-swu}(1+suw) \right\}.$$

Then, setting $s = 1/u$, we have

$$g(u) \leq \frac{G(1/u) - au}{e^{-1} - e^{-w}} + au \frac{2e^{-1} - (1+w)e^{-w}}{e^{-1} - e^{-w}}. \tag{2.9}$$

Taylor's theorem provides $e^{-1} - e^{-w} = (w-1)\exp\left[-\{1 + \theta_1(w-1)\} \right]$ and $2e^{-1} - (1+w)e^{-w} = (w-1)\{1 + \theta_2(w-1)\}\exp\left[-\{1 + \theta_2(w-1)\} \right]$ with $0 < \theta_1, \theta_2 < 1$, where $e^{-1} - e^{-w}$ and $2e^{-1} - (1+w)e^{-w}$ are evaluated as functions of w around $w = 1$. Therefore $e^{-1} - e^{-w} \geq (w-1)\exp(-w)$ and $2e^{-1} - (1+w)e^{-w} \leq (w-1)we^{-1}$. This modifies inequality (2.9) to the form

$$g(u) \leq \frac{G(1/u) - au}{(w-1)e^{-w}} + auwe^{-1+w}.$$

This completes the proof.

Proposition 2.4.1 with $g(u) = E\{N(u)\}$ and $a = E(X_1)$ implies

$$\frac{1}{E(X_1)} \leq \frac{E\{N(u)\}}{u} \leq \frac{G(1/u) - u/E(X_1)}{(w-1)u} e^w + \frac{1}{E(X_1)} we^{w-1},$$

where, in a similar manner to the analysis of $\psi(t) = \int_0^\infty e^{itu} d[E\{N(u)\}] = q/(1-q)$

shown above, we have $G(1/u) = \sum_{j=1}^\infty E\left\{ \exp\left(-\sum_{i=1}^j X_i / u \right) \right\} = v/(1-v)$,

$v = E\left(e^{-X_1/u} \right) = 1 - E(X_1)/u + o(1/u)$ as $u \to \infty$ and $E(X_1^2) < \infty$. This means that

$$\frac{1}{E(X_1)} \leq \lim_{u \to \infty} \frac{E\{N(u)\}}{u} \leq \frac{1}{E(X_1)} we^{w-1}.$$

Considering $w \to 1$, we conclude that $\lim_{u \to \infty} \frac{1}{u} E\{N(u)\} = \{E(X_1)\}^{-1}$.

The asymptotic result $E\{N(H)\} \sim H / E(X_1)$, as $H \to \infty$, is called the *elementary renewal theorem.* Naïvely, taking into account that $E\left(\sum_{i=1}^{n} X_i\right) = nE(X_1)$ and the definition $N(H) = \min\left\{n \geq 1 : \sum_{i=1}^{n} X_i \geq H\right\}$, one can decide that it is obvious that $E\{N(H)\} \sim H/E(X_1)$. However, we invite the reader to employ probabilistic arguments in a different manner to that mentioned above in order to prove this approximation, recognizing a simplicity and structure of the proposed analysis. Proposition 2.4.1 provides non-asymptotically a very accurate upper bound of the renewal function. Perhaps, this proposition can be found only in this book. The demonstrated proof scheme can be extended to more complicated cases with, e.g., dependent random variables as well as improved to obtain more accurate results, e.g., regarding the expression $\lim_{u\to\infty}\left[u^{-\omega}\left[E\{N(u)\} - \{E(X_1)\}^{-1} u\right]\right]$ with $0 \leq \omega \leq 1$ (for example, in Proposition 2.4.1 one can define $w = 1 + u^{-\omega}\log(u)$). The stopping time $N(H)$ will also be studied in several forthcoming sections of this book.

Warning: Tauberian-type propositions should be applied very carefully. For example, define the function $v(x) = \sin(x)$. The corresponding Laplace transformation is $J(s) = \int_{0}^{\infty} e^{-su} d\sin(u) = s/(1+s^2), s > 0$. This does not lead us to conclude that since $J(s) \underset{s\to 0}{\to} 0$, we have $v(x) \underset{x\to\infty}{\to} 0$. In this case we remark that $v(x)$ is not an increasing function for $x \in (-\infty, \infty)$.

2.4.2 Risk-Efficient Estimation

An interesting problem in statistical estimation is that of constructing an estimate for minimizing a *risk function*, which is typically defined as a sum of the estimate's mean squared error cost of sampling. Robbins (1959) initiated the study of such *risk-efficient* estimates and the idea of assessing the performance of sequential estimates using a risk function became extremely popular in statistics. Certain developments in this area of estimation are summarized in Lai (1996).

Let $\hat{\theta}_n$ denote an estimate of an unknown parameter θ computed from a sample of fixed size n. Assume that $nE\left(\hat{\theta}_n - \theta\right)^2 \to \sigma^2$, as $n \to \infty$. If the cost of taking a single observation equals C, then the risk function associated with $\hat{\theta}_n$ is given by

$$R_n(C) = E\left(\hat{\theta}_n - \theta\right)^2 + Cn.$$

Thus we want to minimize the mean squared error of the estimate balanced by the attempt to request larger and larger sets of data points, which is restricted by the requirement to pay for each observation. For example, consider the simple estimator of the mean $\theta = E(X_1)$ based on iid observations $X_i, i = 1, ..., n$ is $\hat{\theta}_n = \bar{X}_n = \sum_{i=1}^{n} X_i/n$. In this case $R_n(C) = \sigma^2/n + Cn$ with $\sigma^2 = \text{var}(X_1)$.

Making use of the definition of the risk function one can easily show that $R_n(C)$ is minimized when $n = n_C^* = \{\sigma/C^{1/2}\}$. Since the optimal fixed sample size n_C^* depends on σ, which is commonly unknown, one can resort to sequential sampling and consider the stopping rule within the estimation procedure of the form

$$N(C) = \inf\left\{n \geq n_0 : n \geq \hat{\sigma}_k/C^{1/2}\right\},$$

where $n_0 \geq 1$ is an initial sample size and $\hat{\sigma}_k$ is a consistent estimate of $\sigma > 0$. We sample the observations sequentially (one by one) and will stop buying data points at $N(C)$, obtaining our final estimate $\hat{\theta}_{N(C)}$. The method presented in Section 2.4.1 can be adopted to show that the expected sample size $E\{N(C)\}$ is asymptotically equivalent to the optimal fixed sample size n_C^* in the sense that $E\{N(C)\}/n_C^* \to 1$ as $C \to 0$ (Vexler and Dmitrienko, 1999).

Consider, for another example, iid observations $X_i > 0, i = 1, ..., n$, from an exponential distribution with the density function $f(u) = \theta^{-1}\exp(-u\theta^{-1})$, $\theta > 0$. In this case, the *maximum likelihood estimator* of the parameter $\theta = E(X_1)$ is $\hat{\theta}_n = \bar{X}_n = \sum_{i=1}^{n} X_i/n$ and $E(\hat{\theta}_n - \theta)^2 = \theta^2/n$. Assume, depending on parameter values, it is required to pay $\theta^4 H$ for one data point. Then $R_n(H) = \theta^2/n + H\theta^4 n$ and we have $R_n(H) - R_{n-1}(H) = -\theta^2/\{(n-1)n\} + H\theta^4$. The equation $R_n(H) - R_{n-1}(H) = 0$ gives the optimal fixed sample size $n_H^* \approx \{\theta^{-1}/H^{1/2}\}$, where θ is unknown. In this framework, the stopping rule is

$$N(H) = \inf\left\{n \geq n_0 : n \geq \left(\hat{\theta}_n\right)^{-1}/H^{1/2}\right\} = \min\left\{n \geq n_0 : \sum_{i=1}^{n} X_i \geq 1/H^{1/2}\right\}$$

and the estimator is $\hat{\theta}_{N(H)} = \sum_{i=1}^{N(H)} X_i/N(H)$. It is straightforward to apply the technique mentioned in Section 2.4.1 to evaluate $E\{N(H)\}$ where the fact that $E(e^{-sX_1}) = \theta^{-1}\int_0^\infty e^{-su}e^{-u/\theta}\,du = \{1 + \theta s\}^{-1}$ can be taken into account.

Note that naïvely one can estimate n_C^* using the estimator $\hat{\sigma}/C^{1/2}$. This is very problematic, since in order to obtain the estimator $\hat{\sigma}$ of σ we need a sample with the size we try to approximate.

2.4.3 Khinchin's (or Hinchin's) Form of the Law of Large Numbers

In this section we assume that random variables $\xi_1,...,\xi_n$ are iid with $E(\xi_1) = \theta$. The average $\bar{\xi}_n = n^{-1}S_n$, $S_n = \sum_{i=1}^{n} \xi_i$, can be considered as a simple estimator of θ. For all $\varepsilon > 0$, *Chebyshev's inequality* states

$$\Pr\left(\left|\bar{\xi}_n - \theta\right| > \varepsilon\right) = \Pr\left(\left|\bar{\xi}_n - \theta\right|^k > \varepsilon^k\right) \le \frac{E\left\{\left|\bar{\xi}_n - \theta\right|^k\right\}}{\varepsilon^k}, \quad k > 0.$$

Consider for example $k = 2$. It may be verified that

$$\begin{aligned}
E\left\{(S_n - n\theta)^2\right\} &= E\left[\left(\sum_{i=1}^{n}(X_i - \theta)\right)^2\right] = E\left\{\sum_{i=1}^{n}\sum_{j=1}^{n}(X_i - \theta)(X_j - \theta)\right\} \\
&= E\left\{\sum_{i=1}^{n}(X_i - \theta)^2\right\} + E\left\{\sum_{i=1}^{n}\sum_{j=1,j\ne i}^{n}(X_i - \theta)(X_j - \theta)\right\} \\
&= \sum_{i=1}^{n}E(X_i - \theta)^2 + \sum_{i=1}^{n}\sum_{j=1,j\ne i}^{n}E(X_i - \theta)(X_j - \theta) \\
&= nE(X_1 - \theta)^2.
\end{aligned}$$

This yields that $\Pr\left(\left|\bar{\xi}_n - \theta\right| > \varepsilon\right) \le E(X_1 - \theta)^2/(n\varepsilon^2) \to 0$ as $n \to \infty$, proving the *law of large numbers,* $\bar{\xi}_n \xrightarrow{p} \theta$ as $n \to \infty$.

It is clear that to conduct proofs in a manner similar to the algorithm above, it is required that $E\left(\left|\xi_1\right|^{1+\delta}\right) < \infty$ for some $\delta > 0$. Let us apply a method based on characteristic functions to prove the property $\bar{\xi}_n \xrightarrow{p} \theta$ as $n \to \infty$. We have the characteristic function of $\bar{\xi}_n$ in the form

$$\varphi_{\bar{\xi}}(t) = E\left(e^{itS_n/n}\right) = \left\{E\left(e^{it\xi_1/n}\right)\right\}^n = \exp\left(n\ln\left(E\left(e^{it\xi_1/n}\right)\right)\right).$$

Define the function $l(t) = \ln\left(E\left(e^{it\xi_1}\right)\right)$, rewriting

$$\varphi_{\bar{\xi}}(t) = \exp\left(nl(t/n)\right) = \exp\left(t\left(\frac{l(t/n) - l(0)}{t/n}\right)\right),$$

where $l(0) = 0$. The derivate $dl(t)/dt$ is $\left\{E\left(e^{it\xi_1}\right)\right\}^{-1}\left\{E\left(i\xi e^{it\xi_1}\right)\right\}$ and then $dl(u)/du\big|_{u=0} = iE(\xi) = i\theta$. By the definition of the derivate

$$\left(\frac{l(t/n) - l(0)}{t/n}\right) \to \frac{dl(u)}{du}\bigg|_{u=0} = i\theta \text{ as } n \to \infty.$$

Thus $\varphi_{\bar\xi_n}(t) \to e^{it\theta}$ as $n \to \infty$, where $e^{it\theta}$ corresponds to a degenerate distribution function of θ. This justifies that $\bar\xi_n \xrightarrow{p} \theta$ as $n \to \infty$ requiring only that $\left|E(\xi_1)\right| < \infty$.

2.4.4 Analytical Forms of Distribution Functions

Characteristic functions can be employed in order to derive analytical forms of distribution functions. Consider the following examples.

1. Let independent random variables $\xi_1, ..., \xi_n$ be normally distributed. The sum $S_n = \xi_1 + ... + \xi_n$ is normally distributed with $E(S_n) = \sum_{i=1}^{n} E(\xi_i)$ and $\text{var}(S_n) = \sum_{i=1}^{n} \text{var}(\xi_i)$. Lemma 2.3.1 shows this fact, since the characteristic function of S_n satisfies

$$\varphi_{S_n}(t) = \prod_{i=1}^{n} E\left(e^{it\xi_i}\right) = \prod_{i=1}^{n} \exp\left(itE(\xi_i) - \text{var}(\xi_i)t^2/2\right)$$

$$= \exp\left(it\sum_{i=1}^{n} E(\xi_i) - \frac{t^2}{2}\sum_{i=1}^{n} \text{var}(\xi_i)\right).$$

2. *Gamma distributions:* Let ξ have the density function

$$f(u) = \begin{cases} \gamma^\lambda u^{\lambda-1} e^{-\gamma u} / \left(\displaystyle\int_0^\infty x^{\gamma-1} e^{-x}\, dx\right), & u \ge 0, \\ 0, & u < 0 \end{cases}$$

with the parameters $\lambda > 0$ (a shape) and $\gamma > 0$ (a rate = 1/scale). In a similar manner to the proof of Lemma 2.3.1, using integration by parts, we have that the characteristic function of ξ satisfies $d\left(\ln\left(\varphi_\xi(t)\right)\right)/dt = d\left(-\lambda \ln(\gamma - it)\right)/dt$. Then, taking into account $\varphi_\xi(0) = 1$, we obtain $\varphi_\xi(t) = (1 - it/\gamma)^{-\lambda}$.

3. By virtue of the definition of the χ_n^2 distribution function with n degrees of freedom, the random variable $\zeta_n = \sum_{i=1}^{n} \xi_i^2$ has a χ_n^2 distribution if iid random variables $\xi_1,...,\xi_n$ are $N(0,1)$ distributed. Note that

$$\Pr(\zeta_1 < u) = \Pr(|\xi_1| < \sqrt{u}) = \frac{2}{\sqrt{2\pi}} \int_0^{\sqrt{u}} e^{-x^2/2}\, dx.$$

Thus, the density function of ζ_1 is $(2\pi)^{-1/2} e^{-u/2} u^{-1/2}$ that corresponds to the gamma distribution from Example 2 above with parameters $\lambda = 1/2$ and $\gamma = 1/2$. This means the characteristic function of ζ_n is $(1 - 2it)^{-n/2}$. Therefore we conclude that ζ_n is gamma distributed with parameters $\lambda = n/2$ and $\gamma = 1/2$.

2.4.5 Central Limit Theorem

Let $\xi_1,...,\xi_n$ be iid random variables with $a = E(\xi_1)$ and $0 < \sigma^2 = \text{var}(\xi_1) < \infty$. Define the random variables $S_n = \sum_{i=1}^{n} \xi_i$ and $\zeta_n = (\sigma^2 n)^{-1/2}(S_n - an)$. The *central limit theorem* states that ζ_n has asymptotically (as $n \to \infty$) the $N(0,1)$ distribution. We will prove this theorem using characteristic functions. Toward this end, we begin with the representation of ζ_n in the form $\zeta_n = (n)^{-1/2} \left\{ \sum_{i=1}^{n} (\xi_i - a)/\sigma \right\}$, where $E(\xi_1 - a)/\sigma = 0$ and $\text{var}\{(\xi_1 - a)/\sigma\} = 1$, which allows us to assume $a = 0, \sigma = 1$ without loss of generality. In this case, we should show that the characteristic function of ζ_n, say $\varphi_{\zeta_n}(t)$, converges to $e^{-t^2/2}$. It is clear that $\varphi_{\zeta_n}(t) = E\left(e^{it\sum_{i=1}^{n}\xi_i/\sqrt{n}}\right) = \prod_{i=1}^{n} E\left(e^{it\xi_i/\sqrt{n}}\right) = \left\{\varphi_\xi(t/\sqrt{n})\right\}^n$, that is, $\ln(\varphi_{\zeta_n}(t)) = n \ln(\varphi_\xi(t/\sqrt{n}))$. When $n \to \infty$, $t/\sqrt{n} \to 0$ that leads us to apply the Taylor theorem to the following objects: (1) $\varphi_\xi(t/\sqrt{n})$, considering $t/\sqrt{n}$ around 0 and (2) the logarithm function, considering its argument around 1. That is

$$\ln(\varphi_{\zeta_n}(t)) = n \ln\left(1 - \frac{t^2}{2n} + o\left(\frac{t^2}{n}\right)\right) = n\left\{-\frac{t^2}{2n} + o\left(\frac{t^2}{n}\right)\right\} \to -\frac{t^2}{2}, n \to \infty.$$

The proof is complete.

The simple proof scheme shown above can be easily adapted when ζ_n has more complicated structure or $\xi_1,...,\xi_n$ are not iid. For example, when

$\xi_1,...,\xi_n$ are independent but not identically distributed, we have $\ln\left(\varphi_{\zeta_n}(t)\right)=\sum_{i=1}^{n}\ln\left(E\left(e^{it\xi_i/\sqrt{n}}\right)\right)$ and then the asymptotic evaluation of $\ln\left(\varphi_{\zeta_n}(t)\right)$ can be provided in a similar manner to that demonstrated in this section.

2.4.5.1 Principles of Monte Carlo Simulations

The outcomes of the law of large numbers and the central limit theorem yield central techniques applied in a context of *Monte Carlo simulations* (e.g., Robert and Casella, 2004).

Consider the problem regarding calculation of the integral $J=\int_a^b g(u)du$, where g is a known function and the bounds a,b are not necessarily finite. One can rewrite the integral in the form

$$J=\int_{-\infty}^{\infty}\left[\left\{\frac{g(u)}{f(u)}\right\}I\{u\in[a,b]\}\right]f(u)\,du,$$

using a density function f. Then, we have $J=E\left[\left\{\frac{g(\xi)}{f(\xi)}\right\}I\{\xi\in[a,b]\}\right]$ with ξ, which is a random variable distributed according to the density function f. In this case, we can approximate J using $J_n=\frac{1}{n}\sum_{i=1}^{n}\left[\left\{\frac{g(\xi_i)}{f(\xi_i)}\right\}I\{\xi_i\in[a,b]\}\right]$, where $\xi_1,...,\xi_n$ are independent and simulated from f. The law of large numbers provides $J_n\to J$ as $n\to\infty$.

The central limit theorem can be applied to evaluate how accurate this approximation is as well as to define a value of the needed sample size n. That is, we have asymptotically $\sqrt{n}\,(J_n-J)\left[E\left(\left[\left\{\frac{g(\xi_1)}{f(\xi_1)}\right\}I\{\xi_1\in[a,b]\}-J\right]^2\right)\right]^{-1/2}\sim N(0,1)$ and then, for example,

$$\Pr\{|J_n-J|\geq\delta\}=1-\Pr\{J_n-J<\delta\}+\Pr\{J_n-J<-\delta\}$$

$$\approx 1-\Phi\left(\delta\sqrt{n}/\Delta\right)+\Phi\left(-\delta\sqrt{n}/\Delta\right),$$

where $\Phi(u)=\int_{-\infty}^{u}e^{-x^2/2}\,dx/\sqrt{2\pi}$ and Δ is an estimator of

$$\left[E\left(\left[\left\{\frac{g(\xi_1)}{f(\xi_1)}\right\}I\{\xi_i\in[a,b]\}-J\right]^2\right)\right]^{1/2}$$ obtained, e.g., by generating, for a relatively

large integer M, iid random variables $\eta_1, ..., \eta_M$ with the density function f, and defining

$$\Delta^2 = \frac{1}{M} \sum_{i=1}^{M} \left[\left\{ \frac{g(\eta_i)}{f(\eta_i)} \right\} I\{\eta_i \in [a,b]\} - \frac{1}{M} \sum_{j=1}^{M} \left\{ \frac{g(\eta_j)}{f(\eta_j)} \right\} I\{\eta_j \in [a,b]\} \right]^2$$

$$= \frac{1}{M} \sum_{i=1}^{M} \left[\left\{ \frac{g(\eta_i)}{f(\eta_i)} \right\} I\{\eta_i \in [a,b]\} \right]^2 - \left[\frac{1}{M} \sum_{j=1}^{M} \left\{ \frac{g(\eta_j)}{f(\eta_j)} \right\} I\{\eta_j \in [a,b]\} \right]^2 .$$

Thus, denoting presumed values of the errors δ_1 and δ_2, we can derive the sample size n that satisfies

$$\Pr\{|J_n - J| \geq \delta_1\} \approx 1 - \Phi(\delta_1 \sqrt{n} / \Delta) + \Phi(-\delta_1 \sqrt{n} / \Delta) \leq \delta_2.$$

Note that, in order to generate random samples from any density function f, we can use the following lemma.

Lemma 2.4.1. Let F denote a continuous distribution function of a random variable ξ. Then the random variable $\eta = F(\xi)$ is uniformly [0,1] distributed.

Proof. Consider the distribution function

$$\Pr(\eta \leq u) = \Pr\{0 \leq F(\xi) \leq u\} = \Pr\{\xi \leq F^{-1}(u)\} I(0 \leq u \leq 1) + I(u > 1)$$

$$= F(F^{-1}(u)) I(0 \leq u \leq 1) + I(u > 1) = u I(0 \leq u \leq 1) + I(u > 1),$$

where F^{-1} defines the inverse function. This completes the proof of Lemma 2.4.1.

From this result, it is apparent that generating $\eta \sim Uniform[0,1]$ we can compute a ξ that is a root of the equation $\eta = F(\xi)$ to obtain the random variable ξ distributed according to F. We remark that an R function (R Development Core Team, 2014), *uniroot* (or *optimize* applied to minimize the function $\{\eta - F(\xi)\}^2$), can be easily used to find numerical solutions for $\eta = F(\xi)$ with respect to ξ.

In many cases, the choice of the density function f in the approximation to J given above is intuitional and a form of f can be close to that of the integrated function g. The function f is assumed to be well-behaved over the support $[a,b]$. For example, to approximate $J = \int_{-1}^{1} g(u)du$, we might select f

associated with the *Uniform*[−1,1] distribution; to approximate $J = \int_{-\infty}^{\infty} g(u)du$, we might select f associated with a normal distribution.

As an alternative to the approach shown above we can employ the Newton–Raphson method, which is a technique for calculating integrals numerically. In several scenarios, the Newton–Raphson method can outperform the Monte Carlo strategy. However, it is known that in various multidimensional cases, e.g., related to $\iiint g(u_1, u_2, u_3)du_1\,du_2\,du_3$, the Monte Carlo approach is simpler, more accurate and faster than Newton–Raphson type algorithms. Regarding multivariate statistical simulations we refer the reader to the book of Johnson (1987).

Example

Assume $T(X_1,..,X_n)$ denotes a statistic based on n iid observations $X_1,..,X_n$ with a known distribution function. In various statistical investigations it is required to evaluate the probability $p = \Pr\{T(X_1,...,X_n) > H\}$ for a fixed threshold, H. This problem statement is common in the context of testing statistical hypotheses when examining the **Type I error** rate and the **power** of a statistical decision-making procedure (e.g., Vexler et al., 2016a). In order to employ the Monte Carlo approach, one can generate $X_1,..,X_n$ from the known distribution, calculating $v_1 = I\{T(X_1,...,X_n) > H\}$. This procedure can be repeated M times to in turn generate the iid variables $v_1,...,v_M$. Then the probability p can be estimated as $\hat{p} = \sum_{i=1}^{M} v_i/M$. The central limit theorem concludes that for large values of M we can expect

$$\Pr\left\{p \in \left[\hat{p} - 1.96\{\hat{p}(1-\hat{p})/M\}^{0.5}, \hat{p} + 1.96\{\hat{p}(1-\hat{p})/M\}^{0.5}\right]\right\} \approx 0.95,$$

where it is applied that $\text{var}(v_1) = p(1-p)$ and the standard normal distribution function $\Phi(1.96) = \int_{-\infty}^{1.96} e^{-x^2/2}\,dx/\sqrt{2\pi} \approx 0.975$. Thus, for example, when p is anticipated to be around 0.05 (e.g., in terms of the Type I error rate analysis), it is reasonable to require $1.96(0.05(1-0.05)/M)^{0.5} < 0.005$ and then we can choose $M > 8000$, whereas, when p is anticipated to be around 0.5 (e.g., in terms of an analysis of the power of a test), it is reasonable to require $1.96(0.5(1-0.5)/M)^{0.5} < 0.05$ and then we can recommend choosing $M > 500$.

For example, to evaluate the Type I error rate of the t-test for H_0: $E(X_1) = 0$ versus H_1: $E(X_1) \neq 0$ (e.g., Vexler et al., 2016a), one can apply the following simple R code:

```
MC<-10000 #the number of the Monte Carlo generations
n<-25
Decision<-array()
TestStatistic<-array()
for(i in 1:MC)
```

```
{
X<-rnorm(n)
TestStatistic[i]<-t.test(X,alternative = c("two.sided")) $'statistic'
Decision[i]<-1*(TestStatistic[i]>qt(0.95,n))
}
mean(Decision)
```

In this code we can change *MC<-10000* to *MC<-1000* and *X<-rnorm(n)* to *X<-rnorm(n,0.1,1)* in order to obtain the **Monte Carlo power**, when the alternative parameter is assumed to be $E(X_1) = 0.1$. Note that, assuming a value of the alternative parameter and a target value of the power, we can employ the R code above to determine n. This statement corresponds to the problem of the **power calculation** (or the **sample size calculation**) that is a common issue of **study designs**.

2.4.5.2 That Is the Question: Do Convergence Rates Matter?

Sums of random variables play vital roles in statistics. For example, logarithms of likelihood functions considered in later chapters have forms of sums of random variables. The law of large numbers as well as the central limit theorem are partial solutions to a general problem of analyzing asymptotic behaviors of sums of random variables. For example, when $\xi_1,...,\xi_n$ are iid random variables with $E(\xi_1) = a$, $\text{var}(\xi_1) = 1$, we have $(\xi_1 +...+\xi_n)/n \to a$ and $(\xi_1 +...+\xi_n - an)/n^{1/2} \to \zeta$ as $n \to \infty$, where a is the constant, but ζ is a $N(0,1)$ random variable. Informally, one can say: "the sum $(\xi_1 +...+\xi_n)$ grows approximately at the same rate as an." The question is what is happening "in between" the law of large numbers (when we divide the sum by n) and the central limit theorem (when we divide the sum by $n^{1/2}$). Specifically, if we consider $\omega_n = (\xi_1 +...+\xi_n - an)/b_n$, where b_n is intermediate in size between $n^{1/2}$ and n, is ω_n asymptotically a constant or a random variable? This is a nontrivial question. We invite the reader to think about this problem that will be discussed in several forthcoming sections of this book.

2.4.6 Problems of Reconstructing the General Distribution Based on the Distribution of Some Statistics

In various practical applications, researchers aim to estimate the distribution function of iid random variables, say $X_1,..,X_n$, observing only statistics based on $X_1,..,X_n$, e.g., in the forms $\sum_{i=1}^{m} X_i$, $X_i + \varepsilon_i$ or $\max(X_i)$. Consider, for example, the following practical problem. One of the main issues of epidemiological research for the last several decades has been the relationship between biological markers (**biomarkers**) and disease risk. Commonly, a measurement process yields operating characteristics of biomarkers. However, the high cost associated with evaluating these biomarkers as well as **measurement errors** corresponding to a measurement process can prohibit further epidemiological applications (e.g., Armstrong, 2015: Chapter 31). When, for example, analysis is restricted by the high cost of assays, following

Pooling

Individual specimens

• Physically combining
several individual
specimens, to create a
single mixed sample

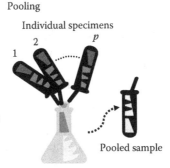

• Pooled samples are the
averages of the
individual specimens

Pooled sample

FIGURE 2.2
Pooling.

Schisterman et al. (2011), we suggest applying an efficient *pooling design* to collection of data (see Figure 2.2 for an illustrative purpose).

In order to allow for the instrument sensitivity problem corresponding to measurement errors, we formulate models with additive measurement errors. Obviously, these issues require assumptions on a biomarker distribution, under which operating characteristics of a biomarker can be evaluated.

The existence of measurement error in exposure data potentially affects any inferences regarding variability and uncertainty because the distribution representing the observed data set deviates from the distribution that represents an error-free data set. Methodologies for improving the characterization of variability and uncertainty with measurement errors in data are proposed by many biostatistical manuscripts. Thus, the model, which corresponds to observing a biomarker of interest plus a measurement error, is not in need of extensive describing. However, note that, since values of a biomarker are functionally convolute with noisy measurement errors, usually distribution functions of measurement errors are assumed to be known. Moreover, on account of the complexity of extracting the biomarker distribution from observed convoluted data (say *deconvolution*), practically, normality assumptions related to the biomarker distribution are assumed. Under these assumptions parameters of an error distribution can be evaluated by applying an auxiliary reliability study of biospecimens (e.g., a cycle of remeasuring of biospecimens) (Schisterman et al. 2001b).

Another stated problem dealing with the deconvolution is the exploration based on pooled data. Without focusing on situations where pooled data is an organic output of a study, we touch on pooling in the context of study design. The concept of a pooling-based design is extensively dealt with in the statistical literature starting with publications related to cost-efficient testing of World War II recruits for syphilis. In order to reduce cost or labor intensiveness of a study, a pooling strategy may be employed, whereby 2 or more (say p) individual specimens are physically combined into a single "pooled" unit for analysis. Thus, applying pooling design provides a p-fold decrease of the number of measured assays. Each pooled sample test result is assumed to be the average of the individual unpooled samples; this is most often the case because many tests are expressed per unit of volume.

Thus, assuming that iid unobserved variables $X_1, X_2, \ldots$ represent measurements of a biomarker of interest, one can consider scenarios in which the distribution function of X_1 should be estimated based on the observations $Z_j = \left(p^{-1}\right) \sum_{i=p(j-1)+1}^{pj} X_i$ (pooling) or $W_j = X_j + \varepsilon_j$ (measurement error), where $\varepsilon_1, \varepsilon_2, \ldots$ are iid random variables with a known distribution function, see for details, e.g., Vexler et al. (2008b, 2010a). In these cases the following idea can be used. The characteristic functions of Z_1 and W_1 satisfy $\varphi_Z(t) = \{\varphi_X(t/p)\}^p$ and $\varphi_W(t) = \varphi_X(t)\varphi_\varepsilon(t)$, respectively, where $\varphi_X(t)$ is the characteristic function of X_1 and $\varphi_\varepsilon(t)$ is the known characteristic function of ε_1. The empirical estimators of $\varphi_Z(t)$ or $\varphi_W(t)$ based on samples $\{Z_j\}_{j\geq 1}$ or $\{W_j\}_{j\geq 1}$ can be easily obtained (e.g., Feuerverger and Mureika, 1977), which yields a possibility to estimate $\varphi_X(t)$ under certain assumptions regarding the distribution function of X_1 (Vexler et al., 2008b, 2010a), e.g., $\hat{\varphi}_X(t) = \hat{\varphi}_W(t)/\varphi_\varepsilon(t)$, where $\hat{\varphi}_W(t)$ is the empirical estimator of $\varphi_W(t)$. Theorem 2.3.2 can be applied to develop an estimator of the distribution function of X_1, using an estimated $\varphi_X(t)$. For example, the estimator of the density function of X_1 can be presented as $\hat{f}(x) = \frac{1}{2\pi}\int_{-T}^{T} e^{-itx}\hat{\varphi}_X(t)dt$, for a fixed $T > 0$. In practice, values of T can be chosen to be 0.6, 0.7, 1.2, 1.3, 1.66, 1.7, etc.

Note that, in several situations, we observe $Z_j = \max_{p(j-1)+1\leq i\leq pj} (X_i)$. A method for reconstructing the distribution function of X_1 based on $\{Z_j\}_{j\geq 1}$ is considered in Belomestnyi (2005).

2.4.7 Extensions and Estimations of Families of Distribution Functions

Relatively simple forms of characteristic functions can represent sets of families of distribution functions. For example, in Chapter 1 we introduce the notation $N(\mu, \sigma^2)$ to define a family of normally distributed random variables with the parameters μ and σ^2 that correspond to the mean and variance of the random variables. Consider, for instance, the parametric characteristic function

$$\varphi(t; \alpha, \beta, \gamma, a) = \exp\left\{iat - \gamma|t|^\alpha \left(1 + i\beta t\omega(|t|, \alpha)/|t|\right)\right\}, \quad t \in (-\infty, \infty),$$

$$\omega(|t|, \alpha) = \begin{cases} \tan(\pi\alpha/2), & \text{if } \alpha \neq 1 \\ 2\ln(|t|)/\pi, & \text{if } \alpha=1 \end{cases}$$

$$\gamma \geq 0, \quad \alpha \in (0, 2], \quad |\beta| \leq 1, \quad a \in (-\infty, \infty).$$

We note that $\omega(|t|, 2) = 0$ so that the class of distribution functions associated with $\varphi(t; \alpha, \beta, \gamma, a)$ covers normal distribution functions for $\alpha = 2$. The parameters α, β, γ, and a are called the characteristic exponent, a measure of skewness, the scale parameter and the location parameter, respectively. The definition of $\varphi(t; \alpha, \beta, \gamma, a)$ is quite general and corresponds to many practical distributions, for example, the normal, $\alpha = 2$; the Cauchy, $\alpha = 1$ and the stable law of characteristic exponent, $\alpha = 1/2$. Thus, changing values of the parameters we can provide a modification of the classical type of a density function corresponded to $\varphi(t; \alpha, \beta, \gamma, a)$. In cases with unknown α, β, γ, a, one can use Theorem 2.3.2 to construct their maximum likelihood estimation (Vexler et al., 2008b).

Although we consider the parametric approach to describe the characteristic function, estimation of the unknown parameters by using directly density functions corresponding to $\varphi(t; \alpha, \beta, \gamma, a)$ is difficult; it is complicated by the fact that their densities are not generally available in closed analytical forms for all possible values of α, β, γ, a, making it difficult to apply conventional estimation methods.

Schematic R codes: The characteristic function $\varphi(t; \alpha, \beta, \gamma, a)$ can be coded in the form

```
fi<- function(t,alpha,beta,gamma,a){
if (alpha==1) w<-2*log(abs(t))/pi else w<-tan(pi*alpha/2)
return(exp(1i*a*t-(gamma*abs(t)^(alpha))*(1+1i*beta*sign(t)*w))) }
```

where (alpha,beta,gamma,a) are the parameters. The corresponding density function is

```
fs<-function(u,alpha,beta,gamma,a){
integ1<-function(t) exp(-1i*u*t)*fi(t,alpha,beta,gamma,a)
integ1R<-function(t) Re(integ1(t))
integrate(integ1R,-Inf,Inf)[[1]]/(2*pi) }
```

Consider the following scenarios to be left for the reader's imagination. Suppose, for example, we estimate α as 1.1 or 1.2, or 1.5. Is this a "drift" from one classical parametric family to other one, e.g., from *Cauchy* to *Normal*, or a "stay" between the families? Suppose we assume data follow a normal $N(\mu, \sigma^2)$ distribution and estimate the parameters (μ, σ^2). In this case, it can be a vital mistake if the real data follow a Cauchy distribution. Perhaps, we can suggest to involve the $\varphi(t; \alpha, \beta, \gamma, a)$-based inference to reduce this risk.

3

Likelihood Tenet

3.1 Introduction

When the forms of data distributions are assumed to be known, the likelihood principle plays a prominent role in statistical methods research for developing powerful statistical inference tools. The *likelihood method*, or simply the *likelihood*, is arguably the most important concept for inference in parametric modeling when the underlying data are subject to various assumed stochastic mechanisms and restrictions related to biomedical and epidemiological studies.

Without loss of generality, consider a situation in which n data points $X_1, ..., X_n$ are distributed according to the joint density function $f(x_1, ..., x_n; \theta)$ with the parameter θ, where $x_1, ..., x_n$ are arguments of f. Various useful modern statistical concepts are focused on the *likelihood function* of θ, $L(\theta) = f(X_1, ..., X_n; \theta)c$, where c can depend on $X_1, ..., X_n$ but not on θ (usually $c = 1$). If $X_1, ..., X_n$ are discrete then for each θ, $L(\theta)$ is defined as the probability of observing a realization of $X_1, ..., X_n$. The likelihood function measures the relative plausibility of the range of values for θ given observations $X_1, ..., X_n$, i.e., the likelihood informs us as to which θ most likely generated the observed data provided that model assumptions are correctly stated.

Beginning from the mid-1700s the problem of determining the *most probable* position for the object of observations, including determining the most likely parameter from a distribution that generated the data, was extensively treated in terms of mathematical descriptions by such historical figures as Thomas Simpson, Thomas Bayes, Johann Heinrich Lambert, and Joseph Louis Lagrange. Statistical literature has credited past figures with their contributions to likelihood theory, in particular Thomas Bayes in terms of the well-known Bayes theorem. However, it was not until Ronald Fisher (1922) revisited the likelihood principle via groundbreaking mathematical arguments that the approach exploded onto the statistical research landscape. Fisher suggested comparing various competing values of θ relative to their likelihood ratios, which in turn provides a measure of the relative plausibility of the parameter. The essence of the modern argument of Fisher can be described in terms of *sufficiency*.

In modern statistical developments a statistic is defined as sufficient with respect to a model and its corresponding unknown parameter if "no other statistic that can be calculated from the same sample provides any additional information as to the value of the parameter" (Fisher, 1922). The function $L(\theta)$ provides a sufficient statistic with respect to θ. Assume that there are two estimates of θ from $L(\theta)$, say $\hat{\theta}_S$ and $\hat{\theta}_A$. Let $\hat{\theta}_S$ be a sufficient statistic. Roughly, we can anticipate that $\hat{\theta}_S$ and $\hat{\theta}_A$ are approximately normal given large samples (in Section 3.3 we rigorously attend to the asymptotic normality of a $L(\theta)$-based estimator of θ). In accordance with Fisher (1922), we can consider the situation when $\hat{\theta}_S$ and $\hat{\theta}_A$ have a bivariate normal distribution (e.g., Balakrishnan and Lai, 2009; Borovkov, 1998, p. 109) with parameters that correspond to the following statements: $E(\hat{\theta}_S) = E(\hat{\theta}_A) = \theta$, $\mathrm{var}(\hat{\theta}_S) = \sigma_S^2, \mathrm{var}(\hat{\theta}_A) = \sigma_A^2$ and $E\{(\hat{\theta}_S - \theta)(\hat{\theta}_A - \theta)\}/(\sigma_S \sigma_A) = \rho$. Intuitively, the assumption $E(\hat{\theta}_S) = E(\hat{\theta}_A) = \theta$ represents our aim to provide the *consistency* of the estimates: $\hat{\theta}_S \to \theta$ and $\hat{\theta}_A \to \theta$ with large samples. Then the classical property of the bivariate normal distribution shows that the conditional expectation is given as $E(\hat{\theta}_A \mid \hat{\theta}_S = u) = \theta + \rho(\sigma_A/\sigma_S)(u - \theta)$. This statistic cannot be associated with θ, since $\hat{\theta}_S$ is sufficient. Thus $\rho(\sigma_A/\sigma_S) = 1$ or $\sigma_S = \rho\sigma_A \leq \sigma_A$, that is, $\hat{\theta}_S$ cannot have a larger mean squared error than any other such estimate $\hat{\theta}_A$ (if we accept the use of "approximate normality" of the estimators, in an informal manner). Thus, Fisher concluded that "Sufficiency implies optimality, at least when combined with consistency and asymptotic normality."

In this book, for clarity of explanation, we will assume $c = 1$ in the definition of the likelihood function and provide our own arguments (see, for example, Section 3.5) to position the likelihood function as an essential and optimal tool in biostatistical inference. We suggest that the reader who is interested in more details regarding likelihood methodology and its epic story consult fundamental guides presented in many publications, including Berger et al. (1988), Reid (2000) and Stigler (2007).

Likelihood methodology is addressed extensively in the literature. There are multitudes of books that consider different likelihood-based methods and their applications to biostatistical problems. In this chapter, we briefly introduce several principles and aspects of the maximum likelihood estimation and its applications (Sections 3.2 and 3.3), likelihood ratio–based procedures and their optimality (Sections 3.4 and 3.5), and maximum likelihood ratio tests and their properties (Section 3.6). In Section 3.7 we introduce an example related to correct model-based likelihood formations.

3.2 Why Likelihood? An Intuitive Point of View

Let us assume that we observe $X_1, ..., X_n$. Then the widely used least squares method for finding the likely parameter b that corresponds to the observed data is via the estimate of b given as $\hat{b} = \arg\min_\beta \sum_{i=1}^{n} (X_i - \beta)^2$. The idea behind this estimation method is clear and easily understandable in the context of minimization of the distances between data points and the estimated parameter location. While focusing on $L(\theta)$, statisticians measure how "likely" θ is relative to generating the observations, oftentimes aiming to detect values of θ that maximize $L(\theta)$. Avoiding considerations based on Bayesian perspectives (e.g., Bickel and Doksum, 2007, p. 114; Carlin and Louis, 2011 as well as Section 5.1), one can ponder the following questions: Why does the concept of $\max_\theta L(\theta)$ seem to be a simple and widely applicable idea? Why maximize the joint density over the parameter space? Why is maximizing the likelihood often the optimal strategy as compared to other methods such as least squares or the method of moments? Why not rise to argue in favor of a method of minimum likelihood or even mediocre likelihood? Even though conceptually the likelihood principle is straightforward on the face of it, the history of the topic shows that this "simple idea" is really anything but simple.

In most likelihood-based procedures it is anticipated that true values of the parameter are located around a maximum of the likelihood function. For pathological cases where the likelihood method fails we refer the reader to Smith (1985). To get some intuition about the likelihood principle we first consider the expectation of the *log likelihood ratio* given as $E_{\theta_0} \{\log(L(\theta_1) / L(\theta_0))\}$, where the operator E_{θ_0} means that the expectation should be derived provided that θ_0 reflects a true value of θ. In this case, Jensen's inequality yields the following inequality:

$$E_{\theta_0}\{\log(L(\theta_1)/L(\theta_0))\} = E_{\theta_0}\{\log(f(X_1,...,X_n;\theta_1)/f(X_1,...,X_n;\theta_0))\}$$

$$\leq \log\left(E_{\theta_0}\left[f(X_1,...,X_n;\theta_1)/f(X_1,...,X_n;\theta_0)\right]\right)$$

$$= \log \int ... \int \frac{f(x_1,...,x_n;\theta_1)}{f(x_1,...,x_n;\theta_0)} f(x_1,...,x_n;\theta_0) dx_1 \cdots dx_n$$

$$= \log \int ... \int f(x_1,...,x_n;\theta_1) dx_1 \cdots dx_n = \log(1)$$

$$= 0.$$

Similarly,

$$E_{\theta_1}\left\{\log\left(L(\theta_1)/L(\theta_0)\right)\right\} = -E_{\theta_1}\left\{\log\left(f(X_1,...,X_n;\theta_0)/f(X_1,...,X_n;\theta_1)\right)\right\}$$

$$\geq -\log\left(E_{\theta_1}\left[f(X_1,...,X_n;\theta_0)/f(X_1,...,X_n;\theta_1)\right]\right)$$

$$= \log\int...\int\frac{f(x_1,...,x_n;\theta_0)}{f(x_1,...,x_n;\theta_1)}f(x_1,...,x_n;\theta_1)dx_1...dx_n$$

$$= \log\int...\int f(x_1,...,x_n;\theta_0)dx_1...dx_n = \log(1)$$

$$= 0.$$

Moreover,

$$E_{\theta_0}\left\{L(\theta_1)/L(\theta_0)\right\} = \log\int...\int\frac{f(x_1,...,x_n;\theta_1)}{f(x_1,...,x_n;\theta_0)}f(x_1,...,x_n;\theta_0)dx_1...dx_n = 1,$$

whereas

$$E_{\theta_1}\left\{L(\theta_1)/L(\theta_0)\right\} = E_{\theta_1}\left\{\frac{1}{L(\theta_0)/L(\theta_1)}\right\} \geq \frac{1}{E_{\theta_1}\left\{L(\theta_0)/L(\theta_1)\right\}}$$

$$= \left[\int...\int\frac{f(x_1,...,x_n;\theta_0)}{f(x_1,...,x_n;\theta_1)}f(x_1,...,x_n;\theta_1)dx_1...dx_n\right]^{-1} = 1.$$

In a probability context, these results support the evaluation of $\Pr_{\theta_0}\left\{L(\theta_0)\leq L(\theta_1)\right\}$, where the subscript θ_0 shows that the probability is considered provided that the true value of θ is θ_0. Toward this end, we remark that $L(\theta) = \prod_{i=1}^{n}f(X_i;\theta)$ when n data points $X_1,...,X_n$ are iid and X_1 is distributed according to the density function $f(x_1;\theta)$ with the parameter θ. Note that in the general case the function $L(\theta)$ can also be presented in the product-type chain rule form

$$L(\theta) = f(X_1,...,X_n;\theta) = f(X_n\mid X_1,...,X_{n-1};\theta)f(X_1,...,X_{n-1};\theta)$$

$$= f(X_n\mid X_1,...,X_{n-1};\theta)f(X_{n-1}\mid X_1,...,X_{n-2};\theta)f(X_1,...,X_{n-2};\theta) = ...$$

$$= \prod_{i=1}^{n}f(X_i\mid X_1,...,X_{i-1};\theta).$$

We highlight this form since commonly theoretical evaluations of statistical procedures employ propositions related to sums of random variables due to their relative theoretical tractability. In this case a convenient form to work with is the *log likelihood function* $l(\theta) = \log(L(\theta))$, which is a sum.

Consider the case with iid observations, in which

$$\Pr_{\theta_0}\left\{L(\theta_0) \leq L(\theta_1)\right\} = \Pr_{\theta_0}\left\{\frac{1}{n}\sum_{i=1}^{n}\left(\log\left(f(X_i;\theta_1)\right) - \log\left(f(X_i;\theta_0)\right)\right) \geq 0\right\}$$

$$= \Pr_{\theta_0}\left\{\frac{1}{n}\sum_{i=1}^{n}\left(\left(\log\left(f(X_i;\theta_1)\right) - a_1\right) - \left(\log\left(f(X_i;\theta_0)\right) - a_0\right)\right) \geq a_0 - a_1\right\},$$

where, for $k = 0, 1$, $\log\left(f(X_i;\theta_k)\right), i = 1,...,n$ are iid random variables with $E_{\theta_0}\left\{\log\left(f(X_1;\theta_k)\right)\right\} = a_k$. Since $a_0 \geq a_1$ as shown above, it is clear that the analysis mentioned in Section 2.4.3, where Chebyshev's inequality is applied, leads to $\Pr_{\theta_0}\left\{L(\theta_0) \leq L(\theta_1)\right\} \to 0$ as $n \to 0$.

Thus, it is "most likely" "on average" and in probability that the true value θ_0 of the parameter θ satisfies $L(\theta_0) \approx \max_{\theta} L(\theta)$.

3.3 Maximum Likelihood Estimation

When the likelihood depends on an unknown parameter (or unknown parameters), it can be suggested that ranges of plausible values for the parameter (or parameters) can be directly obtained from the likelihood function, first by determining the *maximum likelihood estimate*. For n iid observations $X_1,...,X_n$ the maximum likelihood estimate is any value $\hat{\theta}_n$ such that $\prod_{i=1}^{n} f(X_i;\hat{\theta}_n) = \max_{\theta} L(\theta)$. Note that such a $\hat{\theta}_n$ need not exist, and when it does, it usually depends on what form of the density $f(x;\theta)$ was assumed. In this section we assert that in regular cases $\hat{\theta}_n$ is asymptotically normal. We begin by first outlining the following regularity conditions necessary for the asymptotic normality of the parameter estimates to hold. In order to consider $\hat{\theta}_n$ we need its existence and uniqueness, then let

(i) possible values of θ belong to an open interval (not necessarily finite), where the term "open interval" means an interval that has no minimum and maximum, e.g., $(1, 2)$, $(-\infty, 0)$, and

(ii) the set $A = \left\{x : f(x;\theta) > 0\right\}$ be independent of θ.

For example, we cannot determine a maximum likelihood estimator in the situation when $\prod_{i=1}^{n} f(X_i;\theta)$ is 0 for all values of θ.

Chapter 2 introduces tools that can be applied to show the asymptotic normality of likelihood estimators via evaluating sums of iid random variables. The *log maximum likelihood*

$$l(\hat{\theta}_n) = \log\left(\prod_{i=1}^{n} f(X_i;\hat{\theta}_n)\right) = \sum_{i=1}^{n} \log\left(f(X_i;\hat{\theta}_n)\right)$$

is a sum, but its summands are dependent random variables $\log\left(f(X_i;\hat{\theta}_n)\right), i = 1,...,n$. Then tools shown in Chapter 2 cannot be directly applied to analyze the sum $l(\hat{\theta}_n)$. However, Section 3.2 supports that we can anticipate that

(iii) $\hat{\theta}_n \xrightarrow{p} \theta$ as $n \to \infty$, where θ represents a true value of the parameter.

Then Taylor's theorem can be employed to evaluate an $l(\hat{\theta}_n)$-based construction, considering $\hat{\theta}_n$ around θ. Towards this end we should require that

(iv) $\partial^k \log\left(f(x;\theta)\right)/\partial\theta^k, k = 1,..,2$, exist, for all $x \in A$.

Using Taylor's arguments, remainder terms should be taken into account and then the following condition should be satisfied:

(v) There exists a positive number c and a function $M(x)$ such that

$$\left|\partial^3 \log\left(f(x;\theta_0)\right)/\partial\theta_0^3\right| \leq M(x) \text{ for all } x, \ \theta_0 \in (\theta-c,\theta+c) \text{ and } E_\theta\{M(x)\} < \infty.$$

To state that the random variable $\partial\log\left(f(X_1;\theta)\right)/\partial\theta$ has finite positive variance, we denote the *Fisher Information* $I(\theta) = E_\theta\left\{\partial\log\left(f(X_1;\theta)\right)/\partial\theta\right\}^2$, conditioning

(vi) $0 < I(\theta) = E_\theta\left\{\partial\log\left(f(X_1;\theta)\right)/\partial\theta\right\}^2 = -E_\theta\left\{\partial^2 \log\left(f(X_1;\theta)\right)/\partial\theta^2\right\} < \infty.$

A more rigorous and detailed treatment regarding the regularity conditions may be found in Lehmann and Casella (1998, pp. 440–450).

The central limit theorem related to the maximum likelihood estimation has the following form.

Theorem 3.3.1

Assume that $X_1,...,X_n$ are iid and satisfy the conditions *(i–vi)* mentioned above. Then the distribution function of $\sqrt{n}\left(\hat{\theta}_n - \theta\right)$ satisfies

$$\Pr_\theta\left(\sqrt{n}\left(\hat{\theta}_n - \theta\right) < u\right) \to \Pr(\xi < u) \quad \text{as} \quad n \to \infty,$$

where ξ is a normally distributed random variable with $E(\xi) = 0$ and $\text{var}(\xi) = 1 / I(\theta)$.

Proof. The idea of the proof is to apply Taylor's theorem in order to represent a $l(\hat{\theta}_n)$-based statistic as a sum of iid random variables and then use the technique shown in Chapter 2.

Consider the score function given as the derivative $l'(\hat{\theta}_n) = \partial l(u) / \partial u\big|_{u=\hat{\theta}_n}$. Expanding the score function $l'(\hat{\theta}_n)$ about θ, a true value of the unknown parameter, we have

$$l'(\hat{\theta}_n) = l'(\theta) + (\hat{\theta}_n - \theta) l''(\theta) + 0.5(\hat{\theta}_n - \theta)^2 l'''(\tilde{\theta}_n)$$

with $l''(\theta) = \partial^2 l(u) / \partial u^2\big|_{u=\theta}$, $l'''(\tilde{\theta}_n) = \partial^3 l(u) / \partial u^3\big|_{u=\tilde{\theta}_n}$ and $\tilde{\theta}_n$ that lies between θ and $\hat{\theta}_n$. Since $\hat{\theta}_n$ maximizes the log likelihood, $l'(\hat{\theta}_n) = 0$. This provides

$$0 = l'(\theta) + (\hat{\theta}_n - \theta)\{l''(\theta) + 0.5(\hat{\theta}_n - \theta) l'''(\tilde{\theta}_n)\},$$

resulting in

$$\sqrt{n}(\hat{\theta}_n - \theta) = \frac{l'(\theta)/\sqrt{n}}{-l''(\theta)/n - 0.5(\hat{\theta}_n - \theta) l'''(\tilde{\theta}_n)/n}. \tag{3.1}$$

Consider the remainder term $0.5(\hat{\theta}_n - \theta) l'''(\tilde{\theta}_n)/n$. Condition (*v*) implies

$$\left|0.5(\hat{\theta}_n - \theta) l'''(\tilde{\theta}_n) / n\right| \le \left|0.5(\hat{\theta}_n - \theta)\right| \sum_{i=1}^{n} M(X_i)/n,$$

where $M(X_1), ..., M(X_n)$ are iid random variables, and then using the results presented in Section 2.4.3 and condition (*iii*) we obtain that $\left|0.5(\hat{\theta}_n - \theta) l'''(\tilde{\theta}_n)/n\right| = \left|0.5(\hat{\theta}_n - \theta) O_p(1)\right| = o_p(1)$ as $n \to \infty$, since $\sum_{i=1}^{n} M(X_i)/n \overset{p}{\to} E_\theta\{M(X_1)\}$. Similarly, because $l''(\theta)$ is a sum of iid random variables $\{\partial^2 \log(f(X_i;\theta))/\partial\theta^2\}, i = 1,...,n$, we apply condition (*vi*) to conclude that $-l''(\theta)/n \overset{p}{\to} I(\theta)$ as $n \to \infty$, where

$$I(\theta) = E_\theta\{\partial\log(f(X_1;\theta))/\partial\theta\}^2 = -E_\theta\left[\frac{\{\partial f(X_1;\theta)/\partial\theta\}^2 - f(X_1;\theta)\partial^2 f(X_1;\theta)/\partial\theta^2}{\{f(X_1;\theta)\}^2}\right]$$

and

$$E_\theta\left[\frac{f(X_1;\theta)\partial^2 f(X_1;\theta)/\partial\theta^2}{\{f(X_1;\theta)\}^2}\right] = \int \{\partial^2 f(u;\theta)/\partial\theta^2\}du = \frac{\partial^2}{\partial\theta^2}\int f(u;\theta)du = \frac{\partial^2}{\partial\theta^2}1 = 0.$$

Formally speaking, the regularity conditions *(i–vi)* ensure that we can move the operator $\dfrac{\partial^2}{\partial\theta^2}$ outside the integration as was done above.

Thus Equation (3.1) can be rewritten as

$$\sqrt{n}\left(\hat{\theta}_n - \theta\right) = \frac{l'(\theta)/\sqrt{n}}{I(\theta) + o_p(1)},$$

where $l'(\theta)$ is a sum of iid random variables $\{\partial\log(f(X_i;\theta))/\partial\theta\}, i = 1,...,n,$ with

$$
\begin{aligned}
E_\theta\{\partial\log(f(X_1;\theta))/\partial\theta\} &= \int f(u;\theta)\frac{\partial\log(f(u;\theta))}{\partial\theta}du \\
&= \int f(u;\theta)\frac{\partial f(u;\theta)/\partial\theta}{f(u;\theta)}du \\
&= \frac{\partial}{\partial\theta}\int f(u;\theta)du \\
&= \frac{\partial}{\partial\theta}1 = 0.
\end{aligned}
$$

Then by virtue of the central limit theorem (Section 2.4.5) we complete the proof.

The maximum likelihood estimator $\hat{\theta}_n$ is a **point estimator**. One of the statistical applications of Theorem 3.3.1 is related to the construction of large sample **confidence interval estimators**. Towards this end, we consider a situation in which we are interested in obtaining an interval, say $[a,b]$, based on $X_1,...,X_n$ with **coverage probability** given as $\text{Pr}_\theta\{\theta \in [a(X_1,...,X_n), b(X_1,...,X_n)]\} = 1 - \alpha$ for a prespecified level α. In this case, for large n, we have

$$\text{Pr}_\theta\left\{\theta \in \left[\hat{\theta}_n - u_{1-\alpha/2}\sqrt{I(\theta)/n}, \ \hat{\theta}_n + u_{1-\alpha/2}\sqrt{I(\theta)/n}\right]\right\} \approx \Phi(u_{1-\alpha/2}) - \Phi(-u_{1-\alpha/2}),$$

where the constant $u_{1-\alpha/2}$ is given as the root of $\Phi(u_{1-\alpha/2}) = 1 - \alpha/2$, $\Phi(-u_{1-\alpha/2}) = \alpha/2$, and $\Phi(u) = \int_{-\infty}^{u} e^{-x^2/2}dx/\sqrt{2\pi}$ denotes the distribution function of a standard normal random variable. For example, $u_{1-\alpha/2} \approx 1.96$, if $\alpha = 0.05$. Then, calculating a point estimator of $I(\theta)$ as $\hat{I}(\hat{\theta})$, we can obtain the **equal tailed** $(1-\alpha)100\%$ confidence interval estimator given as $\left[a = \hat{\theta}_n - u_{1-\alpha/2}\sqrt{\hat{I}(\hat{\theta})/n}, \ b = \hat{\theta}_n + u_{1-\alpha/2}\sqrt{\hat{I}(\hat{\theta})/n}\right]$.

Theorem 3.3.1 can be used to show that in various scenarios the maximum likelihood method provides asymptotically normal estimators with minimum variances (e.g., Lehmann and Casella, 1998).

Warning: The statement mentioned above is well addressed in textbooks related to elementary courses in statistics. In general, the maximum likelihood estimators might be outperformed by related superefficient estimation procedures. This is almost true for special sets of values of θ with Lebesgue measure zero (Le Cam, 1953). Consider the following example. Let n iid observations $X_1, ..., X_n$ be $N(\theta, 1)$ distributed. In this case, the maximum likelihood estimator $\hat{\theta}_n = \sum_{i=1}^{n} X_i/n$ of θ satisfies $\sqrt{n}(\hat{\theta}_n - \theta) \sim N(0, 1)$. Define an estimator of θ in the form $v_n = \hat{\theta}_n I\left\{|\hat{\theta}_n| \geq n^{-1/4}\right\} + a\hat{\theta}_n I\left\{|\hat{\theta}_n| < n^{-1/4}\right\}$ with $0 < a < 1$. When $\theta \neq 0$, we have that the distribution function $\Pr_{\theta}\left\{\sqrt{n}(v_n - \theta) < u\right\}$ satisfies

$$\Pr_{\theta}\left\{\sqrt{n}(v_n - \theta) < u\right\}$$

$$= \Pr_{\theta}\left\{\sqrt{n}(v_n - \theta) < u, |\hat{\theta}_n| \geq n^{-1/4}\right\} + \Pr_{\theta}\left\{\sqrt{n}(v_n - \theta) < u, |\hat{\theta}_n| < n^{-1/4}\right\}$$

$$= \Pr_{\theta}\left\{\sqrt{n}(\hat{\theta}_n - \theta) < u, |\hat{\theta}_n| \geq n^{-1/4}\right\} + \Pr_{\theta}\left\{\sqrt{n}(a\hat{\theta}_n - \theta) < u, |\hat{\theta}_n| < n^{-1/4}\right\}$$

$$= \Pr_{\theta}\left\{\sqrt{n}(\hat{\theta}_n - \theta) < u\right\} - \Pr_{\theta}\left\{\sqrt{n}(\hat{\theta}_n - \theta) < u, |\hat{\theta}_n| < n^{-1/4}\right\} + \Pr_{\theta}\left\{\sqrt{n}(a\hat{\theta}_n - \theta) < u, |\hat{\theta}_n| < n^{-1/4}\right\}$$

$$\leq \Pr_{\theta}\left\{\sqrt{n}(\hat{\theta}_n - \theta) < u\right\} + \Pr_{\theta}\left\{\sqrt{n}(a\hat{\theta}_n - \theta) < u, |\hat{\theta}_n| < n^{-1/4}\right\}$$

$$\leq \Pr_{\theta}\left\{\sqrt{n}(\hat{\theta}_n - \theta) < u\right\} + \Pr_{\theta}\left\{|\hat{\theta}_n| < n^{-1/4}\right\}$$

as well as

$$\Pr_{\theta}\left\{\sqrt{n}(v_n - \theta) < u\right\} \geq \Pr_{\theta}\left\{\sqrt{n}(\hat{\theta}_n - \theta) < u\right\} - \Pr_{\theta}\left\{|\hat{\theta}_n| < n^{-1/4}\right\}.$$

Since

$$\Pr_{\theta}\left\{|\hat{\theta}_n| < n^{-1/4}\right\} = \Pr_{\theta}\left\{-n^{-1/4} < \sum_{i=1}^{n} X_i/n < n^{-1/4}\right\}$$

$$= \Pr_{\theta}\left\{\sum_{i=1}^{n}(X_i - \theta)/n < n^{-1/4} - \theta\right\} - \Pr_{\theta}\left\{\sum_{i=1}^{n}(X_i - \theta)/n < -n^{-1/4} - \theta\right\}$$

$$= \Pr_{\theta}\left\{\sum_{i=1}^{n}(\theta - X_i) > \theta n - n^{3/4}\right\} - \Pr_{\theta}\left\{\sum_{i=1}^{n}(\theta - X_i) > n^{3/4} + \theta n\right\}$$

and, for large values of n and fixed θ, $\theta n - n^{3/4} > 0$, applying Chebyshev's inequality in a similar manner to that of Section 2.4.3, we obtain $\text{Pr}_\theta\left\{\left|\hat{\theta}_n\right| < n^{-1/4}\right\} \to 0$ as $n \to \infty$. Then asymptotically $\sqrt{n}\,(v_n - \theta) \sim N(0,1)$, if $\theta \neq 0$.

It is clear that when $\theta = 0$ we have

$$\text{Pr}_{\theta=0}\left\{\sqrt{n}\,(v_n - \theta) < u\right\} \leq \text{Pr}_0\left\{\left|\hat{\theta}_n\right| \geq n^{-1/4}\right\} + \text{Pr}_0\left\{\sqrt{n}\,\left(a\hat{\theta}_n\right) < u\right\} \quad \text{and}$$

$$\text{Pr}_{\theta=0}\left\{\sqrt{n}\,(v_n - \theta) < u\right\} \geq -\text{Pr}_0\left\{\left|\hat{\theta}_n\right| \geq n^{-1/4}\right\} + \text{Pr}_0\left\{\sqrt{n}\,\left(a\hat{\theta}_n\right) < u\right\},$$

where $\text{Pr}_0\left\{\left|\hat{\theta}_n\right| \geq n^{-1/4}\right\} = \text{Pr}_0\left\{\left|\sum_{i=1}^{n} X_i\right| \geq n^{3/4}\right\} \to 0$ as $n \to \infty$.

Thus $\sqrt{n}\,(v_n - \theta) \sim N(0, a^2)$, if $\theta = 0$, and $\sqrt{n}\,(v_n - \theta) \sim N(0,1)$, if $\theta \neq 0$, as $n \to \infty$ and $0 < a < 1$. This states that, in this case, the estimator v_n is more efficient asymptotically than the maximum likelihood estimator ($\text{var}(v_n) \leq \text{var}\left(\hat{\theta}_n\right)$, for large n) at least when $\theta = 0$.

Remark 1. In general cases related to different data distributions we need to derive maximum likelihood estimators numerically. For example, consider n iid observations $X_1, ..., X_n$ from the Cauchy distribution with density function $f(u; \theta) = \left[\pi\left\{1 + (u - \theta)^2\right\}\right]^{-1}$. The maximum likelihood estimator $\hat{\theta}_n$ of the shift parameter θ is a root of the equation $l'(\hat{\theta}_n) = 0$, i.e.,

$$\sum_{i=1}^{n} \frac{X_i - \hat{\theta}_n}{1 + \left(X_i - \hat{\theta}_n\right)^2} = 0,$$

that can be solved numerically, e.g., using the Newton–Raphson method (see, e.g., R procedure *uniroot*, R Development Core Team, 2014). In this Cauchy framework, the regularity conditions are satisfied and

$$\frac{\partial \log\left(f(u; \theta)\right)}{\partial \theta} = \frac{2(u - \theta)}{1 + (u - \theta)^2}, \quad E_\theta\left\{\frac{\partial \log\left(f(X_1; \theta)\right)}{\partial \theta}\right\}^2 = \frac{4}{\pi}\int \frac{u^2}{\left\{1 + u^2\right\}^3}\,du = \frac{1}{2}.$$

Thus, following Theorem 3.3.1, we have $\sqrt{n}\left(\hat{\theta}_n - \theta\right) \sim N(0, 2)$ as $n \to \infty$.

Remark 2. In cases of models with several unknown parameters, a multidimensional version of Theorem 3.3.1 can be obtained under appropriate extensions of the regularity conditions in higher dimensions (e.g., Serfling, 2002).

Remark 3. Properties of the maximum likelihood estimation where standard regularity conditions are violated are considered in Borovkov (1998).

3.4 The Likelihood Ratio

Historically the likelihood concept has been associated with the *likelihood ratio* principle, which is the basis for developing powerful statistical inference tools for use in clinical experiments when the forms of data distributions are assumed to be specified.

Let us start by first outlining the likelihood ratio principle applied to statistical decision-making theory. Likelihood ratio–based testing was first proposed and formulated in a series of foundational papers published in the period of 1928–1938 by Neyman and Pearson (1928, 1933, 1938). In 1928, the authors introduced the generalized likelihood ratio test and its association with chi-squared statistics. Five years later, the Neyman–Pearson lemma was introduced, showing the optimality of the likelihood ratio test. These seminal works provided us with the familiar notions of simple and composite hypotheses and errors of the first and second kind, thus defining formal decision-making rules for testing (e.g., Vexler et al., 2016a).

Without loss of generality, the principle idea of the proof of the Neyman–Pearson lemma can be shown by using the following statement: Assume that data points $\{X_i, \ i = 1,\dots,n\}$ are observed presenting for example biomarker measurements. In general, the observations do not need to represent values of iid random variables. We would like to classify $X_1,\dots,X_n$ corresponding to *hypotheses* of the following form: $H_0 : \{X_i, \ i = 1,\dots,n\}$ are from a joint density function f_0, versus $H_1 : \{X_i, \ i = 1,\dots,n\}$ are from a joint density function f_1. For example, one can define $f_k(x_1,\dots,x_n) = f(x_1,\dots,x_n;\theta_k)$, where $k = 0,1$ and θ_0,θ_1 are different values of the parameter of a joint density function f. In this context, in order to construct the *likelihood ratio test statistic*, we should consider the ratio between the joint density function of $\{X_1,\dots,X_n\}$ obtained under H_1 and the joint density function of $\{X_1,\dots,X_n\}$ obtained under H_0. We then define the likelihood ratio (LR) as

$$LR_n = f_1(X_1,\dots,X_n)/f_0(X_1,\dots,X_n).$$

In this case the *likelihood ratio test* based decision rule is to reject H_0 if and only if $LR_n \geq B$, where B is a prespecified test threshold that does not depend on the observations. This test is uniformly most powerful. In order to clarify this fact we note that the term "most powerful" induces us to formally define how to compare statistical tests. According to the Neyman–Pearson concept of testing statistical hypotheses, since the ability to control the *Type I error* rate of statistical test has an essential role in statistical decision-making, we compare tests with equivalent probabilities of the Type I error $\Pr_{H_0}\{\text{test rejects } H_0\} = \alpha$, where the subscript H_0 indicates that we consider the probability given that the null hypothesis is true. The level of significance

α is the probability of making a Type I error. In practice, the researcher should choose a value of α, e.g., $\alpha = 0.05$, before performing the test. Thus, we should compare the likelihood ratio test with δ, any decision rule based on $\{X_i, i = 1, \ldots, n\}$, setting up $\Pr_{H_0}\{\delta \text{ rejects } H_0\} = \alpha$ and $\Pr_{H_0}\{LR_n \geq B\} = \alpha$. This comparison is with respect to the *power* $\Pr_{H_1}\{\text{test rejects } H_0\}$. Notice that to derive the mathematical expectation, in the context of a problem related to testing statistical hypotheses, one must define whether the expectation should be conducted under an H_0- or H_1-regime. For example,

$$E_{H_1}\{\varphi(X_1, X_2, \ldots X_n)\} = \int \ldots \int \varphi(x_1, x_2, \ldots x_n) f_1(x_1, x_2, \ldots x_n) dx_1 dx_2 \ldots dx_n,$$

where the expectation is considered under the alternative hypothesis. In this framework we consider the trivial inequality

$$(A - B)\{I(A \geq B) - v\} \geq 0, \tag{3.2}$$

for all A, B, where $v \in [0, 1]$ and $I(A \geq B)$ denotes the indicator function. Taking into account the comments mentioned above, we derive the expectation under H_0 of inequality (3.2), where $A = LR_n$, B is a test threshold, and $v = \delta = \delta(X_1, \ldots, X_n)$ represents any decision rule based on $\{X_i, i = 1, \ldots, n\}$. One can assume that $\delta = 0, 1$, and when $\delta = 1$ we reject H_0. Thus, we obtain

$$E_{H_0}\{(LR_n - B) I(LR_n \geq B)\} \geq E_{H_0}\{(LR_n - B)\delta\}.$$

And hence,

$$E_{H_0}\left\{\frac{f_1(X_1, \ldots, X_n)}{f_0(X_1, \ldots, X_n)} I(LR_n \geq B)\right\} - B E_{H_0}\{I(LR_n \geq B)\}$$

$$\geq E_{H_0}\left\{\frac{f_1(X_1, \ldots, X_n)}{f_0(X_1, \ldots, X_n)} \delta(X_1, \ldots, X_n)\right\} - B E_{H_0}\{\delta(X_1, \ldots, X_n)\}, \tag{3.3}$$

where $E_{H_0}(\delta) = E_{H_0}\{I(\delta = 1)\} = \Pr_{H_0}\{\delta = 1\} = \Pr_{H_0}\{\delta \text{ rejects } H_0\}$. Since we compare the tests with the fixed level of significance

$$E_{H_0}\{I(LR_n \geq B)\} = \Pr_{H_0}\{LR_n \geq B\} = \Pr_{H_0}\{\delta \text{ rejects } H_0\} = \alpha,$$

inequality (3.3) leads to

$$E_{H_0}\left\{\frac{f_1(X_1,...,X_n)}{f_0(X_1,...,X_n)}I(LR_n \geq B)\right\} \geq E_{H_0}\left\{\frac{f_1(X_1,...,X_n)}{f_0(X_1,...,X_n)}\delta(X_1,...,X_n)\right\}. \quad (3.4)$$

Consider

$$E_{H_0}\left\{\frac{f_1(X_1,...,X_n)}{f_0(X_1,...,X_n)}\delta(X_1,...,X_n)\right\}$$

$$= \int \cdots \int \frac{f_1(x_1,...,x_n)}{f_0(x_1,...,x_n)}\delta(x_1,...,x_n)f_0(x_1,...,x_n)dx_1...dx_n \quad (3.5)$$

$$= \int \cdots \int \delta(x_1,...,x_n)f_1(x_1,...,x_n)dx_1...dx_n = E_{H_1}(\delta) = \Pr_{H_1}\{\delta \text{ rejects } H_0\}.$$

Since δ represents any decision rule based on $\{X_i, i=1,...,n\}$, including the likelihood ratio–based test, Equation (3.5) implies

$$E_{H_0}\left\{\frac{f_1(X_1,...,X_n)}{f_0(X_1,...,X_n)}I(LR_n \geq B)\right\} = \Pr_{H_1}\{LR_n \geq B\}.$$

Applying this equation and Equations (3.5) to (3.4), we complete the proof that the likelihood ratio test is the most powerful statistical decision rule. This simple proof technique was used to show optimal aspects of different statistical decision-making policies based on the likelihood ratio concept (Vexler and Wu, 2009; Vexler et al., 2010b; Vexler and Gurevich, 2009, 2011).

Remark. The approach shown above can be extended to be considered with respect to decision-making procedures that satisfy the requirement $\Pr_{H_1}(\text{reject } H_0) \geq \alpha$ for all levels α's of significance. It is interesting to note that if one proposes a most powerful test, say V, in a set of tests that satisfy $\Pr_{H_1}(\text{reject } H_0) \geq \alpha$ for all α, then it is possible to construct a test, say G, that does not satisfy $\Pr_{H_1}(\text{reject } H_0) \geq \alpha$ for some α, but the power of G outperforms that of V. In this context, we refer the reader to, e.g., Bross et al. (1994), Suissa and Shuster (1984), and Section 9.2.

Warning: *Relativity of Optimality of Statistical Tests.* Commonly, in accordance with a given risk function of hypothesis testing, investigators try to derive an optimal property of a test. Inequality (3.2) helps us to show the optimal property of the likelihood ratio test statistic in terms of maximizing the power at a fixed Type I error rate. However, in the case when we have a given test statistic, say Υ, instead of the likelihood ratio LR_n, inequality (3.2) yields $(\Upsilon - B)\{I(\Upsilon \geq B) - \delta\} \geq 0$, for any decision rule $\delta \in [0,1]$. Therefore, the test rule $\Upsilon > B$ also has an optimal property that can be derived using (3.2). The problem is how to obtain a reasonable interpretation of the optimality? Thus, in scenarios when one wishes to investigate the optimality of a given test in a general context, inequalities similar to (3.2) can be obtained by focusing on the structure of a test. Such inequalities could report an optimal property of the test. However, translation of that property in terms of the quality of tests is the issue. Consider the following simple example. Let iid data points $X_1, \ldots, X_n$ be observed. We would like to test for H_0 versus H_1. Randomly select X_k from the observations and define the test: reject H_0 if $X_k > B$, where the threshold $B > 0$. By virtue of inequality (3.2), we have $(X_k - B)I\{X_k > B\} \geq (X_k - B)\delta$, where $\delta = 0,1$ is any decision rule based on $X_1, \ldots, X_n$ and the event $\{\delta = 1\}$ rejects H_0. Since

$$E_{H_0}\{(X_k - B)I(X_k > B)\} \geq E_{H_0}\{(X_k - B)\delta\},$$

we have

$$E_{H_0}\{X_k I(X_k > B)\} - B\Pr_{H_0}\{X_k > B\} \geq E_{H_0}(X_k\delta) - B\Pr_{H_0}\{\delta \text{ rejects } H_1\}.$$

Thus, considering decision-making procedures that satisfy $E_{H_0}\{X_1 I(\delta \text{ rejects } H_0)\} = \gamma$, for a fixed γ, we conclude that the test based on X_k has the smallest Type I error rate, since the inequality above yields

$$\gamma - B\Pr_{H_0}\{X_k > B\} \geq \gamma - B\Pr_{H_0}\{\delta \text{ rejects } H_1\}.$$

In this instance we would like to preserve the condition that if we incorrectly reject H_0, the expectation of X_k is fixed at a presumed level.

Now, we define the test with the decision rule to reject H_0 if $X_k > -B$. Then $(X_k + B)I\{X_k > -B\} \geq (X_k + B)\delta$ and $E_{H_1}\{X_k I(X_k > -B)\} + B\Pr_{H_1}\{X_k > -B\} \geq E_{H_1}(X_k\delta) + B\Pr_{H_1}\{\delta \text{ rejects } H_1\}$. Then consider tests with $E_{H_1}\{X_k I(\delta \text{ rejects } H_0)\} = \gamma$, for a fixed γ. It follows that the test $X_k > -B$ is the most powerful rule in a set of tests with the fixed characteristic $E_{H_1}\{X_k I(\delta \text{ rejects } H_0)\} = \gamma$. This allows us to consider preserving the conditions such as if we correctly reject H_0, the expectation of X_k is fixed on a presumed level.

The results above demonstrate that criteria for which a given test is optimal can be declared by the structure of this test. Hence, probably almost any reasonable tests are in general optimal.

It is a common situation in statistical practice that we have several outcomes of different tests regarding one test statement. Perhaps, in such cases, it is reasonable to attempt to focus on the optimal aspects of the tests in order to make an appropriate decision.

In this book we will show several examples of determining the optimal properties of test procedures via (3.2)-type inequalities.

3.5 The Intrinsic Relationship between the Likelihood Ratio Test Statistic and the Likelihood Ratio of Test Statistics: One More Reason to Use Likelihood

The Neyman–Pearson testing concept, given by fixing the probability of a Type I error, has come under some criticism by epidemiologists and others. One of the critical points is about the importance of paying attention to **Type II error** rates, $\mathrm{Pr}_{H_1}\{\text{test does not reject } H_0\}$. For example, Freiman et al. (1978) pointed out the results of 71 clinical trials that reported no statistically "significant" differences between the compared treatments. The authors found that in the great majority of these trials, the strong effects of new treatment were clinically significant. It was argued that the investigators in these trials failed to reject the null hypothesis when it appeared the alternative hypothesis was more likely the underlying truth, which probably resulted in an increase in the Type II error. In the context of likelihood ratio–based tests, we present the following result that demonstrates an association between the probabilities of Type I and II errors.

Suppose we would like to test for H_0 versus H_1, employing the likelihood ratio $LR = f_{H_1}(D)/f_{H_0}(D)$ based on data D, where f_H defines a density function that corresponds to the data distribution under the hypothesis H. Say, for simplicity, we reject H_0 if $LR > C$, where C is a presumed threshold. In this case, we can then show the following proposition.

Proposition 3.5.1. Let $f_H^L(u)$ define the density function of the likelihood ratio LR test statistic under the hypothesis H. Then

$$f_{H_1}^L(u) = u f_{H_0}^L(u) \tag{3.6}$$

with $u > 0$.

Proof. In order to obtain the property (3.6), we consider, for nonrandom variables u and s, the probability

$$\mathrm{Pr}_{H_1}\{u - s \le LR \le u\} = E_{H_1}I\{u - s \le LR \le u\} = \int I\{u - s \le LR \le u\} f_{H_1}$$

$$= \int I\{u - s \le LR \le u\}\frac{f_{H_1}}{f_{H_0}} f_{H_0} = \int I\{u - s \le LR \le u\}(LR) f_{H_0}.$$

This implies the inequalities

$$\text{Pr}_{H_1}\{u-s \leq LR \leq u\} \leq \int I\{u-s \leq LR \leq u\}(u)f_{H_0} = u\text{Pr}_{H_0}\{u-s \leq LR \leq u\}$$

and

$$\text{Pr}_{H_1}\{u-s \leq LR \leq u\} \geq \int I\{u-s \leq LR \leq u\}(u-s)f_{H_0} = (u-s)\text{Pr}_{H_0}\{u-s \leq LR \leq u\}.$$

Dividing these inequalities by s and employing $s \rightarrow 0$, we obtain $f_{H_1}^L(u) = f_{H_0}^L(u)u$, where $f_{H_0}^L(u)$ and $f_{H_1}^L(u)$ are the density functions of the statistic $LR = f_{H_1}/f_{H_0}$ under H_0 and H_1, respectively.

The proof is complete.

Thus, we can obtain the probability of a Type II error in the form of Pr {the test does not reject $H_0|H_1$ is true} = $\text{Pr}\{LR \leq C|H_1$ is true} = $\int_0^C f_{H_1}^L(u)du = \int_0^C uf_{H_0}^L(u)du$. Now, if, in order to control the Type I error, the density function $f_{H_0}^L(u)$ is assumed to be known, then the probability of the Type II error can be easily computed.

The likelihood ratio property $f_{H_1}^L(u)/f_{H_0}^L(u) = u$ can be applied to solve different issues related to performing the likelihood ratio test. For example, in terms of the *bias* of the test, one can request to find a value of the threshold C that maximizes

$$\text{Pr}\{\text{the test rejects } H_0 \mid H_1 \text{ is true}\} - \text{Pr}\{\text{the test rejects } H_0 \mid H_0 \text{ is true}\},$$

where the probability $\text{Pr}\{\text{the test rejects } H_0 \mid H_1 \text{ is true}\}$ depicts the *power* of the test. This equation can be expressed as

$$\text{Pr}\{LR > C|H_1 \text{ is true}\} - \text{Pr}\{LR > C|H_0 \text{ is true}\} = \left(1 - \int_0^C f_{H_1}^L(u)du\right) - \left(1 - \int_0^C f_{H_0}^L(u)du\right).$$

Set the derivative of the above formula to be zero and solve the following equation:

$$\frac{d}{dC}\left[\left(1 - \int_0^C f_{H_1}^L(u)du\right) - \left(1 - \int_0^C f_{H_0}^L(u)du\right)\right] = -f_{H_1}^L(C) + f_{H_0}^L(C) = 0.$$

By virtue of the property (3.6), this implies $-Cf_{H_0}^L(C) + f_{H_0}^L(C) = 0$ and then $C = 1$, which provides the maximum discrimination between the power and the probability of a Type I error in the likelihood ratio test.

Likelihood Argument of Optimality: Assume that an investigator provides a test for hypotheses H_0 versus H_1, calculating a test statistic, say T, based on the underlying data. Suppose we would like to improve T in terms of relative efficiency. Towards this end, we made creative efforts to derive the density functions $f_{H_0}^T(u)$ and $f_{H_1}^T(u)$ of the statistic T under H_0 and H_1, respectively. According to Section 3.4, the statistic $f_{H_1}^T(T)/f_{H_0}^T(T)$ should outperform T. In the case when T represents a likelihood ratio, Proposition 3.5.1 shows that one cannot improve the test statistic using only the values of T. In other words, the interesting fact is that the likelihood ratio $f_{H_1}^L/f_{H_0}^L$ based on the likelihood ratio $LR = f_{H_1}/f_{H_0}$ comes to be the likelihood ratio, that is, $f_{H_1}^L(LR)/f_{H_0}^L(LR) = LR$. We leave it to the reader's imagination to interpret this statement in terms of the information that this result provides.

Remark: Change of Measure. In this chapter we apply a very helpful tool for analyzing theoretical characteristics of statistical procedures. This tool is based on a change of measure. Consider for example a test statistic T_n that suggests rejecting H_0 for large values of T_n when n data points are observed. It is reasonable to assume that under the null hypothesis, when n increases, the behavior of T_n is difficult to anticipate, e.g., oftentimes we cannot expect any approximate trend of T_n. Thus, in many situations, the analysis of characteristics similar to $E_{H_0}\{\psi(T_n)\}$, where ψ is a function, including the Type I error rate, is a very complicated issue. Commonly, under the alternative hypothesis H_1, a deterministic trend of T_n can be easily derived for relatively large n, e.g., $T_n \sim cn$, for a constant c, when we could expect the test is power one as $n \to \infty$. Then, to evaluate $E_{H_0}\{\psi(T_n)\}$ one can change the measure

$$E_{H_0}\{\psi(T_n)\} = \int \psi(u) f_{H_0}(u)\, du = \int \psi(u) \frac{f_{H_0}(u)}{f_{H_1}(u)} f_{H_1}(u)\, du = E_{H_1}\left\{\psi(T_n) \frac{f_{H_0}(T_n)}{f_{H_1}(T_n)}\right\},$$

where $f_{H_k}(u)$ is a density function of T_n under the hypothesis H_k, $k = 0, 1$, and focus on properties of T_n under H_1. For example, Taylor's arguments considering $T_n \sim cn$ can be employed.

Formally in this framework we shall use the ***Radon–Nikodym theorem*** (e.g., Chung, 2000; Borovkov, 1998). In this context the likelihood ratio can be referred to as the ***Radon–Nikodym derivative*** of the two measures at time n. An interesting example of an application of the algorithm mentioned above to examine properties of a statistical procedure for change point detection policies can be found in Yakir (1995).

3.6 Maximum Likelihood Ratio

Various real-world data problems require consideration of statistical hypotheses with structures that depend on unknown parameters. In this case, the maximum likelihood method proposes to approximate the most powerful likelihood ratio test, employing a proportion of the maximum likelihoods, where the maximizations are over values of the unknown parameters belonging to distributions of observations under the corresponding null and alternative hypotheses. We shall assume the existence of essential maximum likelihood estimators. The influential *Wilks' theorem* provides the basic rationale as to why the maximum likelihood ratio approach has had tremendous success in statistical applications (Wilks, 1938). Wilks showed that under the regularity conditions, asymptotic null distributions of maximum likelihood ratio test statistics are independent of the nuisance parameters. That is, Type I error rates of the maximum likelihood ratio tests can be controlled asymptotically, and approximations to the corresponding *p-values* can be computed.

In order to present Wilks' theorem we suppose that $X = \{X_1, ..., X_n\}$ are iid observations each with the density function $f(x; \theta)$, where θ is a real-valued vector of parameters. We are interested in testing if the vector θ is in a specified subset Ω_0 of the parametric space Ω, i.e., $H_0 : \theta \in \Omega_0$ versus $H_1 : \theta \in \Omega_0^c$, where Ω_0^c is a complement to Ω_0 in Ω. Let $L(\theta \,|\, x) = \prod_{i=1}^{n} f(X_i; \theta)$ be the likelihood function. In this case, the *maximum likelihood ratio* test statistic is $MLR_n = \sup_{\theta \in \Omega^c} L(\theta \,|\, x) / \sup_{\theta \in \Omega_0} L(\theta \,|\, x)$. Then, under the null hypothesis, the statistic $2 \log(MLR_n)$ follows a χ_d^2 distribution as $n \to \infty$, where the degrees of freedom d equal to the difference in dimensionality of Ω^c and Ω_0. This proposition requires that the *regularity conditions* hold. For simplicity and clarity of exposition, we state Wilks' theorem in the one-dimension case, where we are interested in testing $H_0 : \theta = \theta_0$ versus $H_1 : \theta \neq \theta_0$, where θ is a scalar.

Theorem 3.6.1

Let $l(\theta \,|\, x) = \log(L(\theta \,|\, x))$ and $\hat{\theta}$ be the maximum likelihood estimator of θ under H_1, that is, $\hat{\theta} = \arg\max_\theta l(\theta \,|\, x)$, provided that it exists. Then, under the null hypothesis, the distribution of $2 \log(MLR_n) = 2\{l(\hat{\theta} \,|\, x) - l(\theta_0 \,|\, x)\}$ is asymptotically a $\chi_{d=1}^2$ distribution as $n \to \infty$.

Proof. Expand $l(\theta_0 \,|\, x)$ in a Taylor series around $\hat{\theta}$, that is,

$$l(\theta_0 \,|\, x) = l(\hat{\theta} \,|\, x) + (\theta_0 - \hat{\theta}) \frac{\partial l(\theta \,|\, x)}{\partial \theta}\bigg|_{\theta = \hat{\theta}} + \frac{1}{2}(\theta_0 - \hat{\theta})^2 \frac{\partial^2 l(\theta \,|\, x)}{\partial \theta^2}\bigg|_{\theta = \hat{\theta}} + R,$$

where the remainder term $R = \frac{1}{6}(\theta_0 - \hat{\theta})^3 \left.\frac{\partial^3 l(\theta \mid \mathbf{x})}{\partial \theta^3}\right|_{\theta=\hat{\theta}}$, for some $\tilde{\theta}$ between $\hat{\theta}$

and θ. Based on regularity condition $(v) \mid \partial^3 \log f(x;\theta)/\partial\theta^3 \mid \leq M(x)$ for all $x \in A$, $\theta_0 - c < \theta < \theta_0 + c$ with $E_{\theta_0}\{M(X)\} < \infty$ and the fact that $\mid \theta_0 - \hat{\theta} \mid = O_p(n^{-1/2+\varepsilon})$, $\varepsilon > 0$ (Section 3.3), we can obtain $R = O_p(n^{-3/2+3\varepsilon}n) = O_p(n^{-1/2+3\varepsilon}) = o_p(1)$, where ε can be chosen as $\varepsilon < \frac{1}{6}$. Noting that $\left.\frac{\partial l(\theta \mid \mathbf{x})}{\partial \theta}\right|_{\theta=\hat{\theta}} = 0$, we have

$$l(\theta_0 \mid \mathbf{x}) = l(\hat{\theta} \mid \mathbf{x}) + \frac{1}{2}(\theta_0 - \hat{\theta})^2 \left.\frac{\partial^2 l(\theta \mid \mathbf{x})}{\partial \theta^2}\right|_{\theta=\hat{\theta}} + o_p(1).$$

By substituting $l(\theta_0 \mid \mathbf{x})$ with its corresponding Taylor expansion, we conclude that

$$
\begin{aligned}
2\{l(\hat{\theta} \mid \mathbf{x}) - l(\theta_0 \mid \mathbf{x})\} &= -(\theta_0 - \hat{\theta})^2 \left.\frac{\partial^2 l(\theta \mid \mathbf{x})}{\partial \theta^2}\right|_{\theta=\hat{\theta}} + o_p(1) \\
&= \{\sqrt{n}(\theta_0 - \hat{\theta})\}^2 \left\{-n^{-1}\left.\frac{\partial^2 l(\theta \mid \mathbf{x})}{\partial \theta^2}\right|_{\theta=\hat{\theta}}\right\} + o_p(1) \\
&= \left[\sqrt{n}(\theta_0 - \hat{\theta})\left\{-n^{-1}\left.\frac{\partial^2 l(\theta \mid \mathbf{x})}{\partial \theta^2}\right|_{\theta=\hat{\theta}}\right\}^{1/2}\right]^2 + o_p(1).
\end{aligned}
$$

Under the regularity conditions, we have that $\sqrt{n}(\theta_0 - \hat{\theta}) \to N(0, 1/I(\theta_0))$ (Theorem 3.3.1) and $-n^{-1}\left.\frac{\partial^2 l(\theta \mid \mathbf{x})}{\partial \theta^2}\right|_{\theta=\hat{\theta}} \to I(\theta_0)$ in probability (Chapters 1 and 2 can provide arguments to show this fact). Then $\sqrt{n}(\theta_0 - \hat{\theta})\left\{-n^{-1}\left.\frac{\partial^2 l(\theta \mid \mathbf{x})}{\partial \theta^2}\right|_{\theta=\hat{\theta}}\right\}^{1/2}$

converges to $N(0,1)$ in distribution, and therefore $2\{l(\hat{\theta} \mid \mathbf{x}) - l(\theta_0 \mid \mathbf{x})\}$ converges to χ_1^2 in distribution. (We also suggest the reader consult Slutsky's theorem (Grimmett and Stirzaker, 1992) in this context.)

The proof is complete.

Note that, in the general situation with $MLR_n = \sup_{\theta \in \Omega^c} L(\theta \mid \mathbf{x})$ $\sup_{\theta \in \Omega_0} L(\theta \mid \mathbf{x})$, the proof mentioned above can be easily extended. In this case, under $H_0 : \theta \in \Omega_0$, the statistic $2\log(MLR_n)$ follows asymptotically a χ_d^2 distribution as $n \to \infty$, where the degrees of freedom d equal to the difference in dimensionality of Ω^c and Ω_0 and are clarified by the amount of items

similar to $\left[\sqrt{n}(\theta_0 - \hat{\theta})\left\{-n^{-1}\left.\frac{\partial^2 l(\theta \mid \mathbf{x})}{\partial \theta^2}\right|_{\theta=\hat{\theta}}\right\}^{1/2}\right]^2 \xrightarrow{n \to \infty} \{N(0,1)\}^2$ that should be

presented in the corresponding log likelihood expansion.

Comments: Thus, if certain key assumptions are met, one can show that parametric likelihood methods are very powerful and efficient statistical tools. We should emphasize that the role of the discovery of the likelihood ratio methodology in statistical developments can be compared to the development of the assembly line technique of mass production. The likelihood ratio principle gives clear instructions and technique manuals on how to construct efficient statistical decision rules in various complex problems related to clinical experiments. For example, Vexler et al. (2011) developed a likelihood ratio test for comparing populations based on incomplete longitudinal data subject to instrumental limitations.

Although many statistical publications continue to contribute to the likelihood paradigm and are very important in the statistical discipline (an excellent account can be found in Lehmann and Romano, 2006), several significant questions naturally arise about the general applicability of the maximum likelihood approach. Conceptually, there is an issue specific to classifying maximum likelihoods in terms of likelihoods that are given by joint density (or probability) functions based on data. Integrated likelihood functions, with respect to arguments related to data points, are equal to one, whereas accordingly integrated maximum likelihood functions often have values that are indefinite. Thus, while likelihoods present full information regarding the data, the maximum likelihoods might lose information conditional on the observed data. Consider this simple example: Suppose we observe X_1, which is assumed to be from a normal distribution $N(\mu, 1)$ with mean parameter μ. In this case, the likelihood has the form $(2\pi)^{-0.5} \exp(-(X_1 - \mu)^2 / 2)$ and, correspondingly, $\int (2\pi)^{-0.5} \exp(-(X_1 - \mu)^2 / 2) dX_1 = 1$, whereas the maximum likelihood, i.e., the likelihood evaluated at the estimate of μ, $\hat{\mu} = X_1$, is $(2\pi)^{-0.5}$, which clearly does not represent the data and is not a proper density. This demonstrates that since the Neyman–Pearson lemma is fundamentally founded on the use of the density-based constitutions of likelihood ratios, maximum likelihood ratios cannot be optimal in general cases. That is, the likelihood ratio principle is generally not robust when the hypothesis tests have corresponding nuisance parameters to consider, e.g., testing a hypothesized mean given an unknown variance.

An additional inherent difficulty of the maximum likelihood ratio test occurs when a clinical experiment is associated with an infinite-dimensional problem and the number of unknown parameters is relatively large. In this case, Wilks' theorem should be re-evaluated, and nonparametric approaches should be considered in the contexts of reasonable alternatives to the parametric likelihood methodology (Fan et al., 2001).

The ideas of likelihood and maximum likelihood ratio testing may not be fiducial and applicable in general nonparametric function estimation/testing settings. It is also well known that when key assumptions are not met, parametric approaches may be suboptimal or biased as compared to their robust counterparts across the many features of statistical inferences. For example, in a biomedical application, Ghosh (1995) proved that the maximum likelihood estimators for the Rasch model are inconsistent, as the number of nuisance parameters increases to infinity (Rasch models are often employed in clinical trials that deal with psychological measurements, e.g., abilities, attitudes, and personality traits). Due to the structure of likelihood functions based on products of densities, or conditional density functions, relatively insignificant errors in classifications of data distributions can lead to vital problems related to the applications of likelihood ratio type tests (Gurevich and Vexler, 2010). Moreover, one can note that, given the wide variety and complex nature of biomedical data (e.g., incomplete data subject to instrumental limitations or complex correlation structures), parametric assumptions are rarely satisfied. The respective formal tests are complicated, or oftentimes not readily available.

Author's Note: In this book we will employ *martingale*-based arguments to demonstrate that in general situations the maximum likelihood ratios are vastly different from the likelihood ratio and thus cannot provide optimal non-asymptotic properties similar to those related to the likelihood ratios. Using the idea that commonly in the context of hypothesis testing we do not need to estimate unknown parameters, we only shall decide to reject or not to reject the null hypothesis, we will propose decision-making procedures, applying representative values instead of unknown parameters or more general *Bayes factor* concepts in order to obtain optimal tests based on samples with fixed sizes.

Brief Example of the Maximum Likelihood Ratio MLR_n. Assume that a sample of iid observations $X_1, X_2, ..., X_n$ follow an exponential distribution with the rate parameter λ, that is, $X_1, ..., X_n \sim f(x) = \lambda \exp(-\lambda x)$. We then describe the maximum likelihood ratio test statistic for the composite hypothesis $H_0 : \lambda = 1$ versus $H_1 : \lambda \neq 1$. The log-likelihood function is

$$l(\lambda) = l(\lambda \mid X_1, X_2, ..., X_n) = \sum_{i=1}^{n} \log f(X_i) = n \log \lambda - \lambda \sum_{i=1}^{n} X_i.$$

To calculate the maximum likelihood estimation, we solve the equation $\frac{dl(\lambda)}{d\lambda} = \frac{n}{\lambda} - \sum_{i=1}^{n} X_i = 0$. The maximum likelihood estimator of λ is $\hat{\lambda} = \bar{X}^{-1} = n \Big/ \sum_{i=1}^{n} X_i$. Therefore, the maximum likelihood ratio test statistic is $2 \log(MLR_n) = 2\{l(\hat{\lambda}) - l(1)\} = 2n\{-\log(\bar{X}) - 1 + \bar{X}\}$. The distribution of $2 \log(MLR_n)$ under H_0 is approximately χ_1^2 and $\chi_{1,0.95}^2 = 3.84 \, (\Pr(\chi_1^2 > \chi_{1,0.95}^2) = 0.05)$. We reject H_0 if $2 \log(MLR_n) > 3.84$ at the 0.05 significance level.

Real data examples and their corresponding R codes for implementation are presented in Vexler et al. (2016a).

3.7 An Example of Correct Model-Based Likelihood Formation

Generally speaking, when data are available and model assumptions are fitted, it is not a trivial issue to formulate correctly the corresponding likelihood function. Let us include the following example to illustrate that we need carefully attend to the likelihood statement. Consider n data points $X_1, ..., X_n$ that are assumed to satisfy the **measurement model** with **autoregressive** errors

$$X_i = \mu + \varepsilon_i, \quad \varepsilon_i = \beta \varepsilon_{i-1} + \xi_i, \quad \varepsilon_0 = 0, \quad i = 1, ..., n,$$

where μ and β are parameters, the errors $\varepsilon_1, ..., \varepsilon_n$ are unobserved and dependent corresponding to the model $\varepsilon_i = \beta \varepsilon_{i-1} + \xi_i$, that is called as autoregression with iid noise $\xi_1, ..., \xi_n$ from a specified density function f_ξ.

By virtue of the model assumption, we have

$$\xi_1 = X_1 - \mu, \quad \xi_i = X_i - \mu(1-\beta) - \beta X_{i-1}, \quad i = 2, ..., n.$$

Then one can write the likelihood function in the form

$$L(\mu, \beta) = f_\xi(X_1 - \mu) \prod_{i=2}^{n} f_\xi(X_i - \mu(1-\beta) - \beta X_{i-1}).$$

Although this form is correct, the approach applied above might lead to incorrect likelihood forms in several general scenarios, since by definition the likelihood function should be constructed using distribution functions of observations that are $X_1, ..., X_n$ in this example.

Let us demonstrate the formal exercise to derive the likelihood function. To this end we start by noting that

$$L(\mu, \beta) = f(X_1, ..., X_n) = \prod_{i=1}^{n} f(X_i \mid X_1, ..., X_{i-1}).$$

Taking into account the autoregressive form of the model, we obtain

$$L(\mu,\beta) = f(X_1)\prod_{i=2}^{n} f(X_i \mid X_{i-1}).$$

Now we derive the joint density function of (X_i, X_{i-1}), $f_{X_i, X_{i-1}}(u,v)$, that is

$$
\begin{aligned}
f_{X_i, X_{i-1}}(u,v) &= \frac{\partial^2}{\partial u \partial v} \Pr(X_i < u, X_{i-1} < v) \\
&= \frac{\partial^2}{\partial u \partial v} \Pr(\xi_i + \mu(1-\beta) + \beta X_{i-1} < u, X_{i-1} < v) \\
&= \frac{\partial^2}{\partial u \partial v} \int_{-\infty}^{\infty} \Pr(\xi_i + \mu(1-\beta) + \beta X_{i-1} < u, X_{i-1} < v \mid X_{i-1} = t) f_{X_{i-1}}(t)\, dt \\
&= \frac{\partial^2}{\partial u \partial v} \int_{-\infty}^{\infty} \Pr(\xi_i + \mu(1-\beta) + \beta t < u, t < v \mid X_{i-1} = t) f_{X_{i-1}}(t)\, dt \\
&= \frac{\partial^2}{\partial u \partial v} \int_{-\infty}^{v} \Pr(\xi_i + \mu(1-\beta) + \beta t < u \mid X_{i-1} = t) f_{X_{i-1}}(t)\, dt \\
&= \frac{\partial^2}{\partial u \partial v} \int_{-\infty}^{v} \Pr(\xi_i + \mu(1-\beta) + \beta t < u) f_{X_{i-1}}(t)\, dt \\
&= \frac{\partial}{\partial u} \Pr(\xi_i < u - \mu(1-\beta) - \beta v) f_{X_{i-1}}(v) = f_\xi(u - \mu(1-\beta) - \beta v) f_{X_{i-1}}(v),
\end{aligned}
$$

where the convolution principle (see Chapter 2) is used and $f_{X_{i-1}}(v) = \frac{d}{dv} \Pr(X_{i-1} < v)$. Thus using conditional probability theory we conclude that

$$f(X_i \mid X_{i-1}) = f_\xi(X_i - \mu(1-\beta) - \beta X_{i-1}), \; i \geq 2,$$

and then $L(\mu,\beta) = f_\xi(X_1 - \mu)\prod_{i=2}^{n} f_\xi(X_i - \mu(1-\beta) - \beta X_{i-1}).$

An example of a potential use of the method shown above is related to a likelihood function that implements the autoregressive process of outcomes, incorporating the characteristics of the problematic longitudinal data in bio-medical research, e.g., regarding mouse tumor experiments (Vexler et al.,

2011). For example, one can consider a study with l treatment groups. For treatment group k ($k = 1,...,l$), there are n_k experimental units. Each experimental unit is followed by m equally spaced time points by a prespecified schedule. Let X_{ijk} denote the jth measurement of the ith unit in group k ($j = 1,...,m; i = 1,...,n_k; k = 1,...,l$). The variable X_{ijk} may reflect a tumor size in a tumor development model with mice. We can model successive measurements within an experimental unit as

$$X_{ijk} = \mu_{jk} + \varepsilon_{ijk}, \quad \varepsilon_{ijk} = \sum_{v=1}^{r} \beta_v \varepsilon_{i,j-v,k} + \xi_{ijk},$$

for some integer $r < j$, where ξ_{ijk} are iid with the mean of 0 and the β_v's describe the relationship between ε_{ijk}'s. This model depicts the rth order of autoregressive associations between the observations.

4

Martingale Type Statistics and Their Applications

4.1 Introduction

Probability theory has several fundamental branches that have been dealt with extensively in the theoretical literature associated with *martingale* techniques. Oftentimes, modern concepts of stochastic processes analysis are presented in the framework of martingale constructions. Historically, gambling theory and econometrics have employed martingale theory to model fair stochastic games when information regarding past events does not provide us the ability to predict the mean of future winnings.

There are a multitude of books that cover different martingale based methods. In this chapter, we will focus on the following three aspects that have straightforward connections with biostatistical theory and its applications: (1) A martingale can represent a statistic, say M_n, based on n data points such that the expectation of a future outcome M_{n+1}, which is calculated given knowledge regarding the present statistic M_n, is equal to the observed value M_n. For example, intuitively, if a test statistic, say T_n, based on n observations satisfies this martingale property, under the null hypothesis H_0, then on average T_n values are relatively stable under H_0 (T_n does not increase on average, $E_{H_0}\left(T_{n+1} \mid T_1, ..., T_n\right) = T_n$, with respect to sizes of underlining data). Thus, this can reduce the chances that the test statistic $T_k, k > n$, will overshoot a corresponding test threshold when more data points are available and H_0 is true. (2) In previous chapters, we demonstrated that propositions based on sums of iid random variables can provide general proof schemes in the evaluation of various statistical procedures. The martingale machinery can extend different concepts based on sums of iid summands by taking into account things such as dependency structures between observations. (3) Martingale methodology plays a crucial role in the development and examination of various statistical *sequential procedures*. Common sequential statistical schemes involve random numbers of observations according to random *stopping times (rules)* for surveying data (see, e.g., Chapter 2 for examples of sequential statistical procedures). In this context, martingales present a rather wide class of statistics, which are invariant relative to such operations as a continuous change of a measure and random change of time. Thus, we can extend statistical procedures based on statistics with a fixed number of data points to approaches based on statistics with random numbers of observations.

We suggest that the reader who is interested in further details regarding martingales to consult the essential works of Chow et al. (1971), Chung (1974, 2000), Edgar and Sucheston (2010), Liptser and Shiryayev (1989) and Williams (1991).

This chapter will outline the following topics: Definitions and examples of martingale related components, including σ-algebras, conditional expectations with respect to σ-algebras, martingale type objects and stopping times (Section 4.2); The optional stopping theorem and its corollaries in the forms of Wald's lemma and Doob's inequality (Section 4.3); Applications of martingale theory for developing the principles of efficient retrospective and sequential statistical procedures, including decision-making schemes, adaptive estimators, and change point detection policies (Section 4.4). The material presented in Section 4.5 is optional to be demonstrated when Chapter 4 is to be used in a course text development. The reader can consider Section 4.5 as an advanced example of a scholarly statistical research presentation. We emphasize that Section 4.5 displays a novel discovery in martingale transformations of testing strategies and martingale based comparisons between decision-making procedures. The authors are indebted to Professor Moshe Pollak and Dr. Aiyi Liu for many helpful discussions and comments related to the results shown in Section 4.5.

4.2 Terminology

To begin our chapter we need to first provide some of the key definitions used throughout its development.

In Section 4.1 we referred to the terms "information regarding past events" and "given knowledge regarding the present statistic." In order to formalize these, we provide the following series of fundamental definitions:

Definition 4.2.1: Let **A** be a class of subsets. Then **A** defines an algebra if it satisfies the following conditions:

(*i*) the set of elementary events Ω (see Section 1.3, taking into account that we require $\Pr(\Omega) = 1$) belongs to **A**, $\Omega \subseteq$ **A**;

(ii) the facts $A \subseteq \mathbf{A}$ and $B \subseteq \mathbf{A}$ imply $A \cup B \subseteq \mathbf{A}$ and $A \cap B \subseteq \mathbf{A}$;

(iii) if $A \subseteq \mathbf{A}$ then $A^c \subseteq \mathbf{A}$, where A^c is the complement to A.

Definition 4.2.2: The class of subsets $\Im$ is a σ-algebra if $\Im$ is an algebra such that wherever $F_n \subseteq \Im$ then $\bigcap_{n=1} F_n \subseteq \Im$.

Note that in Definition 4.2.1 using condition *(iii)*, we can require that $A \cup B \subseteq \mathbf{A}$ or $A \cap B \subseteq \mathbf{A}$, since $(A \cup B)^c = A^c \cap B^c$. Similarly, in Definition 4.2.2, one can apply $\bigcup_{n=1} F_n \subseteq \Im$ instead of $\bigcap_{n=1} F_n \subseteq \Im$.

We shall associate the term "knowledge" mentioned above with information provided by a statistic. Toward this end let us define a σ-algebra generated by a random variable X or simply based on X.

Definition 4.2.3: If the σ-algebra $\Im$ consists of subsets A's in the form of $A = \{\omega : X(\omega) \in B\}$, where B's are Borel sets, then $\Im$ is a σ-algebra generated by the random variable X.

In general, the elements of B can be quite complicated. However, if the random variable X is a statistic with real values we often can employ Definition 4.2.3 to denote the σ-algebra based on X, noting it as $\sigma(X)$. In an intuitive manner (not a standard notation), it is very easy to understand that $\Im = \sigma(X)$ corresponds to a collection of all possible analytical functions of X. Similarly, if we have m statistics $X_1, ..., X_m$ the σ-algebra $\Im_m = \sigma(X_1, ..., X_m)$ includes all possible analytic operations based upon $X_1, ..., X_m$. Some examples are given as: $1 = (X_1)^0 \in \Im_m$; $X_1 + X_m \in \Im_m$; $X_{m-1} X_m \in \Im_m$; $\exp(t_1 X_1 + t_2 X_2) \in \Im_m$, where $m \geq 2$ and t_1, t_2 are constants. However, in this setting we should be very careful with, e.g., $X_1 + X_{m+1}$, since in general if X_{m+1} cannot be calculated using only $X_1, ..., X_m$, we have $X_1 + X_{m+1} \notin \Im_m$. More formally the symbols "$\in$" and "$\notin$" should be interpreted in terms of *measurability*, i.e., for example the notation $X_1 + X_m \in \Im_m$ means $X_1 + X_m$ is $\Im_m$-*measurable* for all subsets $A \subset \Im_m$ and here the symbol "$\subset$" indicates that $\Im_m$ includes A. Actually the "confusion" regarding the terms "to belong $\in$" and "to be measurable" is not vital in the context of the materials presented in this chapter and we guess the meaning of, e.g., $X_1 + X_m \in \Im_m$ is more understandable than that of $X_1 + X_m$ is $\Im_m$-measurable for all subsets $A \subset \Im_m$, in the framework of this book.

Martingale methodology employs the conditional expectation concept. Consider, for example, a scenario where we observe data points $\xi_1, ..., \xi_n$ and a statistic X is calculated using values of $\xi_1, ..., \xi_n$, i.e., $X = X(\xi_1, ..., \xi_n)$. Then the conditional expectation $E\{X \mid \sigma(\xi_1, ..., \xi_k)\}, 1 \leq l \leq k \leq n$ can be considered in intuitive fashion as a derivative of the expectation $E\{X\}$ at the moment when we condition on $\xi_l, ..., \xi_k$ to be fixed with respect to this expectation.

This leads us to conclude that $E\{X \mid \sigma(\xi_l,...,\xi_k)\} \in \sigma(\xi_l,...,\xi_k)$, since in $E\{X \mid \sigma(\xi_l,...,\xi_k)\}$ values of $\xi_1,...,\xi_{l-1}$ and $\xi_{k+1},...,\xi_n$ are integrated out with respect to their joint distribution. For example, $E\{\xi_l \mid \sigma(\xi_l,...,\xi_k)\} = \xi_l \in \sigma(\xi_l,...,\xi_k); \quad E\{\xi_1\xi_2 \mid \sigma(\xi_1)\} = \xi_1 E\{\xi_2 \mid \sigma(\xi_1)\} \in \sigma(\xi_1)$, where $E\{\xi_2 \mid \sigma(\xi_1)\} = E(\xi_2) \in \sigma(\xi_1)$ if ξ_1 and ξ_2 are independent; $E\left\{\sum_{i=1}^{n} \xi_i \mid \sigma(\xi_1,...,\xi_k)\right\} = \sum_{i=1}^{k} \xi_i + E\left\{\sum_{i=k+1}^{n} \xi_i \mid \sigma(\xi_1,...,\xi_k)\right\} \in \sigma(\xi_1,...,\xi_k)$. Note that, to be a bit formal, since, in general, $E\{X \mid \sigma(\xi_l,...,\xi_k)\}$ is a $\sigma(\xi_l,...,\xi_k)$ -*measurable random variable*, it would be "elegant" to write "almost sure" (see Section 1.7.2) in the examples shown above, e.g., $E\{\xi_1\xi_2 \mid \sigma(\xi_1)\} = \xi_1 E\{\xi_2 \mid \sigma(\xi_1)\}$ a.s. Nevertheless we shall omit such obvious "a.s." from now on. A general formal definition of a conditional expectation has the form shown below.

Definition 4.2.4: Let X be a random variable with $E|X| < \infty$ and $\Im$ denote a σ-algebra. The conditional expectation of X with respect to $\Im$ is the random variable $Y = E(X \mid \Im)$, which has the following properties: *(i)* $Y \in \Im$; *(ii)* for each $A \subset \Im_m$, we have $E\{Y \, I(A)\} = E\{X \, I(A)\}$, where $I(.)$ is the indicator function.

Property *(ii)* of Definition 4.2.4 leads to a very useful rule of Probability Theory that oftentimes is called as *the law of total expectation* or *the law of iterated expectation* and formulated as

$$E(X) = E\{E(X \mid \Im)\}. \tag{4.1}$$

For example, consider the simple scenarios when (1) $X \in \Im$ then $E(X \mid \Im) = X$ and it is clear that $E\{E(X \mid \Im)\} = E(X)$, and (2) X is independent of $\Im$ then $E(X \mid \Im) = E(X)$ and it is clear that $E\{E(X \mid \Im)\} = E\{E(X)\} = E(X)$. Note that one can show that the *convolution* principle (2.1) shown in Chapter 2 is a corollary of Equation (4.1).

Now, given our background material above, we can define a martingale in an appropriate manner relative to the main purpose of this chapter.

Definition 4.2.5: Let M_n denote a statistic based on n data points and $\Im_1,...,\Im_n$ be a sequence of σ-algebras such that $\Im_1 \subset \Im_2 \subset ... \subset \Im_n$, and $E|M_n| < \infty$. The couple $(M_n, \Im_n)$ is called

   a *martingale*, if it satisfies $E(M_n \mid \Im_{n-1}) = M_{n-1}$;

   a *submartingale*, if it satisfies $E(M_n \mid \Im_{n-1}) \geq M_{n-1}$;

   a *supermartingale*, if it satisfies $E(M_n \mid \Im_{n-1}) \leq M_{n-1}$.

It is clear that if $(M_n, \Im_n)$ is a martingale then, for example, $(M_n^2, \Im_n)$ is a submartingale, whereas $(\log(M_n), \Im_n)$ is a supermartingale, since $E(M_n^2 | \Im_{n-1}) \geq \{E(M_n | \Im_{n-1})\}^2 = M_{n-1}^2$ and $E(\log(M_n) | \Im_{n-1}) \leq \log(E(M_n | \Im_{n-1})) = \log(M_{n-1})$. In these cases *Jensen's inequality* was used.

Warning: It is very important to draw the reader's attention to Definition 4.2.5, which focuses on the pair $(M_n, \Im_n)$. Consider the example where we define M_n as the sum $\sum_{i=1}^{n} \xi_i$ of iid random variables $\xi_1, ..., \xi_n$ with $E(\xi_1) = 0$ and let $\Im_n = \sigma(\xi_1, ..., \xi_n)$. Then $E(M_n | \Im_{n-1}) = \sum_{i=1}^{n-1} \xi_i + E(\xi_n | \Im_{n-1}) = \sum_{i=1}^{n-1} \xi_i + E(\xi_n) = M_{n-1} + 0$. This implies that $(M_n, \Im_n)$ is a martingale. However, defining $\Im'_n = \sigma(y_1, ..., y_n)$, where iid random variables $y_1, ..., y_n$ are independent of $\xi_1, ..., \xi_n$, we obtain $E(M_n | \Im'_{n-1}) = \sum_{i=1}^{n} E(\xi_i) = 0$ and then $(M_n, \Im'_n)$ is not a martingale.

In a general aspect, one can consider martingale type statistics to extend the notion of a statistic consisting of a sum of iid random variables. For example, assume that $\xi_0, ..., \xi_n$ are iid random variables with $E(\xi_1) = a$. In this case, it is clear that $\left(\sum_{i=1}^{n} \xi_i - an, \sigma(\xi_1, ..., \xi_n) \right) = \left(\sum_{i=1}^{n} (\xi_i - a), \sigma(\xi_1, ..., \xi_n) \right)$ is a martingale as shown above. It turns out that by defining the statistic $M_n = \sum_{i=1}^{n} (\xi_{i-1} - a)(\xi_i - a)$ we obtain

$$
\begin{aligned}
E\{M_n | \sigma(\xi_0, ..., \xi_{n-1})\} &= E\left\{ \sum_{i=1}^{n} (\xi_{i-1} - a)(\xi_i - a) | \sigma(\xi_0, ..., \xi_{n-1}) \right\} \\
&= \sum_{i=1}^{n-1} (\xi_{i-1} - a)(\xi_i - a) + E\{(\xi_{n-1} - a)(\xi_n - a) | \sigma(\xi_0, ..., \xi_{n-1})\} \\
&= \sum_{i=1}^{n-1} (\xi_{i-1} - a)(\xi_i - a) + (\xi_{n-1} - a) E(\xi_n - a) \\
&= \sum_{i=1}^{n-1} (\xi_{i-1} - a)(\xi_i - a) = M_{n-1}
\end{aligned}
$$

and then $(M_n, \sigma(\xi_0, ..., \xi_{n-1}))$ is a martingale, where M_n represents a sum of dependent random variables (certainly, we assumed that $E|\xi_1| < \infty$ to apply Definition 4.2.5.). As another example, via taking into account Section 3.7, we propose analyzing observations $\varepsilon_1, ..., \varepsilon_n$ that satisfy the autoregression model $\varepsilon_i = \beta \varepsilon_{i-1} + \xi_i, i = 1, ..., n$, with the iid noise $\xi_1, ..., \xi_n$ and $E(\xi_1) = 0$, $\varepsilon_0 = 0$.

In this case we have $\varepsilon_k = \xi_k + \beta(\xi_{k-1} + \beta\varepsilon_{k-2}) = ... = \sum_{j=1}^{k} \beta^{k-j}\xi_j$, which yields

$$
\begin{aligned}
E\{\beta^{-k}\varepsilon_k \mid \sigma(\xi_1,...,\xi_{k-1})\} &= \beta^{-k}\left[\sum_{j=1}^{k-1}\beta^{k-j}\xi_j + E\{\xi_k \mid \sigma(\xi_1,...,\xi_{k-1})\}\right] \\
&= \beta^{-k}\left\{\sum_{j=1}^{k-1}\beta^{k-j}\xi_j + E(\xi_k)\right\} = \beta^{-k}\sum_{j=1}^{k-1}\beta^{k-j}\xi_j \\
&= \beta^{-(k-1)}\sum_{j=1}^{k-1}\beta^{(k-1)-j}\xi_j = \beta^{-(k-1)}\varepsilon_{k-1}, \ k > 1.
\end{aligned}
$$

This implies that $\left(\beta^{-n}\varepsilon_n, \sigma(\xi_1,...,\xi_n)\right)$ is a martingale, where the observations $\varepsilon_1,...,\varepsilon_n$ are sums of independent and not identically distributed random variables.

Chapter 2 introduced statistical strategies that employ random numbers of data points. In forthcoming sections of this book we will introduce several procedures based on non *retrospective* mechanisms as *statistical sequential schemes*. In order to extend retrospective statistical tools based on data with fixed sample sizes to procedures stopped at random times we introduce the following definition:

Definition 4.2.6: A random variable τ is a *stopping time* with respect to σ-algebra $\Im_n$ $(\Im_1 \subset \Im_2 \subset ... \subset \Im_n)$ if it satisfies (i) $\{\tau \le n\} \subset \Im_n$, for all $n \ge 1$; (ii) $\Pr(\tau < \infty) = 1$.

In the statistical interpretation, the idea is that only information in $\Im_n$ at time n should lead us to stop without knowledge of the future, whether or not time τ has arrived. For example, assume τ is a stopping time. Then $\tau + 1$ is a stopping time, since we can stop at τ observing $\Im_n$ and decide finally to stop our procedure at the next stage $\tau + 1$, i.e., by the definition of τ and the σ-algebra, we have $\{\tau + 1 \le n\} = \{\tau \le n - 1\} \subset \Im_{n-1} \subset \Im_n$. However $\tau - 1$ is not a stopping time, since we cannot stop at τ observing $\Im_n$ and decide that we should stop our procedure at the previous stage $\tau - 1$, i.e., $\{\tau - 1 \le n\} = \{\tau \le n + 1\} \subset \Im_{n+1} \not\subset \Im_n$.

Examples:

1. It is clear that a fixed integer N is a stopping time.
2. Suppose τ and ν are stopping times. Then $\min(\tau, \nu)$ and $\max(\tau, \nu)$ are stopping times. Indeed, $\min(\tau, \nu)$ and $\max(\tau, \nu)$ satisfy condition *(ii)* of Definition 4.2.6, since τ and ν are stopping times. In this case, the events $\{\min(\tau, \nu) \le n\} = \{\tau \le n\} \cup \{\nu \le n\} \subset \Im_n$ and $\{\max(\tau, \nu) \le n\} = \{\tau \le n\} \cap \{\nu \le n\} \subset \Im_n$.

3. Let integers τ and v define stopping times. Then $\tau + v$ is a stopping time, since $\{\tau + v \leq n\} = \{\tau \leq n - v\} = \bigcap_{i=1}^{\infty} \{\tau \leq n - v\} \cap \{v = i\} = \bigcap_{i=1}^{n} \{\tau \leq n - i\} \cap \{v = i\} \subset \mathfrak{I}_n$

where $\{\tau \leq 0\} = \emptyset$.

4. In a similar manner to the example above, one can show that $\tau - v$ is not a stopping time.

5. Consider the random variable $\varpi = \inf\{n \geq 1 : X_n \geq a_n\}$, where $X_1, X_2, X_3, \ldots$ are independent and identically uniformly $[0,1]$ distributed random variables and $a_i = (1 - 1/(i+1)^2), i \geq 1$. Defining $\mathfrak{I}_n = \sigma(X_1, \ldots, X_n)$, we have $\{\varpi \leq n\} = \{\max_{1 \leq k \leq n}(X_k - a_k) \geq 0\} \subset \mathfrak{I}_n$. Let us examine, for a nonrandom N,

$$
\begin{aligned}
\Pr(\varpi > N) &= \Pr\{\max_{1 \leq k \leq N}(X_k - a_k) \leq 0\} \\
&= \Pr\{(X_1 - a_1) \leq 0, \ldots, (X_N - a_N) \leq 0\} \\
&= \prod_{k=1}^{N} \Pr\{(X_k - a_k) \leq 0\} = \prod_{k=1}^{N} \Pr\{X_k \leq a_k\} \\
&= \prod_{k=1}^{N} a_k.
\end{aligned}
$$

In this case,

$$
\log\left(\prod_{k=1}^{N} a_k\right) = \sum_{k=1}^{N} \log(1 - 1/(k+1)^2) \approx \sum_{k=1}^{N} \{-1/(k+1)^2\},
$$

where we apply the Taylor argument to represent $\log(1 - s) = -s + s^2/2 + O(s^3)$ with $s = 1/(k+1)^2$. Thus $\Pr(\varpi > N)$ not $\to 0$ as $N \to \infty$ and then $\Pr(\varpi < \infty) < 1$. This means ϖ is not a stopping time.

6. Defining $a_i = (1 - 1/(i+1)), i \geq 1$, in Example (5) above, we obtain

$$
\log\left(\prod_{k=1}^{N} a_k\right) = \sum_{k=1}^{N} \log(1 - 1/(k+1)) \approx \sum_{k=1}^{N}(-1/(k+1)) \approx -\log(N) \to -\infty
$$

as $N \to \infty$ and then $\Pr(\varpi > N) \to 0$ that implies ϖ is a stopping time, in this case.

7. Consider the random variable $W = \inf\{n \geq 1 : S_n \geq 2n^2(n+1)\}$, where $S_n = \sum_{i}^{n} X_i$ and $X_1 > 0, X_2 > 0, X_3 > 0, \ldots$ are iid random variables with $E(X_1) < 1$. Let us examine

$$\Pr(W < \infty) = \sum_{n=1}^{\infty} \Pr(W = n)$$

$$= \sum_{n=1}^{\infty} \Pr\{S_1 < 4, \ldots, S_{n-1} < 2(n-1)^2 n, S_n \geq 2n^2(n+1)\}$$

$$\leq \sum_{n=1}^{\infty} \Pr\{S_n \geq 2n^2(n+1)\} \leq \sum_{n=1}^{\infty} \frac{E(S_n)}{2n^2(n+1)}$$

$$= \sum_{n=1}^{\infty} \frac{E(X_1)}{2n(n+1)}$$

$$= \frac{1}{2} E(X_1) < 1,$$

where Chebyshev's inequality is used. Thus, although $(W \leq n) \subset \mathfrak{S}_n = \sigma(X_1, \ldots, X_n)$, W is not a stopping time.

4.3 The Optional Stopping Theorem and Its Corollaries: Wald's Lemma and Doob's Inequality

Historically, martingale type objects were associated with Monte Carlo roulette games. Suppose X_n shows our capital obtained at a stage n while we are playing the Monte Carlo roulette game without any arbitrage, i.e., no one outside monitors the roulette wheel and provides us more money.

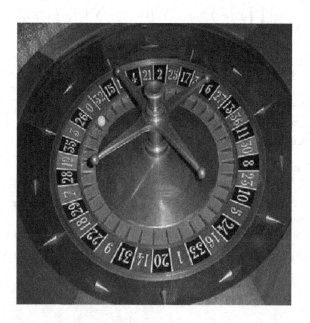

It turns out that, in a fair game, $\left(X_n, \Im_n = \sigma\left(X_1, ..., X_n\right)\right)$ is a martingale. Then on average $E\left(X_n\right) = E\left\{E\left(X_n \mid \Im_{n-1}\right)\right\} = E\left(X_{n-1}\right) = E\left\{E\left(X_{n-1} \mid \Im_{n-2}\right)\right\} = ... = E\left(X_1\right),$ where the rule (4.1) is applied and X_1 displays our initial capital. One can wonder about a "smart" strategy, when the game will be stopped depending on the history of the game, e.g., at the time $\min\left\{N, \inf\left(n \geq 1 : X_n \geq \$100\right)\right\}$, where N is a fixed integer. Towards this end, consider the following result:

Proposition 4.3.1 (*The Optional Stopping Theorem*). Let $\left(M_n, \Im_n\right)$ be a martingale and $\tau \geq 1$ be a stopping time that corresponds to $\Im_n$. Assume that $E\left(\tau\right) < \infty$ and, for all $n \geq 1$ on the set $\left\{\tau \geq n\right\} \subset \Im_{n-1}$, $E\left(\left|M_n - M_{n-1}\right| \mid \Im_{n-1}\right) \leq c,$ where c is a constant. Then $E\left(M_\tau\right) = E\left(M_1\right)$.

Proof. For an integer N, define the stopping time $\tau_N = \min(N, \tau)$. It is clear that

$$
\begin{aligned}
E\left(M_{\tau_N}\right) &= E\left\{\sum_{i=1}^N M_i \, I\left(\tau_N = i\right)\right\} \\
&= E\left[\sum_{i=1}^N M_i \left\{I\left(\tau_N \leq i\right) - I\left(\tau_N \leq i-1\right)\right\}\right] \\
&= \sum_{i=1}^N E\left\{M_i \, I\left(\tau_N \leq i\right)\right\} - \sum_{i=1}^N E\left\{M_i \, I\left(\tau_N \leq i-1\right)\right\}.
\end{aligned}
$$

In this equation, by virtue of property (4.1) and the martingale and stopping time definitions, we have

$$
\begin{aligned}
E\left\{M_i \, I\left(\tau_N \leq i-1\right)\right\} &= EE\left\{M_i \, I\left(\tau_N \leq i-1\right) \mid \Im_{i-1}\right\} \\
&= E\left\{I\left(\tau_N \leq i-1\right) E\left(M_i \mid \Im_{i-1}\right)\right\} \\
&= E\left\{M_{i-1} I\left(\tau_N \leq i-1\right)\right\}.
\end{aligned}
$$

Thus

$$
\begin{aligned}
E\left(M_{\tau_N}\right) &= \sum_{i=1}^N E\left\{M_i \, I\left(\tau_N \leq i\right)\right\} - \sum_{i=1}^N E\left\{M_{i-1} \, I\left(\tau_N \leq i-1\right)\right\} \\
&= E\left\{M_N \, I\left(\tau_N \leq N\right)\right\} \\
&= E\left(M_N\right), \text{ where } M_0 I\left(\tau_N \leq 0\right) = 0.
\end{aligned}
$$

Since $E\left(M_N\right) = E\left\{E\left(M_N \mid \Im_{N-1}\right)\right\} = E\left(M_{N-1}\right) = E\left\{E\left(M_{N-1} \mid \Im_{N-2}\right)\right\} = ... = E\left(M_1\right),$ we conclude with that $E\left(M_{\tau_N}\right) = E\left(M_1\right)$. Now, considering $N \to \infty$, we complete the proof.

In Section 2.4.1 we applied *Wald's lemma* to evaluate the expectation of the *renewal function*. Now we present Wald's lemma in the following form:

Proposition 4.3.2. Assume that $\xi_1, ..., \xi_n$ are iid random variables with $E(\xi_1) = a$ and $E|\xi_1| < \infty$. Let $\tau \geq 1$ be a stopping time with respect to $\mathfrak{I}_n = \sigma(\xi_1, ..., \xi_n)$. If $E(\tau) < \infty$, then

$$E\left(\sum_{i=1}^{\tau} \xi_i\right) = aE(\tau).$$

Proof. Consider

$$E\left(\sum_{i=1}^{n} \xi_i - an \mid \mathfrak{I}_{n-1}\right) = \sum_{i=1}^{n-1} \xi_i - an + E(\xi_n \mid \mathfrak{I}_{n-1})$$

$$= \sum_{i=1}^{n-1} \xi_i - an + a$$

$$= \sum_{i=1}^{n-1} \xi_i - a(n-1).$$

This implies that $\left(\sum_{i=1}^{n} \xi_i - an, \mathfrak{I}_n\right)$ is a martingale. Therefore the use of Proposition 4.3.1 provides $E\left(\sum_{i=1}^{\tau} \xi_i - a\tau\right) = E(\xi_1 - a) = 0$ and then $E\left(\sum_{i=1}^{\tau} \xi_i\right) = aE(\tau)$, which completes the proof.

As has been mentioned previously, *Chebyshev's inequality* plays a very useful role in theoretical statistical analysis. The next proposition can be established as an aspect of extending Chebyshev's approach.

Proposition 4.3.3 (Doob's Inequality). Let $(M_n \geq 0, \mathfrak{I}_n)$ be a martingale. Then, for all $\varepsilon > 0$,

$$\Pr\left(\max_{1 \leq k \leq n} M_k \geq \varepsilon\right) \leq \frac{E(M_1)}{\varepsilon}.$$

Proof. Define the random variable $v = \inf\{n \geq 1 : M_n \geq \varepsilon\}$. Since it is possible that $\Pr(v < \infty) < 1$, v may not be a stopping time, whereas $v_n = \min(v, n)$ defines a stopping time with respect to $\mathfrak{I}_n$. Next, consider the probability

$$\Pr\left(M_{v_n} \geq \varepsilon\right) = \Pr\left(M_{v_n} \geq \varepsilon, v \leq n\right) + \Pr\left(M_{v_n} \geq \varepsilon, v > n\right).$$

It is clear that $v_n = v$, if $v \leq n$; $v_n = n$, provided that $v > n$. Thus

$$\Pr\left(M_{v_n} \geq \varepsilon\right) = \Pr\left(M_v \geq \varepsilon, v \leq n\right) + \Pr\left(M_n \geq \varepsilon, v > n\right),$$

where, by the definition of v, $M_v \geq \varepsilon$ a.s. and the event $\{M_n \geq \varepsilon, v > n\} = \varnothing$, since $\{M_n \geq \varepsilon\}$ means $\{v > n\}$ is not true. This provides

$$\Pr\left(M_{v_n} \geq \varepsilon\right) = \Pr(v \leq n) = \Pr\left(\max_{1 \leq k \leq n} M_k \geq \varepsilon\right).$$

That is $\Pr\left(\max_{1 \leq k \leq n} M_k \geq \varepsilon\right) = \Pr\left(M_{v_n} \geq \varepsilon\right) = E\{I(M_{v_n} \geq \varepsilon)\}$, where the indicator function $I(a \geq b)$ satisfies the inequality $I(a \geq b) \leq a/b$, where a and b are positive. Then $\Pr\left(\max_{1 \leq k \leq n} M_k \geq \varepsilon\right) \leq E(M_{v_n})/\varepsilon$ and the use of Proposition 4.3.1 completes the proof.

Note that Proposition 4.3.3 displays a nontrivial result: for $M_n \geq 0$ one could anticipate that $\max_{1 \leq k \leq n} M_k$ increases, providing $\Pr\left(\max_{1 \leq k \leq n} M_k \geq \varepsilon\right) = 1$ at least for large values of n, however Doob's inequality bounds $\max_{1 \leq k \leq n} M_k$ in probability. We might expect that by using Proposition 4.3.3, an accurate bound for $\Pr\left(\max_{1 \leq k \leq n} M_k \geq \varepsilon\right)$ can be obtained. While evaluating $\Pr\left(\max_{1 \leq k \leq n} M_k \geq \varepsilon\right)$, we could directly employ Chebyshev's approach, obtaining $\Pr\left(\max_{1 \leq k \leq n} M_k \geq \varepsilon\right) \leq E\left(\max_{1 \leq k \leq n} M_k\right)/\varepsilon$, but that is probably not useful.

4.4 Applications

The main theme of this section is to demonstrate that the martingale methodology has valuable substance when it is applied in developing and examining statistical procedures.

4.4.1 The Martingale Principle for Testing Statistical Hypotheses

Suppose we have a set of n observations $X_1, \ldots, X_n$ which are planned to be employed for testing hypotheses H_0 versus H_1. In this case, Section 3.4 suggests applying the likelihood ratio $LR_n = f_1(X_1, \ldots, X_n)/f_0(X_1, \ldots, X_n)$ if the joint density functions f_1, under H_1, and f_0, under H_0, are available. Defining $\Im_n = \sigma(X_1, ..., X_n)$, we use the material of Section 3.2 to derive

$$E_{H_0}(LR_{n+1} \mid \Im_n) = E_{H_0}\left\{\frac{\prod_{i=1}^{n+1} f_1(X_i \mid X_1, ..., X_{i-1})}{\prod_{i=1}^{n+1} f_0(X_i \mid X_1, ..., X_{i-1})} \mid \Im_n\right\}$$

$$= \frac{\prod_{i=1}^{n} f_1(X_i \mid X_1, ..., X_{i-1})}{\prod_{i=1}^{n} f_0(X_i \mid X_1, ..., X_{i-1})} E_{H_0}\left\{\frac{f_1(X_{n+1} \mid X_1, ..., X_n)}{f_0(X_{n+1} \mid X_1, ..., X_n)} \mid \Im_n\right\}$$

$$= \frac{\prod_{i=1}^{n} f_1(X_i \mid X_1, ..., X_{i-1})}{\prod_{i=1}^{n} f_0(X_i \mid X_1, ..., X_{i-1})} \int \frac{f_1(u \mid X_1, ..., X_n)}{f_0(u \mid X_1, ..., X_n)} f_0(u \mid X_1, ..., X_n) du$$

$$= \frac{\prod_{i=1}^{n} f_1(X_i \mid X_1, ..., X_{i-1})}{\prod_{i=1}^{n} f_0(X_i \mid X_1, ..., X_{i-1})} = LR_n,$$

where the subscript H_0 indicates that we consider the expectation given that the hull hypothesis is correct. Then, following Section 4.2, the pair $(LR_n, \Im_n)$ is an H_0-martingale and the pair $(\log(LR_n), \Im_n)$ is an H_0-supermartingale. This says—at the moment in intuitive fashion—that while increasing the amount of observed data points under H_0, we do not enlarge chances to reject H_0 for large values of the likelihood ratio, in average.

Now, under H_1, we consider

$$E_{H_1}(LR_{n+1} \mid \Im_n) = \frac{\prod_{i=1}^{n} f_1(X_i \mid X_1, ..., X_{i-1})}{\prod_{i=1}^{n} f_0(X_i \mid X_1, ..., X_{i-1})} E_{H_1}\left\{\frac{f_1(X_{n+1} \mid X_1, ..., X_n)}{f_0(X_{n+1} \mid X_1, ..., X_n)} \mid \Im_n\right\}$$

$$= \frac{\prod_{i=1}^{n} f_1(X_i \mid X_1, ..., X_{i-1})}{\prod_{i=1}^{n} f_0(X_i \mid X_1, ..., X_{i-1})} E_{H_1}\left\{\frac{1}{f_0(X_{n+1} \mid X_1, ..., X_n)/f_1(X_{n+1} \mid X_1, ..., X_n)} \mid \Im_n\right\}$$

$$\geq \frac{\prod\limits_{i=1}^{n} f_1(X_i \mid X_1,...,X_{i-1})}{\prod\limits_{i=1}^{n} f_0(X_i \mid X_1,...,X_{i-1})} \frac{1}{E_{H_1}\{f_0(X_{n+1} \mid X_1,...,X_n)/f_1(X_{n+1} \mid X_1,...,X_n)\mid \Im_n\}}$$

$$= \frac{\prod\limits_{i=1}^{n} f_1(X_i \mid X_1,...,X_{i-1})}{\prod\limits_{i=1}^{n} f_0(X_i \mid X_1,...,X_{i-1})} \left\{\int \frac{f_0(u \mid X_1,...,X_n)}{f_1(u \mid X_1,...,X_n)} f_1(u \mid X_1,...,X_n)du\right\}^{-1} = LR_n,$$

where Jensen's inequality is used and the subscript H_1 indicates that we consider the expectation given that the alternative hypothesis is true. Regarding $\log(LR_{n+1})$, we have

$$E_{H_1}\{\log(LR_{n+1})\mid \Im_n\}$$

$$= -E_{H_1}\left\{\log\left(\frac{\prod\limits_{i=1}^{n+1} f_0(X_i \mid X_1,...,X_{i-1})}{\prod\limits_{i=1}^{n+1} f_1(X_i \mid X_1,...,X_{i-1})}\right)\mid \Im_n\right\}$$

$$\geq -\log\left(E_{H_1}\left(\frac{\prod\limits_{i=1}^{n+1} f_0(X_i \mid X_1,...,X_{i-1})}{\prod\limits_{i=1}^{n+1} f_1(X_i \mid X_1,...,X_{i-1})}\mid \Im_n\right)\right)$$

$$= -\log\left(\frac{\prod\limits_{i=1}^{n} f_0(X_i \mid X_1,...,X_{i-1})}{\prod\limits_{i=1}^{n} f_1(X_i \mid X_1,...,X_{i-1})} E_{H_1}\left(\frac{f_0(X_{n+1} \mid X_1,...,X_n)}{f_1(X_{n+1} \mid X_1,...,X_n)}\mid \Im_n\right)\right)$$

$$= \log(LR_n).$$

Then the pairs $(LR_n, \Im_n)$ and $(\log(LR_n), \Im_n)$ are H_1-submartingales. Thus, intuitively, under H_1, this shows that by adding more observations to be used in the test procedure, we provide more power to the likelihood ratio test.

Conclusion: The likelihood ratio test statistic is most powerful given all of the assumptions are met. *Therefore, generally speaking, it is reasonable to consider developing test statistics or their transformed versions that could have properties of H_0-martingales (supermartingales) and H_1-submartingales, anticipating an optimality of the corresponding test procedures.* Note that in many testing scenarios the alternative hypothesis H_1 is "not H_0" and hence does not have a specified form. For example, the **composite** statement regarding a parameter θ can be stated as $H_0 : \theta = \theta_0$ versus $H_1 : \theta \neq \theta_0$, where θ_0 is known. In this case, E_{H_1}-type objects do not have unique shapes. Then we can aim to preserve only the H_0-martingale (supermartingales) property of a corresponding rational test statistic, following the Neyman–Pearson concept of statistical tests, in which H_0-characteristics of decision-making strategies are vital (e.g., Vexler et al., 2016a).

4.4.1.1 Maximum Likelihood Ratio in Light of the Martingale Concept

In Section 3.6 we pointed out a significant difference between the likelihood ratio and the maximum likelihood ratio test statistics. In order to provide a martingale interpretation of this fact, we assume that observations $X_1, ..., X_n$ are from the density function $f(x_1, ..., x_n; \theta)$ with a parameter θ. We are interested in testing the hypothesis $H_0 : \theta = \theta_0$ versus $H_1 : \theta \neq \theta_0$, where θ_0 is known. The maximum likelihood ratio is

$$MLR_n = f(X_1, ..., X_n; \hat{\theta}_n) / f(X_1, ..., X_n; \theta_0), \text{ where } \hat{\theta}_n = \arg\max_\theta f(X_1, ..., X_n; \theta).$$

Noting that $\hat{\theta}_{n+1}$ should maximize $f(X_1, ..., X_{n+1}; \theta)$, i.e., $f(X_1, ..., X_n; \hat{\theta}_{n+1}) \geq f(X_1, ..., X_n; \hat{\theta}_n)$, where $\hat{\theta}_n \in \Im_n = \sigma(X_1, ..., X_n)$, we obtain

$$E_{H_0}\left\{ MLR_{n+1} \mid \Im_n = \sigma(X_1, ..., X_n) \right\}$$

$$= E_{H_0}\left\{ \frac{\prod_{i=1}^{n+1} f(X_i \mid X_1, ..., X_{i-1}; \hat{\theta}_{n+1})}{\prod_{i=1}^{n+1} f(X_i \mid X_1, ..., X_{i-1}; \theta_0)} \mid \Im_n = \sigma(X_1, ..., X_n) \right\}$$

$$\geq E_{H_0}\left\{ \frac{\prod_{i=1}^{n+1} f(X_i \mid X_1, ..., X_{i-1}; \hat{\theta}_n)}{\prod_{i=1}^{n+1} f(X_i \mid X_1, ..., X_{i-1}; \theta_0)} \mid \Im_n \right\}$$

$$= \frac{\prod_{i=1}^{n} f(X_i \mid X_1, ..., X_{i-1}; \hat{\theta}_n)}{\prod_{i=1}^{n} f(X_i \mid X_1, ..., X_{i-1}; \theta_0)} E_{H_0} \left\{ \frac{f(X_{n+1} \mid X_1, ..., X_n; \hat{\theta}_n)}{f(X_{n+1} \mid X_1, ..., X_n; \theta_0)} \mid \Im_n \right\}$$

$$= \frac{\prod_{i=1}^{n} f(X_i \mid X_1, ..., X_{i-1}; \hat{\theta}_n)}{\prod_{i=1}^{n} f(X_i \mid X_1, ..., X_{i-1}; \theta_0)} \int \frac{f(u \mid X_1, ..., X_n; \hat{\theta}_n(X_1, ..., X_n))}{f(u \mid X_1, ..., X_n; \theta_0)} \; f(u \mid X_1, ..., X_n; \theta_0) du$$

$$= MLR_n.$$

Thus the pair $(MLR_n, \Im_n)$ is an H_0-submartingale (not a martingale as wanted). This reinforces a concern that, in general, the maximum likelihood ratio statistic can provide an optimal decision-making strategy based on data with fixed sample sizes. It follows that while increasing the amount of observed data points under H_0, we do increase the chances to reject H_0 on average for large values of the maximum likelihood ratio. One may then conclude that the violation of the H_0-martingale principle shown above yields that maximum likelihood–based testing procedures are not very useful when sample sizes are very large. Almost no null hypothesis is exactly true in practice. Consequently, when sample sizes are large enough, almost any null hypothesis will have a tiny *p-value*, and hence will be rejected at conventional levels (Marden, 2000).

4.4.1.2 Likelihood Ratios Based on Representative Values

Let us repeat the idea that oftentimes in the context of hypothesis testing we do not need to estimate unknown parameters when we only are interested in the decision to reject or not to reject the null hypothesis. In this section we consider decision-making procedures based upon representative values that can substitute for unknown parameters.

Without loss of generality, we consider a straightforward example that introduces the basic ingredients for further explanations in this book.

Assume that we observe iid data points $X_1, ..., X_n$ and are interested in testing the hypothesis

$$H_0 : X_1 \sim f_0(x) \quad \text{versus} \quad H_1 : X_1 \sim f_1(x) = f_0(x) \exp(\theta_1 x + \theta_2), \qquad (4.2)$$

where f_0 is a density function (known or unknown), and quantities θ_1, θ_2 are unknown, θ_2 can depend on θ_1. Let the sign of θ_1 be known, e.g., $\theta_1 > 0$.

The statement of the problem above is quite general. For example, when $X_1 \sim N(\mu, \sigma^2)$ with unknown σ^2, the considered hypothesis could have the form of $H_0 : \mu = 0, \sigma = \eta$ versus $H_1 : \mu \neq 0, \sigma = \eta$, for some unknown $\eta > 0$. In this case, we have $f_0(x) = \exp\left(-x^2/(2\eta^2)\right)/\sqrt{2\pi\eta^2}$ and $f_1(x) = f_0(x)\exp(\theta_1 x + \theta_2)$ with $\theta_1 = \mu/(\eta^2)$ and $\theta_2 = -\mu^2/(2\eta^2)$, respectively.

By virtue of the statement (4.2), the likelihood ratio test statistic is

$$LR_n = \exp\left(\theta_1 \sum_{i=1}^{n} X_i + n\theta_2\right).$$

Since θ_1, θ_2 are unknown, we denote the statistic

$$T_n = \exp\left(a \sum_{i=1}^{n} X_i + b\right),$$

where a and b can be chosen arbitrarily and a is of the same sign of θ_1, i.e., $a > 0$ in this example, e.g., $a = 7, b = 0$. The decision-making policy is to reject H_0 if $T_n > C$, where $C > 0$ is a test threshold.

Suppose, only for the following theoretical exercise, that $c = \int f_0(u)\exp(au+b)\,du < \infty$. Then

$$E_{H_0}\left(\frac{1}{c^{n+1}}T_{n+1}\mid \mathfrak{I}_n = \sigma(X_1,...,X_n)\right) = \frac{1}{c^{n+1}}E_{H_0}\left\{\frac{\prod_{i=1}^{n+1} f_0(X_i)\exp(aX_i+b)}{\prod_{i=1}^{n+1} f_0(X_i)}\mid \mathfrak{I}_n\right\}$$

$$= \frac{T_n}{c^{n+1}}E_{H_0}\left\{\frac{f_0(X_{n+1})\exp(aX_{n+1}+b)}{f_0(X_{n+1})}\right\}$$

$$= \frac{T_n}{c^{n+1}}\int \frac{f_0(u)\exp(au+b)}{f_0(u)}f_0(u)\,du$$

$$= \frac{T_n}{c^n},$$

i.e., $\left(T_n/c^n, \mathfrak{I}_n\right)$ is an H_0-martingale, where c^n is independent of the underlying data. Thus we can anticipate that the test statistic T_n can be optimal. This is displayed in the following result:

The statistic T_n provides *the most powerful test of the hypothesis testing* at (4.2).

Proof. Note again that the likelihood ratio test statistic $LR_n = \exp\left(\theta_1 \sum_{i=1}^{n} X_i + n\theta_2\right)$ is most powerful. Following the Neyman–Pearson concept, in order to compare the test statistics LR_n and T_n, we define test thresholds C_α^T and C_α^{LR} to satisfy $\alpha = \Pr_{H_0}(LR_n > C_\alpha^{LR}) = \Pr_{H_0}(T_n > C_\alpha^T)$ for a prespecified significance level α, since the Type I error rates of the tests should be equivalent. In this case, using the definitions of the test statistics, we have

$$\alpha = \Pr_{H_0}\left[\sum_{i=1}^{n} X_i > \left\{\log\left(C_\alpha^{LR}\right) - n\theta_2\right\}\Big/\theta_1\right] = \Pr_{H_0}\left[\sum_{i=1}^{n} X_i > \left\{\log\left(C_\alpha^{T}\right) - b\right\}\Big/a\right], \theta_1 > 0, a > 0.$$

That is, $\left\{\log\left(C_\alpha^{LR}\right) - n\theta_2\right\}\big/\theta_1 = \left\{\log\left(C_\alpha^{T}\right) - b\right\}\big/a$ and then $\log\left(C_\alpha^{T}\right) = a\left\{\log\left(C_\alpha^{LR}\right) - n\theta_2\right\}\big/\theta_1 + b$.

Therefore, under H_1, the power

$$\begin{aligned}
\Pr_{H_1}(T_n > C_\alpha^{T}) &= \Pr_{H_1}\left[\sum_{i=1}^{n} X_i > \left\{\log\left(C_\alpha^{T}\right) - b\right\}\Big/a\right] \\
&= \Pr_{H_1}\left[\sum_{i=1}^{n} X_i > \left\{\log\left(C_\alpha^{LR}\right) - n\theta_2\right\}\Big/\theta_1\right] \\
&= \Pr_{H_1}(LR_n > C_\alpha^{LR}),
\end{aligned}$$

i.e., the statistic T_n is the most powerful test statistic. (In this book, the notation $\Pr_{H_k}(A)$ means that we consider the probability of (A) given that the hypothesis H_k is true, $k = 0, 1$.) This completes the proof.

Since θ_1 and θ_2 are unknown, one can propose to estimate θ_1 and θ_2 by using the maximum likelihood method in order to approximate the likelihood ratio test statistic. In this case, the efficiency of the maximum likelihood ratio test may be lost completely. The optimal method based on the test statistic $\exp\left(a\sum_{i=1}^{n} X_i + b\right)$ can be referred as a simple *representative method*, since we employ arbitrarily chosen numbers to represent the unknown parameters θ_1 and θ_2.

In this section, we present the simple representative method, which can be easily extended by integrating test statistics through variables that represent unknown parameters with respect to functions that can display weights corresponding to values of the variables. This approach can be referred to as a *Bayes factor* type decision-making mechanism that will be described formally in forthcoming sections of this book. For example, observing $X_1, ..., X_n$, one can denote the test statistic

$$BF_n = \frac{\int f_1(X_1, ..., X_n; \theta)\pi(\theta)\,d\theta}{f_0(X_1, ..., X_n; \theta_0)}$$

to test for $H_0 : X_1, ..., X_n \sim f_0(x_1, ..., x_n; \theta_0)$ versus $H_1 : X_1, ..., X_n \sim f_1(x_1, ..., x_n; \theta_1)$, $\theta_1 \neq \theta_0$ with known θ_0 and unknown θ_1, where $\pi(\theta)$ represents our level of belief (probability-based weights) on the possible consequences of the decisions and/or the possible values of θ under the alternative hypothesis. In this case, it is clear that $\left(BF_n, \mathfrak{I}_n = \sigma(X_1, ..., X_n)\right)$ is an H_0-martingale.

4.4.2 Guaranteed Type I Error Rate Control of the Likelihood Ratio Tests

As shown in Section 4.4.1 the pair $\left(LR_n > 0, \Im_n = \sigma(X_1, ..., X_n)\right)$ is an H_0-martingale. Thus Proposition 4.3.3 implies $\Pr_{H_0}\left(\max_{1 \le k \le n} LR_k > C\right) \le C^{-1}$, since $E_{H_0}(LR_1) = \int \left\{f_1(u) / f_0(u)\right\} f_0(u) \, du = 1$. This result insures that we can non-asymptotically control maximum values of the likelihood ratio test statistic in probability. For example, setting the test threshold $C = 20$, we guarantee that the Type I error rate of the likelihood ratio test does not exceed 5%, for all fixed $n \ge 1$. This result could be conservative, however, we should note that the inequality $\Pr_{H_0}\left(\max_{1 \le k \le n} LR_k > C\right) \le C^{-1}$ was obtained without any requirements on the data density functions, e.g., we did not restrict the observations to be iid. It is clear that when the form of LR_n is specified (in general, this form can be very complicated) one can try to obtain an accurate evaluation of the corresponding Type I error rates, e.g., via Monte Carlo approximations (see Section 2.4.5.1). In this case, Doob's inequality suggests the initial values for the evaluations.

Assume we observe sequentially (one-by-one) iid data points $X_1, X_2, X_3, ...$ and need to decide $X_1, X_2, X_3, ... \sim f_0$ or $X_1, X_2, X_3, ... \sim f_1$, provided that if $X_1, X_2, X_3, ... \sim f_0$ it is not required to stop the sampling. In this case, we can define the stopping time $\tau(C) = \min\left(k \ge 1 : LR_k \ge C\right)$. Then an error is to stop the sampling under $X_1, X_2, X_3, ... \sim f_0$ with the rate $\Pr\left(\tau \le n \mid X_1 \sim f_0\right) = \Pr\left(\max_{1 \le k \le n} LR_k > C \mid X_1 \sim f_0\right) \le C^{-1}$, for all $n \ge 1$. This determines the Type I error rate of the sequential procedure $\tau(C)$ to be C^{-1}-bounded. (In this context, see Section 4.4.4 and the forthcoming material of the book related to sequential statistical procedures.)

4.4.3 Retrospective Change Point Detection Policies

Change point problems originally arose in quality control applications, when one typically observes the output of production processes and should indicate violations of acceptable specifications. In general, the problem of detecting changes is found in quite a variety of experimental sciences. For example, in epidemiology one may be interested in testing whether the incidence of a disease has remained constant over time, and if not, in estimating the time of change in order to suggest possible causes, e.g., increases in asthma prevalence due to a new factory opening.

In health studies there may be a distributional shift, oftentimes in terms of a shift in location either due to random factors or due to some known factors at a fixed point in time that is either known or needs to be estimated. For example, biomarker levels may be measured differently between two laboratories and a given research organization may switch laboratories. Then there may be a shift in mean biomarker levels simply due to differences in sample processing. As another example, the speed limit on many expressways in the

United States was increased from 55 miles per hour to 65 miles per hour in 1987. In order to investigate the effect of this increased speed limit on highway traveling, one may study the change in the traffic accident death rate after the modification of the 55 mile per hour speed limit law. Problems closely related to the example above are called *change point* problems in the statistical literature.

We will concentrate in this section on *retrospective* change point problems, where inference regarding the detection of a change occurs *retrospectively*, i.e., after the data has already been collected. Various applications, e.g., in the areas of biological, medical and economics, tend to generate retrospective change point problems. For example, in genomics, detecting chromosomal DNA copy number changes or copy number variations in tumor cells can facilitate the development of medical diagnostic tools and personalized treatment regimens for cancer and other genetic diseases; e.g., see Lucito et al. (2000). The retrospective change point detection methods are also useful in studying the variation (over time) of share prices on the major stock exchanges. Various examples of change point detection schemes and their applications are introduced in Csörgö and Horváth (1997) and Vexler et al. (2016a).

Let $X_1, X_2, ..., X_n$ be independent continuous random variables with fixed sample size n. In the formal context of hypotheses testing, we state the change point detection problem as testing for

$$H_0 : X_1, X_2, ..., X_n \sim f_0 \text{ versus } H_1 : X_i \sim f_0, X_j \sim f_1, i = 1, ..., v-1, j = v, ..., n,$$

where $f_0 \neq f_1$ are density functions. Note that $v \in (1, n]$ is an unknown parameter. This simple change point model is termed a so-called *at most one change-point* model. In the parametric fashion, efficient detection methods for the classical simple change point problem include the *cumulative sum (CUSUM)* and *Shiryayev–Roberts* approaches (e.g., Vexler et al., 2016a).

4.4.3.1 The Cumulative Sum (CUSUM) Technique

When the parameter v can be assumed to be known, the likelihood ratio statistic Λ_v^n provides the most powerful test by virtue of the proof shown in Section 3.4, where

$$\Lambda_k^n = \frac{\Pi_{i=k}^n f_1(X_i)}{\Pi_{i=k}^n f_0(X_i)}.$$

We refer the reader to Chapter 3 for details regarding likelihood ratio tests. When the parameter v is unknown, the maximum likelihood estimator $\hat{v} = \arg\max_{1 \leq k \leq n} \Lambda_k^n$ of the parameter v can be applied. By plugging the maximum likelihood estimator $\hat{v}$ of the change point location v, we have

$$\Lambda_n = \Lambda_{\hat{v}} = \max_{1 \le k \le n} \Lambda_k^n,$$

which has the maximum likelihood ratio form. Note that $\log(\Lambda_n) = \max_{1 \le k \le n} \sum_{i=k}^{n} \log(f_1(X_i) / f_0(X_i))$, which corresponds to the well-known cumulative sum (CUSUM) type test statistic. The null hypothesis is rejected for large values of the CUSUM test statistic Λ_n. It turns out that, even in this simple case, evaluations of H_0-properties of the CUSUM test are very complicated tasks.

Consider the σ-algebra $\mathfrak{I}_k^n = \sigma(X_k, ..., X_n)$ and the expectation

$$
\begin{aligned}
E_{H_0}\left(\Lambda_{k-1}^n \mid \mathfrak{I}_k^n\right) &= E_{H_0}\left(\frac{\Pi_{i=k-1}^n f_1(X_i)}{\Pi_{i=k-1}^n f_0(X_i)} \mid \mathfrak{I}_k^n\right) \\
&= \frac{\Pi_{i=k}^n f_1(X_i)}{\Pi_{i=k}^n f_0(X_i)} E_{H_0}\left(\frac{f_1(X_{k-1})}{f_0(X_{k-1})} \mid \mathfrak{I}_k^n\right) \\
&= \Lambda_k^n.
\end{aligned}
$$

This shows that $\left(\Lambda_k^n, \mathfrak{I}_k^n\right)$ is an H_0-martingale that can be called an H_0-nonnegative *reverse martingale*. Then a simple modification of Proposition 4.3.3 (Gurevich and Vexler, 2005) implies

$$\Pr_{H_0}(\Lambda_n > C) \le E_{H_0}\left(\Lambda_n^n\right) / C = 1/C$$

that provides an upper bound of the corresponding Type I error rate. The arguments mentioned below Proposition 4.3.3 support that the bound $1/C$ might be very close to the actual Type I error rate. The non-asymptotic Type I error rate monitoring via $1/C$ was obtained without any requirements on the density functions f_0, f_1. In several scenarios with specified f_0, f_1-forms, complex asymptotic propositions can be used to approximate $\Pr_{H_0}(\Lambda_n > C)$ (Csörgö and Horváth, 1997) as well as one can also employ Monte Carlo approximations to the Type I error rate. In these cases, the bound $1/C$ suggests the initial values for the evaluations.

4.4.3.2 The Shiryayev–Roberts (SR) Statistic-Based Techniques

In the previous subsection, we considered the case where the change point location is maximum likelihood estimated, which leads to the CUSUM scheme. Alternatively taking into account Section 4.4.1.2, we can propose the statistic $\Lambda_j^n = \dfrac{\Pi_{i=j}^n f_1(X_i)}{\Pi_{i=j}^n f_0(X_i)}$, where an integer j can be chosen arbitrarily.

Extending this approach, we obtain the test statistic $SR_n = \sum_{j=1}^{n} w_j \Lambda_j^n$, where the deterministic weights $w_j \geq 0, j = 1, ..., n$, are known. For simplicity and clarity of exposition, we redefine

$$SR_n = \sum_{j=1}^{n} \Lambda_j^n.$$

The statistic SR_n can be considered in the context of a Bayes factor type testing, when we integrate the unknown change point with respect to the uniform prior information regarding a point where the change is occurred. In this change point problem, the integration will correspond to simple summation. This approach is well-addressed in the change point literature as the Shiryayev–Roberts (SR) scheme (Vexler et al., 2016a). The null hypothesis is rejected if $SR_n / n > C$, for a fixed test threshold $C > 0$.

Noting that $SR_n = \dfrac{f_1(X_n)}{f_0(X_n)}(SR_{n-1} + 1)$, we consider the pair $(SR_n - n, \Im_n = \sigma(X_1, ..., X_n))$ that satisfies

$$E_{H_0}(SR_n - n \mid \Im_{n-1}) = (SR_{n-1} + 1)E_{H_0}\left\{\frac{f_1(X_n)}{f_0(X_n)}\right\} - n = SR_{n-1} - (n-1).$$

Then $(SR_n - n, \Im_n)$ is an H_0-martingale. Similarly, since

$$E_{H_1}\left\{\frac{f_1(X_n)}{f_0(X_n)}\right\} \geq \frac{1}{E_{H_1}\{f_0(X_n) / f_1(X_n)\}} = 1,$$

one can show that $(SR_n - n, \Im_n)$ is an H_1-submartingale. Thus, according to Section 4.4.1, it is reasonable to attempt deriving an optimal property of the retrospective SR change point detection policy. (In this context, we would like to direct the reader's attention again to the "Warning" in Section 3.4.)

It turns out that the retrospective change point detection policy based on the SR statistic is non-asymptotically optimal in the sense of average most powerful (via $v = 1, ..., n$).

Proof. To prove this statement, one can use in equality (3.2) in the form

$$\left(\frac{1}{n}SR_n - C\right)\left\{I\left(\frac{1}{n}SR_n \geq C\right) - \delta\right\} \geq 0,$$

where $\delta = \delta(X_1, \ldots, X_n)$ represents any decision rule based on $\{X_i, i = 1, \ldots, n\}$, $\delta = 0, 1$, and when $\delta = 1$ we reject H_0. Then in a similar manner to the analysis of the likelihood ratio statistic shown in Section 3.4, we obtain

$$\frac{1}{n}\sum_{k=1}^{n} E_{H_0}\left\{\frac{\Pi_{i=1}^{k-1} f_0(X_i)\Pi_{i=k}^{n} f_1(X_i)}{\Pi_{i=1}^{n} f_0(X_i)} I\left(\frac{1}{n}SR_n \geq C\right)\right\}\left(\frac{1}{n}SR_n \geq C\right)$$

$$\geq \frac{1}{n}\sum_{k=1}^{n} E_{H_0}\left\{\frac{\Pi_{i=1}^{k-1} f_0(X_i)\Pi_{i=k}^{n} f_1(X_i)}{\Pi_{i=1}^{n} f_0(X_i)} I\left(\delta(X_1, \ldots, X_n) \text{ rejects } H_0\right)\right\} - C\,\mathrm{Pr}_{H_0}\left(\delta(X_1, \ldots, X_n) \text{ rejects } H_0\right),$$

$$\frac{1}{n}\sum_{k=1}^{n}\int \cdots \int I\left(\frac{1}{n}SR_n \geq C\right) f_0(x_1, \ldots, x_{k-1}) f_1(x_k, \ldots, x_n)\prod_{i=1}^{n} dx_i - C\,\mathrm{Pr}_{H_0}\left(\frac{1}{n}SR_n \geq C\right)$$

$$\geq \frac{1}{n}\sum_{k=1}^{n}\int \cdots \int I\left(\delta(x_1, \ldots, x_n) \text{ rejects } H_0\right) f_0(x_1, \ldots, x_{k-1}) f_1(x_k, \ldots, x_n)\prod_{i=1}^{n} dx_i -$$

$$C\,\mathrm{Pr}_{H_0}\left(\delta \text{ rejects } H_0\right).$$

This leads to the conclusion

$$\frac{1}{n}\sum_{i=1}^{n}\mathrm{Pr}_{H_1}\left(\frac{1}{n}SR_n \geq C \mid \nu = i\right) \geq \frac{1}{n}\sum_{i=1}^{n}\mathrm{Pr}_{H_1}\left(\delta \text{ rejects } H_0 \mid \nu = i\right),$$

when the Type I error rates $\mathrm{Pr}_{H_0}\left(SR_n / n \geq C\right)$ and $\mathrm{Pr}_{H_0}\left(\delta \text{ rejects } H_0\right)$ are equal. The proof is complete.

Remark 1. In the considered statement of the problem, the change point parameter $\nu \in (1, n]$ is unknown. In this case, how does one calculate the power of change point detection procedures? It is clear the test power is a function of ν, so is it unknown, in general? Suppose, for example, when $n > 10$ a student defines a test statistic Λ_{10}^n. Then his/her test statistic can be powerless when, e.g., $\nu = 1, 2$, however when $\nu = 10$ no one can outperform the power of Λ_{10}^n, since Λ_{10}^n is the likelihood ratio, in this case. Thus it is interesting to ask the question: what is the sense of "most powerful testing" in the change point problem? In this context, the meaning of the statement "most powerful in average" is clear.

Remark 2. Vexler et al. (2016a) presented a literature review, data examples and relevant R codes in order to compare the CUSUM and SR retrospective change point detection procedures and their extended forms. The authors discussed properties of the maximum likelihood estimator $\hat{\nu} = \arg\max_{1 \leq k \leq n} \Lambda_k^n$

of the change point parameter ν. Section 4.5 introduces a novel martingale based concept to compare the CUSUM and SR statistics.

4.4.4 Adaptive (Nonanticipating) Maximum Likelihood Estimation

In this subsection we introduce modifications of the maximum likelihood estimations that preserve the H_0-martingale properties of test statistics. Consider the following scenarios:

(i) Let $X_1, ..., X_n$ be from the density function $f(x_1, ..., x_n; \theta)$ with a parameter θ. We are interested in testing the hypothesis $H_0 : \theta = \theta_0$ versus $H_1 : \theta \neq \theta_0$, where θ_0 is known.
Define the maximum likelihood estimators of θ as

$$\hat{\theta}_{1,k} = \arg\max_\theta f(X_1, ..., X_n; \theta), \hat{\theta}_{1,0} = \theta_0, \; k = 0, ..., n.$$

In this case, the maximum likelihood ratio test statistic $MLR_n = f(X_1, ..., X_n; \hat{\theta}_{1,n}) / f(X_1, ..., X_n; \theta_0)$ is

$$MLR_n = \frac{\prod\limits_{i=1}^{n} f(X_i \mid X_1, ..., X_{i-1}; \hat{\theta}_n)}{\prod\limits_{i=1}^{n} f(X_i \mid X_1, ..., X_{i-1}; \theta_0)}.$$

Then the adaptive (nonanticipating) maximum likelihood ratio test statistic can be denoted in the form

$$ALR_n = \frac{\prod\limits_{i=1}^{n} f(X_i \mid X_1, ..., X_{i-1}; \hat{\theta}_{1,i-1})}{\prod\limits_{i=1}^{n} f(X_i \mid X_1, ..., X_{i-1}; \theta_0)}.$$

It turns out that $\left(ALR_n > 0, \Im_n = \sigma(X_1, ..., X_n) \right)$ is an H_0-martingale, since $\hat{\theta}_{1,i-1} \in \Im_{i-1}$ and

$$E_{H_0}\left(ALR_{n+1} \mid \Im_n \right) = \frac{\prod\limits_{i=1}^{n} f(X_i \mid X_1, ..., X_{i-1}; \hat{\theta}_{1,i-1})}{\prod\limits_{i=1}^{n} f(X_i \mid X_1, ..., X_{i-1}; \theta_0)} E_{H_0}\left(\frac{f(X_{n+1} \mid X_1, ..., X_n; \hat{\theta}_{1,n})}{f(X_{n+1} \mid X_1, ..., X_n; \theta_0)} \mid \Im_n \right)$$

$$= ALR_n \int \frac{f(u \mid X_1, ..., X_n; \hat{\theta}_{1,n})}{f(u \mid X_1, ..., X_n; \theta_0)} f(u \mid X_1, ..., X_n; \theta_0) du = ALR_n.$$

Thus Proposition 4.3.3 implies $\Pr_{H_0}(\max_{1 \le k \le n} ALR_k > C) \le C^{-1}$.

(ii) Let $X_1, ..., X_n$ be from the density function $f(x_1, ..., x_n; \theta, \lambda)$ with parameters θ and λ. We are interested in testing the hypothesis $H_0 : \theta = \theta_0$ versus $H_1 : \theta \ne \theta_0$, where θ_0 is known. The parameter λ is a nuisance parameter that can have different values under H_0 and H_1, respectively.

A testing strategy, which can be applied in this case, is to try finding *invariant transformations* of the observations, thus eliminating the nuisance parameter from the statement of the testing problem. For example, when we observe the iid data points $X_1, ..., X_n \sim N(\mu, \sigma^2)$ to test for $H_0 : \sigma^2 = 1$ versus $H_1 : \sigma^2 \ne 1$, the observations can be transformed to be $Y_2 = X_2 - X_1, Y_3 = X_3 - X_1 ..., Y_n = X_n - X_1$ and the likelihood ratio statistic based on $Y_2, ..., Y_n$, where $Y_2, ..., Y_n$ are iid given X_1, can be applied without any attention to μ's values. (In this context, one can also use $Y_1 = X_1 - g_k, Y_2 = X_2 - g_k ..., Y_n = X_n - g_k$, where $g_k = \sum_{i=1}^{k} X_i / k$ with a fixed $k < n$ or, for simplicity, $Y_1 = X_2 - X_1, Y_2 = X_4 - X_3, ...$) Testing strategies based on *invariant statistics* are very complicated in general and cannot be employed in various situations, depending on forms of $f(x_1, ..., x_n; \theta, \lambda)$.

It is interesting to note that classical statistical methodology is directed toward the use of decision-making mechanisms with fixed significant levels. Classic inference requires special and careful attention of practitioners relative to the Type I error rate control since it can be defined by different functional forms. In the testing problem with the nuisance parameter λ, for any presumed significance level, α, the *Type I error rate control* may take the following forms:

(1). $\sup_\lambda \Pr_{H_0}(\text{reject } H_0) = \alpha$;

(2). $\sup_\lambda \lim_{n \to \infty} \Pr_{H_0}(\text{reject } H_0 \text{ based on observations} \{X_1, ..., X_n\}) = \alpha$;

(3). $\lim_{n \to \infty} \sup_\lambda \Pr_{H_0}(\text{reject } H_0 \text{ based on observations} \{X_1, ..., X_n\}) = \alpha$;

(4). $\int \Pr_{H_0}(\text{reject } H_0) \pi(\lambda) d\lambda = \alpha, \ \pi > 0: \int \pi(\lambda) d\lambda = 1$.

Form (1) from above is the classical definition (e.g., Lehmann and Romano, 2006). However, in some situations, it may occur that $\sup_\lambda \Pr_{H_0}(\text{reject } H_0) = 1$. If this is the case the Type I error rate is not controlled appropriately. In addition, the formal notation of the supremum is mathematically complicated in terms of derivations and calculations, either analytically or via Monte Carlo approximations. Form (2) above is commonly applied when we deal with maximum likelihood ratio tests as it relates to Wilks' theorem (Wilks, 1938). However, since the form at (2) is an asymptotical large sample consideration, the actual Type I error rate $\Pr_{H_0}(\text{reject } H_0)$ may not be close to the expected level α given small or moderate fixed sample sizes n. The form given above at (3) is rarely applied in practice. The form above at (4) is also introduced in

Lehmann and Romano (2006). This definition of the Type I error rate control depends on the choice of the function $\pi(\theta)$ in general.

Now let us define the maximum likelihood estimators of θ and λ as

$$\left(\hat{\theta}_{1,k}, \hat{\lambda}_{1,k}\right) = \arg\max_{(\theta,\lambda)} f(X_1,...,X_n;\theta,\lambda), \quad \hat{\theta}_{1,0} = \theta_0, \hat{\lambda}_{1,0} = \lambda_{10}, \quad k = 0,...,n \text{ and}$$

$$\hat{\lambda}_{0,1,k} = \arg\max_{\lambda} f(X_1,...,X_n;\theta_0,\lambda), \quad k = 1,...,n,$$

where λ_{10} is a fixed reasonable variable. Then the *adaptive maximum likelihood ratio* test statistic can be denoted in the form

$$ALR_n = \frac{\prod\limits_{i=1}^{n} f(X_i \mid X_1,...,X_{i-1};\hat{\theta}_{1,i-1},\hat{\lambda}_{1,i-1})}{\prod\limits_{i=1}^{n} f(X_i \mid X_1,...,X_{i-1};\theta_0,\hat{\lambda}_{0,1,n})}.$$

By virtue of the definition of $\hat{\lambda}_{0,1,k}$, we have $\prod\limits_{i=1}^{n} f(X_i \mid X_1,...,X_{i-1};\theta_0,\hat{\lambda}_{0,1,n}) \geq$

$\prod\limits_{i=1}^{n} f(X_i \mid X_1,...,X_{i-1};\theta_0,\lambda_{H_0})$, where λ_{H_0} is a true value of λ under H_0. Then

$$ALR_n = \frac{\prod\limits_{i=1}^{n} f(X_i \mid X_1,...,X_{i-1};\hat{\theta}_{1,i-1},\hat{\lambda}_{1,i-1})}{\prod\limits_{i=1}^{n} f(X_i \mid X_1,...,X_{i-1};\theta_0,\hat{\lambda}_{0,1,n})} \leq M_n \text{ with}$$

$$M_n = \frac{\prod\limits_{i=1}^{n} f(X_i \mid X_1,...,X_{i-1};\hat{\theta}_{1,i-1},\hat{\lambda}_{1,i-1})}{\prod\limits_{i=1}^{n} f(X_i \mid X_1,...,X_{i-1};\theta_0,\lambda_{H_0})},$$

where it is clear that $\left(M_n > 0, \mathfrak{S}_n = \sigma(X_1,...,X_n)\right)$ is an H_0-martingale. Thus Proposition 4.3.3 implies

$$\sup\nolimits_{\lambda_{H_0}} \Pr\nolimits_{H_0} \left(\max\nolimits_{1 \leq k \leq n} ALR_k > C\right) \leq \sup\nolimits_{\lambda_{H_0}} \Pr\nolimits_{H_0} \left(\max\nolimits_{1 \leq k \leq n} M_k > C\right) \leq C^{-1}.$$

This result is very general and does not depend on forms of $f(x_1,...,x_n;\theta,\lambda)$.

(iii) Let $X_1,...,X_n$ be from the density function $f(x_1,...,x_n;\theta,\lambda)$ with parameters θ and λ. Assume that we are interested in testing the hypothesis $H_0 : \theta \in (\theta_L,\theta_U)$ versus $H_1 : \theta \notin (\theta_L,\theta_U)$, where θ_L,θ_U are known. The parameter λ is a nuisance parameter that can have different values under H_0 and H_1, respectively.

In this case, the ***adaptive maximum likelihood ratio*** test statistic can be denoted in the form

$$ALR_n = \frac{\prod\limits_{i=1}^{n} f(X_i \mid X_1, ..., X_{i-1}; \hat{\theta}_{1,i-1}, \hat{\lambda}_{1,i-1})}{\prod\limits_{i=1}^{n} f(X_i \mid X_1, ..., X_{i-1}; \hat{\theta}_{0,1,n}, \hat{\lambda}_{0,1,n})},$$

where

$$\left(\hat{\theta}_{1,k}, \hat{\lambda}_{1,k}\right) = \arg\max_{(\theta \notin (\theta_L, \theta_U), \lambda)} f(X_1, ..., X_n; \theta, \lambda), \; \hat{\theta}_{1,0} = \theta_{10}, \hat{\lambda}_{1,0} = \lambda_{10}, \; k = 0, ..., n$$

and

$$\left(\hat{\theta}_{0,1,k}, \hat{\lambda}_{0,1,k}\right) = \arg\max_{(\theta \in (\theta_L, \theta_U), \lambda)} f(X_1, ..., X_n; \theta, \lambda), \quad k = 1, ..., n$$

with $\theta_{10}, \lambda_{10}$ that have fixed reasonable values.

In a similar manner to that shown in Scenario *(ii)* above, we obtain

$$\sup\nolimits_{\{\theta \in (\theta_L, \theta_U), \lambda\}} \Pr\nolimits_{H_0} \left(\max\nolimits_{1 \le k \le n} ALR_k > C\right) \le C^{-1}.$$

(iv) Let $X_1, X_2, ..., X_n$ be independent continuous random variables with fixed sample size n. We state the change point problem as testing for

$$H_0 : X_1, X_2, ..., X_n \sim f_0(u; \theta_0) \text{ versus } H_1 : X_i \sim f_0(u; \theta_0), X_j \sim f_1(u; \theta_1),$$

$$i = 1, ..., v - 1, j = v, ..., n,$$

where θ_0 is an known parameter, θ_1 is an unknown parameter and forms of the density functions f_0, f_1 can be equivalent if $\theta_0 \ne \theta_1$. In many practical situations, we can assume that θ_0 is known, for example, when the stable regime under the null hypothesis has been observed for a long time. Applications of ***invariant data transformations*** (e.g., see Scenario *(ii)* above) can also lead us to a possibility to assume θ_0 is known to be, e.g., zero. In this case, the adaptive CUSUM test statistic is

$$\Lambda_n = \max_{1 \le k \le n} \left\{ \frac{\prod_{i=k}^{n} f_1(X_i; \hat{\theta}_{i+1,n})}{\prod_{i=k}^{n} f_0(X_i; \theta_0)} \right\}, \; \hat{\theta}_{l,n} = \arg\max_{\theta} \left\{ \prod_{i=l}^{n} f_1(X_i; \theta) \right\}, \; \hat{\theta}_{n+1,n} = \theta_0$$

that implies the pair $\left(\Lambda_n, \mathfrak{I}_k^n = \sigma(X_k, ..., X_n)\right)$ is an H_0-nonnegative ***reverse martingale*** (Section 4.4.3.1). Then, by virtue of Proposition 4.3.3, the Type I error rate of the considered change point detection procedure satisfies $\Pr_{H_0}(\Lambda_n > C) \le 1 / C$.

(v) Let $X_1, X_2, ..., X_n$ be independent continuous random variables with fixed sample size n. Assume that the change point problem is to test for

$$H_0 : X_1, X_2, ..., X_n \sim f_0(u; \theta_0) \text{ versus } H_1 : X_i \sim f_0(u; \theta_0), X_j \sim f_1(u; \theta_1),$$

$$i = 1, ..., \nu - 1, j = \nu, ..., n,$$

where θ_0 and θ_1 are unknown.

In this case, the adaptive CUSUM test statistic is

$$\Lambda_n = \max_{1 \le k \le n} \left\{ \frac{\prod_{i=k}^{n} f_1(X_i; \hat{\theta}_{1, i+1, n})}{\prod_{i=k}^{n} f_0(X_i; \hat{\theta}_{0, k, n})} \right\}, \ \hat{\theta}_{s, l, n} = \arg\max_\theta \left\{ \prod_{i=l}^{n} f_s(X_i; \theta) \right\},$$

$$s = 0, 1, \ \hat{\theta}_{1, n+1, n} = \theta_{10},$$

where θ_{10} is a fixed reasonable variable. Then, using the techniques presented in Scenarios *(i)*, *(iii)*, and *(iv)* above, we conclude that the Type I error rate of this change point detection procedure satisfies the very general inequality $\sup_{\theta_0} \Pr_{H_0}(\Lambda_n > C) \le 1/C$.

Remark. In the context of general retrospective change point detection procedures based on martingale type statistics, we refer the reader, e.g., to Vexler (2006, 2008) and Vexler et al. (2009b), where the following issues are presented: multiple change point detection statements, martingale type associations between the CUSUM and SR techniques, martingale type transformations of test statistics, Monte Carlo comparisons related to the CUSUM and SR techniques, and biostatistical data examples associated with change point detection problems.

4.4.5 Sequential Change Point Detection Policies

In previous sections we focused on offline change point detection or retrospective change point analysis, where inference regarding the detection of a change occurs retrospectively, i.e., after the data has already been collected. In contrast to the retrospective change point problem, the so-called online (*sequential*) change point problem or an online surveillance change problem features methods in which a prospective analysis is performed *sequentially*. In this case, in order to detect a change as soon as possible, such that the consequences of such a change can be tackled effectively, the detection method is implemented after every new observation is collected. The online change point problems are widely presented and studied in fields such as statistical quality control, public health surveillance, and signal processing. For instance, in a continuous production process, the quality of the products is expected to remain stable. However, in practice, for some known or unknown reasons, the process may fail to produce products of equal quality. Therefore, one may be interested in investigating when the quality of a product starts to deteriorate. Under such circumstances, online change point analysis can be used in the form of control charts to monitor output of industrial processes. Typically, control charts have a central line (the mean) and upper and lower lines representing control limits, which are usually set at three-sigma (standard deviations) detection limits away from the mean. Any data points that fall outside these limits or unusual patterns (determined by various run tests) on the control chart suggest that systematic causes of variation are present. Under such circumstance, the process is said to be *out of control* and actions are to be taken to find, and possibly eliminate the corresponding causes. A process is declared to be *in control* if all points charted lie randomly within the control limits. In order to illustrate the construction and operation of control charts we consider the following two data examples.

Example 1: We consider a data example containing one-at-a-time measurements of a continuous process variable presented in Gavit et al. (2009). Figure 4.1 shows the X-chart or control chart for the data. The horizontal upper and lower dashed lines represent the upper and lower three-sigma control limits, respectively. The middle solid horizontal

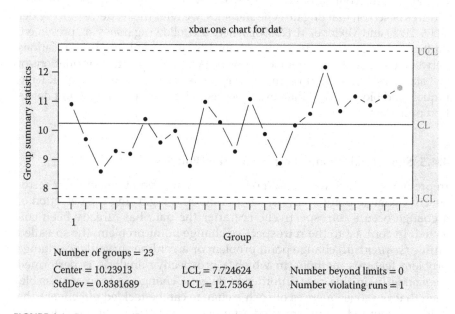

FIGURE 4.1

The X-chart for a data example containing one-at-a-time measurements of a continuous process variable presented in Gavit, P. et al., *BioPharm International*, 22, 46–55, 2009.

line is the mean. Based on the X-chart shown in Figure 4.1, there is no evidence showing that the process is out of control.

Implementation of Figure 4.1 is shown in the following R code:

```
> # install.packages("qcc") # install it for the first time
> library(qcc)
> dat.raw <- c(10.9,9.7,8.6,9.3,9.2,10.4,9.6,10.0,8.8,11.0,10.3,9
.3,11.1,9.9,8.9,10.2,10.6,12.2,10.7,11.2,10.9,11.2,11.5)
> dat <- qcc.groups(dat.raw, sample=1:length(dat.raw))
> obj <- qcc(dat, type="xbar.one",nsigmas = 3)
```

Example 2: We consider another data example obtained from the inside diameter measurements of piston rings for an automotive engine produced by a forging process (Montgomery, 1991). The inside diameter of the rings manufactured by the process is measured on 25 samples, each of size 5, for control phase I.

Figure 4.2 presents the X-bar chart, a type of Shewhart control chart that is used to monitor the arithmetic means of successive samples of constant size, for this calibration data. This control chart shows the center line (CL) as a horizontal solid line and the upper limits (UCL) and lower control limits (LCL) as dashed lines, and the sample group statistics are drawn as points connected with lines.

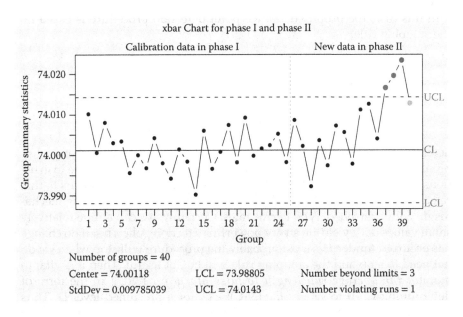

FIGURE 4.2
The Shewhart chart (X-bar chart) for both calibration data and new data, where all the statistics and the control limits are solely based on the calibration data, i.e., the first 25 samples.

Implementation of Figure 4.2 is shown in the following R code:

```
> # install.packages("qcc") # install it for the first time
> library(qcc)
> data(pistonrings)
> diameter <- qcc.groups(pistonrings$diameter,
pistonrings$sample)
>
> # Plot sample means to control the mean level of a continuous variable

> `Phase I` <- diameter[1:25,]
> `Phase II` <- diameter[26:40,]
> obj <- qcc(`Phase I`, type="xbar", newdata=`Phase II`, nsigmas = 3)
```

In contrast to the simple strategies mentioned above, we consider a very efficient sequential change point detection policy based on the Shiryayev–Roberts technique. Assume we sequentially (one-by-one) observe independent continuous random variables $X_1, X_2, \ldots$. The statement of the sequential change point detection problem consists of providing an indication (an *alarm*) regarding a possible change in distribution of the data points. We are interested in a sequential test for

$$H_0 : X_1, X_2, \ldots \sim f_0 \text{ versus } H_1 : X_1, \ldots, X_{v-1} \sim f_0, X_v, X_{v+1}, \ldots \sim f_1,$$

where $f_0 \neq f_1$ are density functions.

In this case, the proposed change point detection procedure is based on the stopping rule:

$$N(C) = \min\{n \geq 1: SR_n > C\}, SR_n = \sum_{j=1}^{n} \Lambda_j^n, \Lambda_j^n = \frac{\Pi_{i=j}^n f_1(X_i)}{\Pi_{i=j}^n f_0(X_i)},$$

$C > 0$ is a test threshold,

determining when one should stop sampling and claim a change has occurred. In order to perform the $N(C)$ strategy, we need to provide instructions regarding how to select values of $C > 0$. This issue is analogous to that related to defining test thresholds in retrospective decision-making mechanisms with controlled Type I error rates. Certainly, we can define relatively small values of C, yielding a very powerful detection policy, but if no change has occurred (under H_0) most probably the procedure will stop when we do not need to stop and the stopping rule will be not useful. Then it is vital to monitor *the average run length to false alarm* $E_{H_0}\{N(C)\}$ in the form of determining $C > 0$ to satisfy $E_{H_0}\{N(C)\} \geq D$, for a presumed level D. Thus defining, e.g., $D = 100$ and stopping at $N(C) = 150$ we could expect that a false alarm is in effect and then just rerun the detection procedure after additional investigations. In this context, we note that $\left(SR_n - n, \Im_n = \sigma(X_1, \ldots, X_n)\right)$ is an H_0-martingale (Section 4.4.3.2) and then Proposition 4.3.1 concludes with $E_{H_0}\{SR_{N(C)} - N(C)\} = E_{H_0}\{SR_1 - 1\} = 0$, i.e., $E_{H_0}\{N(C)\} = E_{H_0}\{SR_{N(C)}\}$. Thus, since, by virtue of the definition of $N(C)$, $SR_{N(C)} \geq C$, we have $E_{H_0}\{N(C)\} \geq C$. This result gives a rule to select values of C, controlling the average run length of the procedure to false alarm. It is clear that Monte Carlo simulation schemes can help us to derive accurate approximations to $E_{H_0}\{N(C)\}$ in specified scenarios of the data distributions. In these cases, the result $E_{H_0}\{N(C)\} \geq C$ is still valuable in the context of initial values that can be applied in terms of the Monte Carlo study.

Note that the techniques described in Section 4.4.4 can be easily applied to extend the statement of the detection problem mentioned above preserving $\left[E_{H_0}\{N(C)\} \geq C\right]$-type properties.

Remark. In order to obtain detailed information regarding sequential change point detection mechanisms and their applications, the reader can consult outstanding publications of Professor Moshe Pollak and Professor Tze Lai (e.g., Pollak, 1985, 1987; Lai, 1995).

4.5 Transformation of Change Point Detection Methods into a Shiryayev–Roberts Form

The Shiryayev–Roberts statistic SR_n for detection of a change has the appealing property that, when the process is *in control*, $SR_n - n$ is a martingale with zero expectation, thus the average run lengths to false alarm $E_{H_0}(N)$ of a stopping time N can be evaluated via $E_{H_0}(N) = E_{H_0}(SR_N)$.

We apply an idea of Brostrom (1997) and show that in certain cases it is possible to transform a surveillance statistic into a Shiryayev–Roberts form. We demonstrate our method with several examples, both parametric as well as nonparametric. In addition, we propose an explanation of the phenomenon that simple CUSUM and Shiryayev–Roberts schemes have similar properties.

The Shiryayev–Roberts change point detection technique is usually based on $N(C) =$ the first crossing time of a certain statistic SR_n over a prespecified threshold C. The statistic SR_n has the property that $SR_n - n$ is a martingale with zero expectation when the process is in control. Therefore, the *average run lengths (ARL) to false alarm* $E_{H_0}\{N(C)\}$ satisfies $E_{H_0}\{N(C)\} = E_{H_0}\{SR_{N(C)}\}$, and since $SR_{N(C)} \geq C$ one easily obtains the inequality $E_{H_0}\{N(C)\} \geq C$. (Renewal-theoretic arguments can be applied often to obtain an approximation $E_{H_0}\{N(C)\} \approx aC$, where a is a constant.) Thus, if a constraint $E_{H_0}\{N(C)\} \geq B$ on the false alarm rate is to be satisfied, choosing $C = B$ (or $C = B/a$) does the job (see Pollak, 1987, and Yakir, 1995, for the basic theory).

Alternative approaches do not have this property. When a method is based on a sequence of statistics $\{T_n\}$ that is an H_0-submartingale when the process is in control (such as CUSUM), we follow Brostrom (1997) in applying **Doob's decomposition** to $\{T_n\}$ and extract the martingale component. (The anticipating component depends on the past and does not contain new information about the future.) We transform the martingale component into a Shiryayev–Roberts form. We apply this procedure to several examples. Among others, we show that our approach can be used to obtain nonparametric Shiryayev–Roberts procedures based on ranks. Another application is to the case of estimation of unknown postchange parameters.

4.5.1 Motivation

To motivate the general method, consider the following example. Suppose that observations $Y_1, Y_2, \ldots$ are independent, $Y_1, \ldots, Y_{v-1} \sim N(0, 1)$ when the process is in control, $Y_v, Y_{v+1}, \ldots \sim N(\theta, 1)$ when the process is out of control, where v is the change point and θ is unknown. Let P_v and E_v denote the probability measure and expectation when the change occurs at v. The value of v is set to ∞ if no change ever takes place in the sequence of observations. Where θ is known, the classical Shiryayev–Roberts procedure would declare a change to be in effect if $SR_n^I \geq C$ for some prespecified threshold C, where

$$SR_n^I = \sum_{k=1}^{n} \exp\left\{ \sum_{i=k}^{n} \left(\theta Y_i - \theta^2 / 2 \right) \right\} \tag{4.3}$$

(e.g., Pollak, 1985, 1987). When θ is unknown, it is natural to estimate θ. In order to preserve the P_∞-martingale structure, Lorden and Pollak (2005) and Vexler (2006) propose to replace θ in the kth term of SR_n^I by $\sum_{j=k}^{i-1} Y_j / (i-k)$. (The same idea appears in Robbins and Siegmund (1973) and Dragalin (1997) in a different context.) A criticism of this approach is that foregoing the use of $Y_k, \ldots, Y_{i-1}$ without $Y_i, \ldots, Y_n$ when estimating θ in the kth term is inefficient (e.g., Lai, 2001, p. 398).

An alternative is to estimate θ in the kth term of SR_n^I by the $P_{v=k}$ maximum likelihood estimator $\hat{\theta}_{k,n} = \sum_{j=k}^{n} Y_j / (n-k+1)$, so that SR_n^I becomes

$$SR_n^I = \sum_{k=1}^{n-1} \exp\left\{ \hat{\theta}_{k,n} \sum_{i=k}^{n} Y_i - (n-k+1)\left(\hat{\theta}_{k,n}\right)^2 / 2 \right\} + 1 \tag{4.4}$$

with the convention that $\sum_1^0 = 0$ (the $k = n$ term is mechanically replaced by 1 in order that $E_{H_0}\left(SR_n^I\right) = E_\infty\left(SR_n^I\right) < \infty$). Note that $\left(SR_n^I, \Im_n = \sigma\left(Y_1, ..., Y_n\right)\right)$ is a P_∞-submartingale, for

$$SR_n^I \geq \sum_{k=1}^{n-1} \exp\left\{\hat{\theta}_{k,n-1}\sum_{i=k}^{n} Y_i - (n-k+1)\left(\hat{\theta}_{k,n-1}\right)^2 / 2\right\} + 1$$

(because the maximum is attained at $\hat{\theta}_{k,n}$), so

$E_\infty\left(SR_n^I \mid \Im_{n-1}\right)$

$$\geq \sum_{k=1}^{n-2} \exp\left\{\hat{\theta}_{k,n-1}\sum_{i=k}^{n-1} Y_i - \frac{1}{2}(n-k)\left(\hat{\theta}_{k,n-1}\right)^2\right\} E_\infty\left(\exp\left\{\hat{\theta}_{k,n-1}Y_n\sum_{i=k}^{n-1} Y_i - \frac{1}{2}\left(\hat{\theta}_{k,n-1}\right)^2\right\} \mid \Im_{n-1}\right)$$

$+1 = SR_{n-1}^I.$

Generally, one can show that applying the maximum likelihood estimation of the unknown postchange parameters to the initial Shiryayev–Roberts statistics of the parametric detection schemes leads to the same submartingale property.

Our goal is to transform SR_n^I into SR_n such that $\left(SR_n - n, \Im_n\right)$ is a P_∞-martingale with zero expectation, in such a manner that relevant information will not be lost. Rather than continue with this example, we present a general theory.

4.5.2 The Method

We assume that initially we have a series $\left\{SR_n^I\right\}$ of test statistics that is a P_∞-submartingale. Let $SR_0^I = 0$ and define recursively

$$W_n = \frac{\left(SR_{n-1}^I\right)W_{n-1} + 1}{E_\infty\left(SR_n^I \mid \Im_{n-1}\right)}, \quad SR_n = \left(SR_n^I\right)W_n, \quad W_0 = 0, \ n = 1, 2, ... \quad (4.5)$$

It is clear that $W_n \in \Im_{n-1}$ and therefore $E_\infty\left(SR_n \mid \Im_{n-1}\right) = SR_n + 1$ so that $\left(SR_n - n, \Im_n\right)$ is a P_∞-martingale with zero expectation. (If $\left(SR_n^I - n, \Im_n\right)$ is a P_∞-martingale with zero expectation, then Equation (4.5) provides $W_n = 1, n \geq 1$.) We will now show that $\{SR_n - n\}$ is a P_∞-martingale transform of the martingale component of SR_n^I. Towards this end, we present the ***Doob's decomposition*** result, representing several notations that appear in this section.

Lemma 4.5.1.

Let S_n be a submartingale with respect to $\Im_n$ then S_n can be uniquely decomposed as $S_n = \langle S \rangle_n^M + \langle S \rangle_n^P$ with the following properties:

$\langle S \rangle_n^M$ *is a martingale component of S_n (i.e., $\left(\langle S \rangle_n^M, \Im_n \right)$ is a martingale);*

$\langle S \rangle_n^P$ *is $\Im_{n-1}$-measurable, having the predictable property, $\langle S \rangle_n^P \geq \langle S \rangle_{n-1}^P$ (a.s.),*
$\langle S \rangle_1^P = 1$ *and* $\langle S \rangle_n^P - \langle S \rangle_{n-1}^P = E\left(S_n - S_{n-1} \mid \Im_{n-1} \right)$.

Now we formulate the widely known definition of ***martingale transforms***. If $\langle G \rangle_n^M$ is a martingale with respect to $\Im_n$, then a martingale transform $\langle G' \rangle_n^M$ of $\langle G \rangle_n^M$ is given by

$$\langle G' \rangle_n^M = \langle G' \rangle_{n-1}^M + a_n \left(\langle G \rangle_n^M - \langle G \rangle_{n-1}^M \right), \tag{4.6}$$

where $a_n \in \Im_{n-1}$. Such transformations have a long history and interesting interpretations in terms of gambling. An interpretation is if we have a fair game, we can choose the size and side of our bet at each stage based on the prior history and the game will continue to be fair. An association of a stochastic game with a change point detection is presented, for example, by Ritov (1990).

Thus, if $\langle SR \rangle_n^M$ is a martingale transform ("transition: martingale-martingale") of $\langle SR^I \rangle_n^M$ ($\langle SR \rangle_n^M \in \Im_n$, but $\langle SR \rangle_n^M \notin \left\{ \Im_{n-1} \cap \left\{ \langle SR^I \rangle_k^M \right\}_{k=1}^{n-1} \right\}$), then this implies that the information in SR_n about a change having or not having taken place is the same as that contained in $\langle SR^I \rangle_n^M$, which in turn is the same as the information contained in the initial sequence $\{ SR_n^I \}$.

Proposition 4.5.1. Let $\left(SR_n^I, \Im_n \right)$ be a nonnegative P_∞-submartingale $\left(SR_0^I = 0 \right)$. Then, under P_∞-regime,

1. $SR_n = \left(SR_n^I \right) W_n$ is a nonnegative submartingale with respect to $\Im_n$;
2. $\langle SR \rangle_n^M$ is a martingale transform of $\langle SR^I \rangle_n^M$, where W_n is defined by (4.5).

Proof. By applying the definition of $W_n \in \mathfrak{S}_{n-1}$, we obtain $E_\infty \left(SR_n \mid \mathfrak{S}_{n-1} \right) = W_{n-1}$ $\left(SR_{n-1}^I \right) + 1 \geq SR_{n-1}$ hence $SR_n = \left(SR_n^I \right) W_n$ is a nonnegative submartingale with respect to $\mathfrak{S}_n$. It now follows from Lemma 4.5.1 that

$$\langle SR \rangle_n^M = SR_n - \langle SR \rangle_n^P = SR_n - n.$$

Therefore,

$$\langle SR \rangle_n^M - \langle SR \rangle_{n-1}^M = SR_n - SR_{n-1} - 1 = \left(SR_n^I \right) W_n - \left(SR_{n-1}^I \right) W_{n-1} - 1,$$

where $\left(SR_{n-1}^I \right) W_{n-1} = \left\{ E_\infty \left(SR_n^I \mid \mathfrak{S}_{n-1} \right) \right\} W_n - 1$ by the definition of W_n. Consequently,

$$\langle SR \rangle_n^M - \langle SR \rangle_{n-1}^M = \left\{ SR_n^I - E_\infty \left(SR_n^I \mid \mathfrak{S}_{n-1} \right) \right\} W_n.$$

On the other hand, by Lemma 4.5.1 one can show that

$$\langle SR^I \rangle_n^M - \langle SR^I \rangle_{n-1}^M = SR_n^I - \sum_{k}^{n} \left\{ E_\infty \left(SR_k^I \mid \mathfrak{S}_{k-1} \right) - SR_{k-1}^I \right\} - SR_{n-1}^I$$

$$- \sum_{k}^{n-1} \left\{ E_\infty \left(SR_k^I \mid \mathfrak{S}_{k-1} \right) - SR_{k-1}^I \right\}$$

$$= SR_n^I - E_\infty \left(SR_n^I \mid \mathfrak{S}_{n-1} \right).$$

Since $W_n \in \mathfrak{S}_{n-1}$, by definition (4.6) the proof of Proposition 4.5.1 is now complete.

Consider an inverse version of Proposition 4.5.1.

Proposition 4.5.2. Assume $v = \infty$ and $a_n \in \mathfrak{S}_{n-1}$ exists, such that

$$\langle SR' \rangle_n^M = \langle SR' \rangle_{n-1}^M + a_n \left(\langle SR' \rangle_n^M - \langle SR' \rangle_{n-1}^M \right),$$

where $SR'_n \in \mathfrak{S}_n$ is a submartingale with respect to $\mathfrak{S}_n$ and $E_\infty \left(SR'_n \mid \mathfrak{S}_{n-1} \right) = SR'_{n-1} + 1$. Then $SR'_n = \left(SR_n^I \right) W_n + \varsigma_n$, where $W_n \in \mathfrak{S}_{n-1}$ is defined by (4.5), $(\varsigma_n, \mathfrak{S}_n)$ is a martingale with zero expectation, and ς_n is a martingale transform of $\langle SR^I \rangle_n^M$.

Proof. We have $SR'_n = \left(SR_n^I\right)W_n + \varsigma_n$, where $\varsigma_n = SR'_n - \left(SR_n^I\right)W_n \in \mathfrak{J}_n$. Consider the conditional expectation

$$
\begin{aligned}
E_\infty\left(SR'_n \mid \mathfrak{J}_{n-1}\right) &= E_\infty\left(\left(SR_n^I\right)W_n \mid \mathfrak{J}_{n-1}\right) + E_\infty\left(\varsigma_n \mid \mathfrak{J}_{n-1}\right) \\
&= \left(SR_{n-1}^I\right)W_{n-1} + 1 + E_\infty\left(\varsigma_n \mid \mathfrak{J}_{n-1}\right) \\
&= SR'_{n-1} - \varsigma_{n-1} + 1 + E_\infty\left(\varsigma_n \mid \mathfrak{J}_{n-1}\right).
\end{aligned}
$$

On the other hand, by the statement of this proposition, $E_\infty\left(SR'_n \mid \mathfrak{J}_{n-1}\right) = SR'_{n-1} + 1$. Therefore, we conclude with $E_\infty\left(\varsigma_n \mid \mathfrak{J}_{n-1}\right) = \varsigma_{n-1}$.

From the basic definitions and Lemma 4.5.1 (in a similar manner to the proof of Proposition 4.5.1) it follows that

$$
\begin{aligned}
\langle SR'\rangle_n^M - \langle SR'\rangle_{n-1}^M &= \left(SR_n^I\right)W_n + \varsigma_n - \left(SR_{n-1}^I\right)W_{n-1} - \varsigma_{n-1} - \langle SR'\rangle_n^P + \langle SR'\rangle_{n-1}^P \\
&= \left(SR_n^I\right)W_n + \varsigma_n - W_n E_\infty\left(SR_n^I \mid \mathfrak{J}_{n-1}\right) + 1 - \varsigma_{n-1} - E_\infty\left(SR'_n - SR'_{n-1} \mid \mathfrak{J}_{n-1}\right) \\
&= \varsigma_n - \varsigma_{n-1} + \left\{SR_n^I - E_\infty\left(SR_n^I \mid \mathfrak{J}_{n-1}\right)\right\}W_n \\
&= \varsigma_n - \varsigma_{n-1} + \left\{\langle SR^I\rangle_n^M - \langle SR^I\rangle_{n-1}^M\right\}W_n.
\end{aligned}
$$

Hence

$$
\varsigma_n - \varsigma_{n-1} = (a_n - W_n)\left\{\langle SR^I\rangle_n^M - \langle SR^I\rangle_{n-1}^M\right\}, \quad (a_n - W_n) \in \mathfrak{J}_{n-1}.
$$

This completes the proof of Proposition 4.5.2.

Interpretation: We set out to extract the martingale component $\langle SR^I\rangle_n^M$ of SR_n^I and to get a martingale transform $\langle SR\rangle_n^M = SR_n - n$ of $\langle SR^I\rangle_n^M$ such that $SR_n - n$ is a P_∞-martingale with zero expectation. However, if we are given any SR'_n with the property that $SR'_n - n$ is a P_∞-martingale with zero expectation, then Proposition 4.5.2 states that $SR'_n = SR_n + \varsigma_n$ where ς_n is a martingale transform of $\langle SR^I\rangle_n^M$. Therefore, note that the information in SR_n and in SR'_n is the same. In other words, from an information point of view, our procedure is equivalent to any other procedure based on a sequence $\left\{SR_n^I\right\}$ that has the same martingale properties as $\{SR_n\}$.

An obvious property of our procedure is:

Corollary 4.5.1. Let $N(C) = \min\{n \geq 1 : SR_n \geq C\}$, where SR_n is defined by (4.5). Then $E_\infty\{N(C)\} \geq C$.

Returning to the example of the previous section, we obtain (from Equation (4.4)) by a standard calculation:

$$SR_n^I = \sum_{k=1}^{n-1} \exp\left\{(n-k+1)\left(\hat{\theta}_{k,n}\right)^2 / 2\right\} + 1,$$

$$E_\infty\left(SR_n^I \mid \Im_{n-1}\right) = \sum_{k=1}^{n-1} \left(\frac{n-k+1}{n-k}\right)^{1/2} \exp\left\{(n-k)\left(\hat{\theta}_{k,n-1}\right)^2 / 2\right\} + 1$$

and $\{W_n\}$, $\{SR_n\}$ are obtained from (4.5).

Additional examples:

1. Let the prechange and postchange distributions of the independent observations $Y_1, Y_2, \dots$ be respectively the standard exponential (i.e., $Y_1, \dots, Y_{v-1} \sim f_0(u) = \exp(-u)$) and the exponential with an unknown parameter $\theta > 0$ (i.e., $Y_v, Y_{v+1}, \dots \sim f_1(u; \theta) = \theta \exp(-\theta u)$). Therefore, $\hat{\theta}_{k,n} = (n-k+1)/\sum_{j=k}^{n} Y_j$ is the maximum likelihood estimator and the initial Shiryayev–Roberts statistic is

$$SR_n^I = \sum_{k=1}^{n-1} \prod_{i=k}^{n} \frac{f_1(Y_i; \hat{\theta}_{k,n})}{f_0(Y_i)} + 1 = \sum_{k=1}^{n-1} \left(\hat{\theta}_{k,n}\right)^{n-k+1} \exp\left\{(n-k+1)\left(\left(\hat{\theta}_{k,n}\right)^{-1} - 1\right)\right\} + 1.$$

Since

$$E_\infty\left(\prod_{i=k}^{n} \frac{f_1(Y_i; \hat{\theta}_{k,n})}{f_0(Y_i)} \mid \Im_{n-1}\right)$$

$$= (n-k+1)^{n-k+1} e^{(n-k)\left(\hat{\theta}_{k,n-1}\right)^{-1} - (n-k+1)} \int_0^\infty \frac{e^u}{\left[u + (n-k)\left(\hat{\theta}_{k,n-1}\right)^{-1}\right]^{n-k+1}} e^{-u} \, du$$

$$= \left(\frac{n-k+1}{n-k}\right)^{n-k+1} \left(\hat{\theta}_{k,n-1}\right)^{n-k} \exp\left\{(n-k)\left(\hat{\theta}_{k,n-1}\right)^{-1} - (n-k+1)\right\},$$

we have

$$E_\infty\left(SR_n^I \mid \Im_{n-1}\right) = \sum_{k=1}^{n-1} \left(\frac{n-k+1}{n-k}\right)^{n-k+1} \left(\hat{\theta}_{k,n-1}\right)^{n-k} \exp\left\{(n-k)\left(\hat{\theta}_{k,n-1}\right)^{-1} - (n-k+1)\right\} + 1$$

and $\{W_n\}$, $\{SR_n\}$ are obtained from (4.5).

2. Consider the simple segmented linear regression model

$$Y_i = \theta x_i I \left(i \geq v\right) + \varepsilon_i, \ i \geq 1. \tag{4.7}$$

where θ is the unknown regression parameter, $x_i, i \geq 1$, are fixed predictors, $\varepsilon_i, i \geq 1$, are independent random disturbance terms with standard normal density and $I(\cdot)$ is the indicator function. In this case, the maximum likelihood estimator of the unknown parameter is

$$\hat{\theta}_{k,n} = \frac{\sum_{j=k}^{n} Y_j x_j}{\sum_{j=k}^{n} x_j^2}. \tag{4.8}$$

Since the conditional expectation of the estimator of the likelihood ratio is

$$E_\infty\left[\prod_{i=k}^{n} \frac{\exp\left\{-\left(Y_i - \hat{\theta}_{k,n} x_i\right)^2/2\right\}}{\exp\left\{-\left(Y_i\right)^2/2\right\}} \,\big|\, \mathfrak{I}_{n-1}\right] = \left(\frac{\sum_{j=k}^{n} x_j^2}{\sum_{j=k}^{n-1} x_j^2}\right)^{1/2} \exp\left\{\frac{\left(\sum_{j=k}^{n-1} Y_j x_j\right)^2}{2\sum_{j=k}^{n-1} x_j^2}\right\},$$

the transformed detection scheme for the model (4.7) has form (4.5), where

$$SR_n^I = \sum_{k=1}^{n-1} \exp\left\{\frac{\left(\sum_{j=k}^{n} Y_j x_j\right)^2}{2\sum_{j=k}^{n} x_j^2}\right\} + 1,$$

$$\tag{4.9}$$

$$E_\infty\left(SR_n^I \,|\, \mathfrak{I}_{n-1}\right) = \sum_{k=1}^{n-1} \left(\frac{\sum_{j=k}^{n} x_j^2}{\sum_{j=k}^{n-1} x_j^2}\right)^{1/2} \exp\left\{\frac{\left(\sum_{j=k}^{n-1} Y_j x_j\right)^2}{2\sum_{j=k}^{n-1} x_j^2}\right\} + 1.$$

Note that, if the parameters of a segmented linear regression similar to (4.7), under regime P_∞ are unknown (e.g., the intercept, under P_∞, is unknown), then the observations can be invariantly transformed into the case considered in this example (e.g., Krieger et al., 2003; Vexler, 2006).

4.5.3 CUSUM versus Shiryayev–Roberts

It is well accepted that the change point detection procedures based on Shiryayev–Roberts statistics and the schemes founded on CUSUM statistics have almost equivalent optimal statistical properties (e.g., Krieger et al., 2003: Section 1). Here we establish an interesting link between the CUSUM and Shiryayev–Roberts detection policies.

We assume that prior to a change the observations $Y_1, Y_2, \ldots$ are iid with density f_0. Post-change they are iid with density f_1. The simple CUSUM procedure stops at

$$M(C) = \min\{n \geq 1: \Lambda_n \geq C\}, \text{ where } \Lambda_n = \max_{1 \leq k \leq n} \prod_{i=k}^{n} \frac{f_1(Y_i)}{f_0(Y_i)}$$

and the simple Shiryayev–Roberts procedure stops at

$$N(C) = \min\{n \geq 1: SR_n \geq C\}, \; SR_n = \sum_{k=1}^{n} \prod_{i=k}^{n} \frac{f_1(Y_i)}{f_0(Y_i)}.$$

In accordance with the proposed methodology, we present the following proposition.

Proposition 4.5.3. The P_∞-martingale component $\langle SR \rangle_n^M$ of the Shiryayev-Roberts statistic SR_n is a martingale transform of $\langle \Lambda \rangle_n^M$, which is the P_∞-martingale component of the CUSUM statistic Λ_n (and vice versa).

Proof. We have

$$
\begin{aligned}
\Lambda_n &= \max \left\{ \prod_{i=1}^{n} \frac{f_1(Y_i)}{f_0(Y_i)}, \prod_{i=2}^{n} \frac{f_1(Y_i)}{f_0(Y_i)}, \ldots, \frac{f_1(Y_n)}{f_0(Y_n)} \right\} \\
&= \max \left[\max \left\{ \prod_{i=1}^{n} \frac{f_1(Y_i)}{f_0(Y_i)}, \prod_{i=2}^{n} \frac{f_1(Y_i)}{f_0(Y_i)}, \ldots, \prod_{i=n-1}^{n} \frac{f_1(Y_i)}{f_0(Y_i)} \right\}, \frac{f_1(Y_n)}{f_0(Y_n)} \right] \\
&= \frac{f_1(Y_n)}{f_0(Y_n)} \max \left[\max \left\{ \prod_{i=1}^{n-1} \frac{f_1(Y_i)}{f_0(Y_i)}, \prod_{i=2}^{n-1} \frac{f_1(Y_i)}{f_0(Y_i)}, \ldots, \prod_{i=n-1}^{n-1} \frac{f_1(Y_i)}{f_0(Y_i)} \right\}, 1 \right] \\
&= \frac{f_1(Y_n)}{f_0(Y_n)} \max(\Lambda_n, 1).
\end{aligned}
\tag{4.10}
$$

Since $E_\infty \{f_1(Y_n)/f_0(Y_n) \,|\, \mathfrak{I}_{n-1}\} = 1$ and $\Lambda_{n-1} \in \mathfrak{I}_{n-1}$, Λ_n is a P_∞-submartingale with respect to $\mathfrak{I}_n$. By applying Lemma 4.5.1, we obtain the P_∞-martingale component of Λ_n in the form

$$\langle \Lambda \rangle_n^M = \Lambda_n - \sum_{k}^{n} \{\max(\Lambda_{k-1}, 1) - \Lambda_{k-1}\}.$$

Hence, by (4.10)

$$\langle \Lambda \rangle_n^M - \langle \Lambda \rangle_{n-1}^M = \Lambda_n - \Lambda_{n-1} - \max(\Lambda_{n-1}, 1) + \Lambda_{n-1}$$

$$= \max(\Lambda_{n-1}, 1) \left\{ \frac{f_1(Y_n)}{f_0(Y_n)} - 1 \right\}.$$

On the other hand, it is clear that SR_n is a P_∞-submartingale with respect to $\Im_n$ and

$$\langle SR \rangle_n^M - \langle SR \rangle_{n-1}^M = SR_n - n - SR_{n-1} + (n-1) = \frac{f_1(Y_n)}{f_0(Y_n)}(SR_{n-1}+1) - (SR_{n-1}+1)$$

$$= (SR_{n-1}+1)\left\{\frac{f_1(Y_n)}{f_0(Y_n)} - 1\right\}.$$

By virtue of $a_n = \max(\Lambda_{n-1}, 1)/(SR_{n-1}+1) \in \Im_{n-1}$ (or $a_n = (SR_{n-1}+1)/\max(\Lambda_{n-1}, 1) \in \Im_{n-1}$), the proof of Proposition 4.5.3 now follows from definition (4.6).

Thus, following our methodology, we can transform the CUSUM method into a martingale-based procedure (i.e., Equation (4.5) with $SR'_n = \Lambda_n$). Here

$$SR'_n = \Lambda_n W_n, \quad W_n = \frac{\Lambda_{n-1}W_{n-1}+1}{\max(\Lambda_{n-1}, 1)}, \quad W_0 = 0, \Lambda_0 = 0. \tag{4.11}$$

where $\max(\Lambda_{n-1}, 1) = E_\infty(\Lambda_n | \Im_{n-1})$. Certainly, in a similar manner to Corollary 4.5.1, the stopping time $N'(C) = \min\{n \geq 1: SR'_n \geq C\}$ satisfies $E_\infty\{N'(C)\} \geq C$. Moreover, we have the following proposition.

Proposition 4.5.4. The classical Shiryayev–Roberts statistic SR_n is the transformed CUSUM statistic (4.11) (and vice versa).

Proof. By substituting (4.10) in (4.11), we obtain

$$SR'_n = \frac{(\Lambda_{n-1}W_{n-1}+1)}{\max(\Lambda_{n-1}, 1)}\Lambda_n$$

$$= \frac{(\Lambda_{n-1}W_{n-1}+1)}{\max(\Lambda_{n-1}, 1)}\frac{f_1(Y_n)}{f_0(Y_n)}\max(\Lambda_{n-1}, 1)$$

$$= (SR'_n+1)\frac{f_1(Y_n)}{f_0(Y_n)}, \quad SR'_0 = 0.$$

Since

$$SR_n = (SR_n+1)\frac{f_1(Y_n)}{f_0(Y_n)}, \quad SR_0 = 0,$$

the proof of Proposition 4.5.4 is now complete.

What this means is that the CUSUM scheme and the Shiryayev–Roberts policy are based on the same information. The difference between them stems from their different predictable components: that of Shiryayev–Roberts is n whereas that of CUSUM is $\sum_{k=1}^{n}\{\max(\Lambda_{k-1}, 1) - \Lambda_{k-1}\}$. In other words, CUSUM makes use of superfluous information contained in the observations.

Note that $\sum_{k=1}^{n}\left\{\max\left(\Lambda_{k-1},1\right)-\Lambda_{k-1}\right\}$ is increasing prior to a change, shortening the ARL to false alarm, but its increase is approximately zero postchange, so that it does not contribute toward shortening the average delay to detection. This explains why Shiryayev–Roberts is somewhat better than CUSUM.

4.5.4 A Nonparametric Example*

Consider the sequential change point problem where nothing is known about both the prechange and postchange distributions other than that they are continuous. In this case, an obvious approach would be to base surveillance on the sequence of sequential ranks of the observations. Several procedures have been constructed for this problem, e.g., Gordon and Pollak (1995). Here we consider a problem of a slightly different nature. Suppose one feels that the prechange observations may be $N\left(0,\sigma^2\right)$ and the postchange observations $N\left(\theta\sigma,\sigma^2\right)$ (θ,σ are possibly unknown), but is not sure of this. If a nonparametric method could be constructed in a way that will be efficient if the observations were truly $N\left(0,\sigma^2\right)$ and $N\left(\theta\sigma,\sigma^2\right)$ as above, one may well prefer the nonparametric scheme, as it promises validity of ARL to false alarm even if the normality assumption is violated. It is this problem that we address here.

Formally, let $Y_1,Y_2,\dots$ be independent random variables. When the process is in control, $\{Y_i, i \geq 1\}$ are iid. If the process goes out of control at time ν, then $\{Y_i, i \geq \nu\}$ are iid and have a distribution deferent from the in-control state. Define

$$r_{j,n} = \sum_{i=1}^{n} I\left(Y_i \leq Y_j\right), \ \rho_n = r_{n,n}/(n+1), \ Z_n = \Phi^{-1}(\rho_n), \ \Im_n = \sigma\left(\rho_1,\dots,\rho_n\right),$$

where Φ^{-1} is the inverse of the standard normal distribution function. Note that the in-control distribution of the sequence $\{\rho_i, i \geq 1\}$ does not depend on the distribution of the Y's as long as it is continuous, and $\rho_1,\dots,\rho_n$ are independent. Clearly, under P_∞, ρ_n converges in distribution to $U[0,1]$ and therefore $Z_n \to N(0,1)$, as $n \to \infty$. Fix $\theta \neq 0$ and define recursively

$$SR_{\theta,n}^I = e^{\theta Z_n - \theta^2/2}\left(SR_{\theta,n-1}^I + 1\right) = \sum_{k=1}^{n} e^{\theta \sum_{i=k}^{n} Z_i - \theta^2(n-k+1)/2}, \ SR_{\theta,0}^I = 0. \quad (4.12)$$

(Note that if $Z_1,Z_2,\dots$ were exactly standard normal, then (4.12) is the same as (4.3).) Applying our methodology, letting $W_{\theta,0} = 0$, define recursively

---

* This subsection was prepared by Professor Moshe Pollak.

$$SR_{\theta,n} = \left(SR_{\theta,n}^{I}\right)W_{\theta,n}, \quad W_{\theta,n} = \frac{\left(SR_{\theta,n-1}^{I}\right)W_{\theta,n-1}+1}{E_{\infty}\left(SR_{\theta,n}^{I} \mid \mathfrak{I}_{n-1}\right)}$$

$$= \frac{\left(SR_{\theta,n-1}^{I}\right)W_{\theta,n-1}+1}{e^{-\frac{1}{2}\theta^2}\frac{1}{n}\sum_{i=1}^{n}\exp\left\{\Phi^{-1}\left(\frac{i}{n+1}\right)\theta\right\}\left(SR_{\theta,n-1}^{I}+1\right)},$$

(4.13)

$$N_{\theta}(C) = \min\left\{n \geq 1: \; SR_{\theta,n} \geq C\right\}$$

and therefore $E_{\infty}\left\{N_{\theta}(C)\right\} \geq C$.

Remark 1. For the sake of clarity, the example above was developed to give a robust detection method if one believes the observations to be approximately normal (and one is on guard against a change of mean). This method can be applied to other families of distributions in a similar manner.

Remark 2. Instead of fixing θ, one can fix a prior G for θ, and define the Bayes factor type procedure

$$SR_n = \left(SR_n^{I}\right)W_n, \quad SR_n^{I} = \int SR_{\theta,n}^{I} \, dG(\theta),$$

$$W_n = \frac{\left(SR_{n-1}^{I}\right)W_{n-1}+1}{\left(SR_{n-1}^{I}+1\right)\frac{1}{n}\sum_{i=1}^{n}\int \exp\left\{\Phi^{-1}\left(\frac{i}{n+1}\right)\theta - \frac{1}{2}\theta^2\right\}dG(\theta)},$$

(4.14)

$$SR_0^{I} = W_0 = 0.$$

Note that if G is a conjugate prior (e.g., $G = N(.,.)$), then the integral in the denominator of W_n can be calculated explicitly. An alternative approach to Equation (4.14) is simply to define $SR_n = \int SR_{\theta,n} \, dG(\theta)$. However, the calculation of $\int SR_{\theta,n} \, dG(\theta)$ involves an arduous numerical integration (after every observation).

4.5.5 Monte Carlo Simulation Study

Proposed transformation versus application of nonanticipating estimation. Let the simulated samples satisfy (4.7) with $x_i = \sin(i)$. In accordance with Krieger et al. (2003) and Lorden and Pollak (2005), denote the stopping rule

$$N^{(1)}(A) = \min\left\{n \geq 1: \; \sum_{k=1}^{n}\prod_{i=k}^{n}\exp\left\{-\frac{1}{2}\left(Y_i - \hat{\theta}_{k,i-1}x_i\right)^2 - \frac{1}{2}\left(Y_i\right)^2\right\} \geq A\right\}$$

based on the application of the nonanticipating estimation $\left\{\hat{\theta}_{k,i-1}\right\}$, where the maximum likelihood estimator 4.8 defines $\hat{\theta}_{k,l}$ ($\hat{\theta}_{k,l} = 0$, if $l < k$). Alternatively, let

$$N^{(2)}(A) = \min\{n \geq 1 : SR_n \geq A\},$$

where SR_n is defined by (4.5) with (4.9).

We ran 15,000 repetitions of the model for each procedure and at each point $A = 50, 75, 100, 125,\ldots$. Figure 4.3 depicts the Monte Carlo averages of $N^{(1)}(A)$ and $N^{(2)}(A)$ in this case, where every simulated observation is from $N(0,1)$ (i.e., $v = \infty$ and this simulation run is independent of θ).

It appears that $E_\infty\{N^{(1)}(A)\}/A$ behaves nonconstantly, for the range of A. Note that, in the case where $x_i = 1$, we have $\lim_{A\to\infty}\left[E_\infty\{N^{(1)}(A)\}/A\right] = const$ (see Lorden and Pollak, 2005). Figure 4.4 corresponds to the definition of the model (4.7), where $v = 1$ and $\theta = 1/4, 1/2$.

In accordance with Figures 4.3 and 4.4, the detecting strategy $N^{(2)}(A)$ tends to be a quicker detecting scheme (with estimated $A_1, A_2 : E_\infty\{N^{(1)}(A_1)\} \simeq E_\infty\{N^{(2)}(A_1)\}$). Moreover, in this experiment $E_1\{N^{(1)}(A)\}$ is not a linear function of $\log(A)$, as it usually is for parametric change point detections.

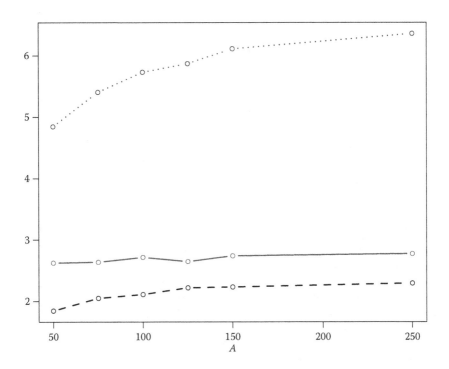

FIGURE 4.3

Comparison between the Monte Carlo estimator of $E_\infty\{N^{(1)}(A)\}/A$ ($\cdots\circ\cdots$) and the Monte Carlo estimator of $E_\infty\{N^{(2)}(A)\}/A$ (—$\circ$—). The curve (--$\circ$--) images the Monte Carlo estimator of $E_\infty\{N^{(1)}(A)\}/E_\infty\{N^{(2)}(A)\}$.

Modification of CUSUM. Next, we investigate one conclusion of Section 4.5.3 regarding the CUSUM detection scheme. In particular, Section 4.5.3 suggests that the stopping rule

$$N'(A) = \min\left[n \geq 0: \ \langle \Lambda \rangle_n^M = \Lambda_n - \sum_{k=1}^{n}\left\{\max(\Lambda_{k-1}, 1) - \Lambda_{k-1}\right\} \geq A\right]$$

is somewhat better than the classical CUSUM stopping time

$$M(A) = \min\{n \geq 1: \ \Lambda_n \geq A\}, \text{ where } \Lambda_n = \max_{1 \leq k \leq n} \prod_{i=k}^{n} \frac{f_1(Y_i)}{f_0(Y_i)}.$$

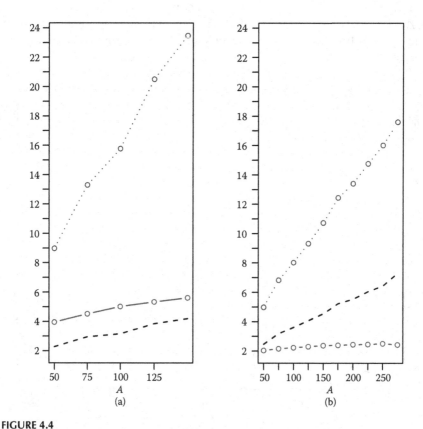

FIGURE 4.4

Comparison between the Monte Carlo estimator of $E_1\{N^{(1)}(A)\}/(5\log(A))$ ($\cdots\circ\cdots$) and the Monte Carlo estimator of $E_1\{N^{(2)}(A)\}/(5\log(A))$ ($\text{---}\circ\text{---}$). The curve (- - - -) images the Monte Carlo estimator of $E_1\{N^{(1)}(A)\}/E_1\{N^{(2)}(A)\}$. The graphs (a) and (b) correspond to the model (4.7), where $\theta = 1/4, 1/2$, respectively.

We executed 15,000 repetitions of independent observations $Y_1, ..., Y_{v-1} \sim f_0 = N(0,1)$; $Y_v, ... \sim f_1 = N(\theta = 0.5, 1)$ for each Monte Carlo simulation. In the case of $v = \infty$ and $A = 50, 100, 150, 200, 250$, the Monte Carlo estimator of $E_\infty \{N'(A)\}/A$ behaves approximately constantly and we evaluate $E_\infty \{N^{(1)}(A)\}/A \approx 768.2$. At that rate, we can conclude with $E_\infty \{M(A)\}/A \approx 13.8$. Figure 4.5 illustrates the accuracy of the considered conclusion of Section 4.5.3.

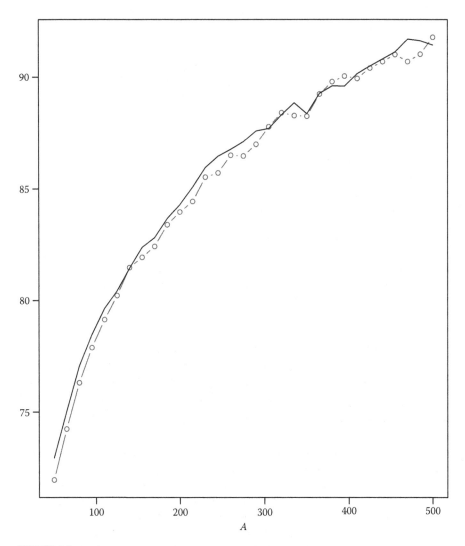

FIGURE 4.5
The curved lines (—∘—) and (——) denote the Monte Carlo estimators of $E_{50}\{N'(A)\}$ and $E_{50}\{M(A)\}$, respectively.

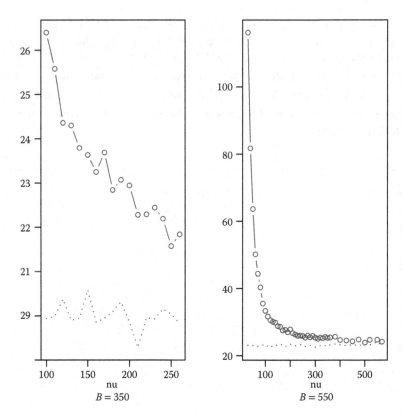

FIGURE 4.6
The curved lines (—o—) and (····) denote the Monte Carlo estimators of $L(N_{\theta=0.5}(B/1.3301), v)$ and $L(N_o(B/1.3316), v)$, respectively, plotted against v.

Nonparametric procedure. Here, by basing on simulations of the process $\{Y_1, ..., Y_{v-1} \sim N(0,1); Y_v, ... \sim f_1 = N(\theta = 0.5, 1)\}$, we evaluate the efficiency of the policy (4.13). We employ the loss function $L(N(A), v) = E_v\{N(A) - v \mid N(A) \geq v\}$ regarding the stopping time $N_\theta(A)$ from (4.13) and the optimal stopping time $N_o(A) = \min\{n \geq 1 : SR_n^l \geq A\}$, where SR_n^l is given by (4.3). Applying the theoretical results by Pollak (1987) and Yakir (1995) leads to the estimated $E_\infty\{N_o(A)\} \simeq 1.3316A$. Running 15,000 repetitions of $N_\theta(A)$ at each point $A = 50$, $75, 100, ..., 550$ (with $v = \infty$) shows that the Monte Carlo estimator of $E_\infty\{N_\theta(A)\}/A$ behaves constantly and $E_\infty\{N_\theta(A)\}/A \simeq 1.3301$.

Fixing $B = 350$ and $B = 550$, we calculate the Monte Carlo estimators of $L(N_o(B/1.3316), v)$ and $L(N_\theta(B/1.3301), v)$ based on 15,000 repetitions of $N_o(B/1.3316)$ and $N_\theta(B/1.3301)$ at each point $v = 30, 40, 50, ...$ We depict the results of these simulations in Figure 4.6.

From these results we conclude that the proposed nonparametric method is asymptotically (as $A \to \infty$ and $v \to \infty$) optimal in the considered case.

5

Bayes Factor

5.1 Introduction

Over the years statistical science has developed two schools of thought as it applies to statistical inference. One school is termed frequentist methodology and the other school of thought is termed *Bayesian methodology*. There has been a decades-long debate between both schools of thought on the optimality and appropriateness of each other's approaches. The fundamental difference between the two schools of thought is philosophical in nature regarding the definition of probability, which ultimately one could argue is axiomatic in nature.

The frequentist approach denotes probability in terms of long run averages, e.g., the probability of getting heads when flipping a coin infinitely many times would be ½ given a fair coin. Inference within the frequentist context is based on the assumption that a given experiment is one realization of an experiment that could be repeated infinitely many times, e.g., the notion of the Type I error rate discussed earlier is that if we were to repeat the same experiment infinitely many times we would falsely reject the null hypothesis a fixed percentage of the time.

The *Bayesian approach* defines probability as a measure of an individual's objective view of scientific truth based on his or her current state of knowledge. The state of knowledge, given as a probability measure, is then updated through new observations. The Bayesian approach to inference is appealing as it treats uncertainty probabilistically through conditional distributions. In this framework, it is assumed that *a priori* information regarding the parameters of interest is available in order to weight the corresponding likelihood functions toward the prior beliefs via the use of *Bayes theorem*.

Although Bayesian procedures are increasingly popular, expressing accurate prior information can be difficult, particularly for nonstatisticians and/or in a multidimensional setting. In practice one may be tempted to use the underlying data in order to help determine the prior through estimation of the prior information. This mixed approach is usually referred to as *empirical Bayes* in the literature (e.g., Carlin and Louis, 2011).

We take the approach that the Bayesian, empirical Bayesian, and frequentist methods are useful and that in general there should not be much disagreement between the scientific conclusions that are drawn in the practical setting. Our ultimate goal is to provide a roadmap for tools that are efficient in a given setting. In general, Bayesian approaches are more computationally intensive than frequentist approaches. However, due to the advances in computing power, Bayesian methods have emerged as an increasingly effective and practical alternative to the corresponding frequentist methods. Perhaps, empirical Bayes methods somewhat bridge the gap between pure Bayesian and frequentist approaches.

This chapter provides a basic introduction to the Bayesian view on statistical testing strategies with a focus on Bayes factor–type principles.

As an introduction to the Bayesian approach, in contrast to frequentist methods, first consider the simple hypothesis test $H_0 : \theta = \theta_0$ versus $H_1 : \theta = \theta_1$, where the parameters θ_0 and θ_1 are known. Given an observed random sample $X = \{X_1, ..., X_n\}$, we can then construct the likelihood ratio test statistic $LR = f(X | \theta_1) / f(X | \theta_0)$ for the purpose of determining which hypothesis is more probable. (Although, in previous chapters, we used the notation $f(X; \theta)$ for displaying density functions, in this chapter we also state $f(X | \theta)$ as the density notation in order to be consistent with the Bayesian aspect that — "the data distribution is conditional on the parameter, where the parameter is a random variable with a prior distribution.") The decision-making procedure is to reject H_0 for large values of LR. In this case, the decision-making rule based on the likelihood ratio test is uniformly most powerful. Although this classical hypothesis testing approach has a long and celebrated history in the statistical literature and continues to be a favorite of practitioners, it can be applied straightforwardly only in the case of simple null and alternative hypotheses, i.e., when the parameter under the alternative hypothesis, θ_1, is known.

Various practical hypothesis testing problems involve scenarios where the parameter under the alternative θ_1 is unknown, e.g., testing the composite hypothesis $H_0 : \theta = \theta_0$ versus $H_1 : \theta \neq \theta_0$. In general, when the alternative parameter is unknown, the parametric likelihood ratio test is not applicable, since it is not well defined. When a hypothesis is composite, Neyman and Pearson suggested replacing the density at a single parameter value with the maximum of the density over all parameters in that hypothesis. As a result of this groundbreaking theory the maximum likelihood ratio test became a key method in statistical inference (see Chapter 3).

It should be noted that several criticisms pertaining to the maximum likelihood ratio test may be made. First, in a decision-making process, we do not generally need to estimate the unknown parameters under H_0 or H_1. We just need to make a binary decision regarding whether to reject or not to reject the null hypothesis. Another criticism is that in practice we rely on the function $f(X | \hat{\theta})$ in place of $f(X | \theta)$, which technically does not yield a likelihood function, i.e., it is not a proper density function. Therefore, the maximum likelihood ratio test may lose efficiency as compared to the likelihood ratio test of interest (see details in Chapters 3 and 4).

Alternatively, one can provide testing procedures by substituting the unknown alternative parameter by variables that do not depend on the observed data (see details in Chapter 4). Such approaches can be extended to provide test procedures within a Bayes factor type framework. We can integrate test statistics through variables that represent the unknown parameters with respect to a function commonly called the *prior* distribution. This approach can be generalized to more complicated hypotheses and models.

A formal Bayesian concept for analyzing the collected data X involves the specification of a prior distribution for all parameters of interest, say θ, denoted by $\pi(\theta)$, and a distribution for X, denoted by $\Pr(X|\theta)$. Then the *posterior distribution* of θ given the data X is

$$\Pr(\theta \mid X) = \frac{\Pr(X \mid \theta)\pi(\theta)}{\int \Pr(X \mid \theta)\pi(\theta)d\theta},$$

which provides a basis for performing formal Bayesian analysis. Note that *maximum likelihood estimation* (Chapter 3) in light of the posterior distribution function, where $\Pr(X|\theta)$ is expressed using the likelihood function based on X, has a simple interpretation as the mode of the posterior distribution, representing a value of the parameter θ that is "most likely" to have produced the data.

Consider an interesting example to illustrate advantages of the Bayesian methodology. Assume we observe a sample $X = \{X_1,...,X_n\}$ of iid data points from a density function $f(x|\theta)$, where θ is the parameter of interest. In order to define the posterior density

$$g(\theta \mid X) = \frac{\prod_{i=1}^{n} f(X_i \mid \theta)\pi(\theta)}{\int \prod_{i=1}^{n} f(X_i \mid \theta)\pi(\theta)d\theta},$$

a parametric form of $f(x|\theta)$ should be known. Let us relax this requirement by assuming that the distribution function F of X_1 is unknown, but $F \in \{F_1,...,F_T\}$, where $F_1,...,F_T$ have known parametric forms and correspond to density functions $f_1,...,f_T$, respectively. Then the posterior joint density function can be written as

$$g(\theta, k \mid X) = \frac{\prod_{i=1}^{n} f_k(X_i \mid \theta)\pi(\theta)G_k}{\sum_{k=1}^{T} G_k \int \prod_{i=1}^{n} f_k(X_i \mid \theta)\pi(\theta)d\theta},$$

where G_k denotes a prior probability weight regarding the event $F = F_k$. Suppose that, for simplicity, $F \in \{\text{Exp}(1/\theta), N(\theta, 1)\}$ and then using the posterior density function we can calculate the posterior probabilities p_1, p_2, p_3, and p_4 of $\{\theta \in (0.1, 0.2), k = 1\}$, $\{\theta \in (0.1, 0.2), k = 2\}$, $\{\theta \in (0.2, 0.25), k = 1\}$ and $\{\theta \in (0.2, 0.25), k = 2\}$, respectively. Assume that $p_1 > p_2$ and $p_3 < p_4$. Thus one can conclude that when $\theta \in (0.1, 0.2)$ we probably have the data from an exponential distribution, whereas when $\theta \in (0.2, 0.25)$ we probably have the data from a normal distribution. For different intervals of θ values we can "prefer" different forms of data distributions. In contrast, the common parametric frequentist approach suggests to fix one distribution function, fitting the data distribution, and to evaluate different values of θ.

We suggest that the reader who is interested in further details regarding Bayesian theory and its applications to consult the essential works of Berger (1985) and Carlin and Louis (2011).

In the following sections, we describe and explore topics regarding the use of Bayes factor principles. Under Bayes factor type statistical decision-making mechanisms, external information is incorporated into the evaluation of evidence about a hypothesis and functions that represent possible parameter values under the alternative hypothesis are considered. These functions can be interpreted in light of our current state of knowledge, such as belief where we would like to be most powerful with regard to the external, or prior information on the parameter of interest under the alternative hypothesis. For example, a physician may expect the median survival rate for a new compound to fall in a certain range with a given degree of probability. Without loss of generality, we focus on basic scenarios of testing that can be easily extended to more complicated situations of statistical decision-making procedures. In Section 5.2 we show an optimality property relative to using Bayes factor statistics for testing statistical hypotheses. In Section 5.3 we introduce Bayes factor principles in general scenarios, including considerations of the relevant computational aspects, asymptotic approximations, prior selection issues and we provide brief illustrations. In Section 5.4 we provide some remarks regarding a relationship between Bayesian (Bayes factor) and frequentist (*p-values*) strategies for statistical testing.

5.2 Integrated Most Powerful Tests

In Section 4.4.1.2 we studied the simple representative method, which can be easily extended by integrating test statistics through variables that represent unknown parameters with respect to a function that links the corresponding weights to the variables. This approach can be applied to develop Bayes factor type decision-making mechanisms that will be described formally below.

Without loss of generality, assume for the purpose of explanation that we have a sample $X = \{X_1, ..., X_n\}$ and are interested in the composite hypothesis $H_0 : \theta = \theta_0$ versus $H_1 : \theta \neq \theta_0$. Frequentist statistics are operationalized solely by the use of sample information (the data obtained from the statistical investigation) in terms of making inferences about θ, without in general employing prior knowledge of the parameter space (i.e., the set of all possible values of the unknown parameter). On the other hand, in decision-making processes attempts are made to combine the sample information with other relevant facets of the problem in order to make an optimal decision.

Typically, two sorts of external information are relevant to Bayesian methodologies. The first source of information is a set of rules regarding the possible cost of any given decision. Usually this information, referred to as the loss function, can be quantified by determining the incurred loss for each possible decision as a function of θ. The second source of information can be termed prior information, that is, prior belief (weights) on the possible values of θ being true under the alternative hypothesis across the parameter space. This is information about the parameter of interest, θ, that is obtained from sources other than the statistical investigation, e.g., information comes from past experience about similar situations involving a similar parameter of interest; see Berger (1980) for more details in terms of *eliciting prior* information. In the clinical trial setting, one may for example gain insight into the behavior of the process in the early phases of clinical investigations and can then apply this information to the later phases of investigation.

More formally, let $\pi(\theta)$ represent our level of belief (probability based weights) for the likely values of θ under the alternative hypothesis satisfying $\int \pi(\theta) d\theta = 1$. One can extend the technique of Section 4.4.1.2 in order to propose the test statistic

$$B_n = \frac{\int f_{H_1}(X_1, ..., X_n \mid \theta) \pi(\theta) d\theta}{f_{H_0}(X_1, ..., X_n \mid \theta_0)},$$

where f_{H_1}, f_{H_0} denote the joint density functions of $\{X_1, ..., X_n\}$ under H_1 and H_0 respectively. The decision rule is to reject the null hypothesis for large values of the test statistic.

It turns out that $(B_n, \mathfrak{I}_n = \sigma(X_1, ..., X_n))$ is an H_0-martingale, since

$$E_{H_0}\left(B_{n+1} \mid \mathfrak{I}_n\right) = \int E_{H_0}\left\{\frac{f_{H_1}(X_1,...,X_{n+1} \mid \theta)}{f_{H_0}(X_1,...,X_{n+1} \mid \theta_0)} \mid \mathfrak{I}_n\right\}\pi(\theta)\,d\theta$$

$$= \int E_{H_0}\left\{\frac{\displaystyle\prod_{i=1}^{n+1} f_{H_1}(X_i \mid X_1,...,X_{i-1},\theta)}{\displaystyle\prod_{i=1}^{n+1} f_{H_0}(X_i \mid X_1,...,X_{i-1},\theta_0)} \mid \mathfrak{I}_n\right\}\pi(\theta)\,d\theta$$

$$= \int \frac{\displaystyle\prod_{i=1}^{n} f_{H_1}(X_i \mid X_1,...,X_{i-1},\theta)}{\displaystyle\prod_{i=1}^{n} f_{H_0}(X_i \mid X_1,...,X_{i-1},\theta_0)} E_{H_0}\left\{\frac{f_{H_1}(X_{n+1} \mid X_1,...,X_n,\theta)}{f_{H_0}(X_{n+1} \mid X_1,...,X_n,\theta_0)} \mid \mathfrak{I}_n\right\}\pi(\theta)\,d\theta$$

$$= \int \frac{\displaystyle\prod_{i=1}^{n} f_{H_1}(X_i \mid X_1,...,X_{i-1},\theta)}{\displaystyle\prod_{i=1}^{n} f_{H_0}(X_i \mid X_1,...,X_{i-1},\theta_0)} \left\{\int \frac{f_{H_1}(u \mid X_1,...,X_n,\theta)}{f_{H_0}(u \mid X_1,...,X_n,\theta_0)} f_{H_0}(u \mid X_1,...,X_n,\theta_0)\,du\right\}\pi(\theta)\,d\theta$$

$$= \int \frac{\displaystyle\prod_{i=1}^{n} f_{H_1}(X_i \mid X_1,...,X_{i-1},\theta)}{\displaystyle\prod_{i=1}^{n} f_{H_0}(X_i \mid X_1,...,X_{i-1},\theta_0)}\pi(\theta)\,d\theta = B_n.$$

Thus, according to Section 4.4.1, we can anticipate that the test statistic B_n can be optimal. This is displayed in the following result: the decision rule based on B_n provides the ***integrated most powerful test with respect to the function*** $\pi(\theta)$.

Proof. Taking into account the inequality $(A - B)\{I(A \geq B) - \delta\} \geq 0$, where δ could be either 0 or 1, described in Section 3.4, we define $A = B_n$ and $B = C$ (C is a test threshold: the event $\{B_n > C\}$ implies one should reject H_0), and δ represents a rejection rule for *any* test statistic based on the observations; if $\delta = 1$ we reject the null hypothesis. Then it follows that

$$E_{H_0}\{B_n I(B_n \geq C)\} - C E_{H_0}\{I(B_n \geq C)\} \geq E_{H_0}(B_n \delta - C\delta),$$

$$E_{H_0}\{B_n I(B_n \geq C)\} - C \Pr{}_{H_0}(B_n \geq C) \geq E_{H_0}(B_n\delta) - C \Pr{}_{H_0}(\delta = 1).$$

Since we control the Type I error rate of the tests to be $\Pr\{\text{Test rejects } H_0 \mid H_0\} = \alpha$, we have

$$E_{H_0}\{B_n I(B_n \geq C)\} \geq E_{H_0}(B_n\delta).$$

Thus

$$\int\cdots\int \frac{\int f_{H_1}(u_1,...,u_n \mid \theta)\pi(\theta)\,d\theta}{f_{H_0}(u_1,...,u_n \mid \theta_0)} f_{H_0}(u_1,...,u_n \mid \theta_0)I(B_n \geq C)\,du_1\cdots du_n$$

$$\geq \int \cdots \int \frac{\int f_{H_1}(u_1,...,u_n \mid \theta)\pi(\theta)d\theta}{f_{H_0}(u_1,...,u_n \mid \theta_0)} f_{H_0}(u_1,...,u_n \mid \theta_0)\delta(u_1,...,u_n)du_1 \cdots du_n.$$

That is,

$$\int \left\{ \int \cdots \int f_{H_1}(u_1,...,u_n \mid \theta)I(B_n \geq C)du_1 \cdots du_n \right\}\pi(\theta)d\theta$$

$$\geq \int \left\{ \int \cdots \int f_{H_1}(u_1,...,u_n \mid \theta)I(\delta(u_1,...,u_n)=1)du_1 \cdots du_n \right\}\pi(\theta)d\theta.$$

This concludes with

$$\int \Pr\{B_n \text{ rejects } H_0 \mid H_1 \text{ with the alternative parameter } \theta=\theta_1\}\pi(\theta_1)\theta_1$$

$$\geq \int \Pr\{\delta \text{ rejects } H_0 \mid H_1 \text{ with the alternative parameter } \theta=\theta_1\}\pi(\theta_1)\theta_1,$$

completing the proof.

Note that the definition of the test statistic B_n corresponding to the point null hypothesis $\theta = \theta_0$ is widely addressed in the Bayesian statistical literature, e.g., Berger (1985, pp. 148–150, Equation 4.15), Bernardo and Smith (1994, pp. 391–392), and Kass (1993).

Following this result, we can reconsider $\pi(\theta)$ with respect to the area under which it would yield the most powerful decision-making rule. For example, if $\pi(\theta) = I\{\theta \in [G_1, G_2]\} / (G_2 - G_1)$, $G_2 > G_1$, where $I\{\cdot\}$ is the indicator function, then B_n will provide the integrated most powerful test with respect to the interval $[G_1, G_2]$. The values of G_1 and G_2 can be set up based on the practical meaning of the parameter θ under the alternative hypothesis.

Remark. The function $\pi(\theta)$ can be chosen in a conservative fashion, oftentimes known as a *flat prior*, or it can be chosen in an anti-conservative fashion such that we put more weight on a narrow range of values for θ or it can be chosen anywhere between. The benefit of the anti-conservative approach is that if our prior belief about the location of θ is corroborated by the observed data values we have a very powerful decision rule. In general, the following principles can be considered: (1) the function $\pi(\theta)$ depicts our belief on how good values of θ represent the unknown parameter, weighting the θ values over the corresponding range of the parameter; (2) $\pi(\theta)$ provides a functional form of the prior information; and (3) the function $\pi(\theta)$ can be chosen depending on the area under which we would like to obtain the most powerful decision rule by virtue of the result regarding the integrated most powerful property of the Bayes factor based test statistics shown above. We also refer the reader to Section 5.3.2 for more details regarding the choice of $\pi(\theta)$.

5.3 Bayes Factor

The Bayesian approach for hypothesis testing was developed by Jeffreys (1935, 1961) as a major part of his program for scientific theory. A large statistical literature has been devoted to the development of Bayesian methods on various testing problems. The **Bayes factor**, as the centerpiece in Bayesian evaluation of evidence, closely integrates human thought processes of decision-making mechanisms into formal statistical tests. In a probabilistic manner, the Bayes factor efficiently combines information about a parameter based on data (or likelihood) with prior knowledge about the parameter.

Assume that the data, X, have arisen from one of the two hypotheses H_0 and H_1 according to a probability density $\Pr(X|H_0)$ or $\Pr(X|H_1)$. Given *a priori* (prior) probabilities $\Pr(H_0)$ and $\Pr(H_1) = 1 - \Pr(H_0)$, the data produce *a posteriori* (posterior) probabilities of the form $\Pr(H_0|X)$ and $\Pr(H_1|X) = 1 - \Pr(H_0|X)$. Based on Bayes theorem, we then have

$$\frac{\Pr(H_1|X)}{\Pr(H_0|X)} = \frac{\Pr(X|H_1)}{\Pr(X|H_0)} \frac{\Pr(H_1)}{\Pr(H_0)}.$$

The transformation from the prior probability to the posterior probability is simply multiplication by

$$B_{10} = \frac{\Pr(X|H_1)}{\Pr(X|H_0)}, \tag{5.1}$$

which is named the **Bayes factor**. Therefore, **posterior odds** (odds = probability/ (1−probability)) is the product of the Bayes factor and the prior odds. In other words, the Bayes factor is the ratio of the posterior odds of H_1 to its prior odds, regardless of the value of the prior odds. When there are unknown parameters under either or both of the hypotheses, the densities $\Pr(X|H_k)$ ($(k = 0,1)$) can be obtained by integrating (not maximizing) over the parameter space, i.e.,

$$\Pr(X|H_k) = \int \Pr(X|\theta_k, H_k)\pi(\theta_k|H_k)d\theta_k, \; k = 0,1,$$

where θ_k is the parameter under H_k, $\pi(\theta_k|H_k)$ is its prior density, and $\Pr(X|\theta_k, H_k)$ is the probability density of X, given the value of θ_k, or the likelihood function of θ_k. Here θ_k may be a vector, and in what follows we will denote its dimension by d_k. When multiple hypotheses are involved, we denote B_{jk} as the Bayes factor for H_k versus H_j. In this case, as a common practice, one of the hypotheses is considered the null and is denoted by H_0. Kass and Raftery's (1995) outstanding paper provided helpful details related to the Bayes factor mechanisms.

5.3.1 The Computation of Bayes Factors

Bayes factors involve computation of integrals usually solved via numerical methods. Many integration techniques have been adapted to problems of Bayesian inference, including the computation of Bayes factors.

Define the density (integral) in the numerator or the denominator of the Bayes factor described in Equation (5.1) as

$$I = \Pr(X \mid H) = \int \Pr(X \mid \theta, H)\pi(\theta \mid H)d\theta.$$

For simplicity and for ease of exposition, the subscript k $(k = 0, 1)$ as the hypothesis indicator is eliminated in the notation H here.

In some cases, the density (integral) I may be evaluated analytically. For example, an exact analytic evaluation of the integral I is possible for exponential family distributions with *conjugate priors*, including normal linear models (DeGroot, 2005; Zellner, 1996). Exact analytic evaluation is best in the sense of accuracy and computational efficiency, but it is only feasible for a narrow class of models.

More often, numerical integration, also called "quadrature," is required when the analytic evaluation of the integral I is intractable. Generally, most relevant software is inefficient and of little use for the computation of these integrals. One reason is that when sample sizes are moderate or large, the integrand becomes *highly peaked* around its maximum, which may be found more efficiently by other techniques. In this instance, general purpose quadrature methods that do not incorporate knowledge of the likely maximum are likely to have difficulty finding the region where the integrand mass is accumulating. In order to demonstrate this intuitively, we first show that an important approximation of the log-likelihood function is based on a quadratic function of the parameter, e.g., θ. We do not attempt a general proof but provide a brief outline in the unidimensional case. Suppose the log-likelihood function $l(\theta)$ is three times differentiable. Informally, consider a Taylor approximation to the log-likelihood function $l(\theta)$ of second order around the *maximum likelihood estimator* (MLE) $\hat{\theta}$, that is,

$$l(\theta) \approx l(\hat{\theta}) + (\theta - \hat{\theta})l'(\hat{\theta}) + \frac{(\theta - \hat{\theta})^2}{2!}l''(\hat{\theta}).$$

Note that at the MLE $\hat{\theta}$, the first derivative of the log-likelihood function $l'(\hat{\theta}) = 0$. Thus, in the neighborhood of the MLE $\hat{\theta}$, the log-likelihood function $l(\theta)$ can be expressed in the form

$$l(\theta) \approx l(\hat{\theta}) + \frac{(\theta - \hat{\theta})^2}{2!} l''(\hat{\theta}).$$

(We required that $l'''(\theta)$ exists, since the remainder term of the approximation above consists of a l''' component.) The following example provides some intuition about the quadratic approximation of the log-likelihood function.

Example

Let $X = \{X_1, ..., X_n\}$ denote a random sample from a gamma distribution with unknown shape parameter θ and known scale parameter κ_0. The density function of the gamma distribution is

$f(x; \theta, \kappa_0) = x^{\theta-1} \exp(-x/\kappa_0)/(\Gamma(\theta)\kappa_0^\theta)$, where the gamma function

$\Gamma(\theta) = \int_0^\infty t^{\theta-1} \exp(-t) dt$. The log-likelihood function of θ is

$$l(\theta) = (\theta - 1) \sum_{i=1}^n \log(X_i) - n \log(\Gamma(\theta)) - n\theta \log(\kappa_0) - \sum_{i=1}^n X_i / \kappa_0.$$

The first and the second derivatives of the log-likelihood function are

$$l'(\theta) = -n\Gamma'(\theta)/\Gamma(\theta) + \sum_{i=1}^n \log(X_i) - n\log(\kappa_0),$$

$$l''(\theta) = -n\frac{d^2}{d\theta^2}\log(\Gamma(\theta)) = n\int_0^1 \frac{t^{\theta-1}\log(t)}{1-t}dt < 0,$$

respectively. In this case, there is no closed-form solution of the MLE of the shape parameter θ, which can be found by solving $l'(\hat{\theta}) = 0$ numerically. Correspondingly, the value of the second derivative of the log-likelihood function at the MLE $l''(\hat{\theta})$ can be computed. Figure 5.1 presents the plot of log-likelihood (solid line) and its quadratic approximation (dashed line) versus values of the shape parameter θ based on samples of sample sizes $n = 10$, 25, 35, 50 from a gamma distribution with the true shape parameter of $\theta = \theta_0 = 2$ and a known scale parameter $\kappa_0 = 2$. It is obvious from Figure 5.1 that as the sample size n increases, the quadratic approximation to the log-likelihood function $l(\theta)$ performs better in the neighborhood of the MLE of θ.

Implementation of Figure 5.1 is shown in the following R code:

```
> n.seq<-c(10,25,35,50)
> N<-max(n.seq)
```

```
> shape0<-2
> scale0<-2
> X<-rgamma(N,shape=shape0,scale = scale0)
>
> #  Quadratic approximation to the log-likelihood function
> par(mar=c(3.5, 4, 3.5, 1),mfrow=c(2,2),mgp=c(2,1,0))
> for (n in n.seq){
+    x<-X[sample(1:N,n,replace=FALSE)]
+    # log-likelihood as a function of the shape parameter theta
+    loglike<-function(theta) (theta-1)*sum(log(x))-n*log(gamma(theta))-n*theta
*log(scale0)-sum(x)/scale0
+    neg.loglike<-function(theta)-loglike(theta)
+
+    # the first derivative of loglikelihoodlog
+    loglike.D<-function(theta) sum(log(x)) - n*digamma(theta)-n*log(scale0)
+    # the second derivative of log-likelihood
+    loglike.DD<-function(theta)  -n*trigamma(theta)
+
+    # one-dimensional optimization that maximize log-likelihood with respect to
the shape parameter
+    init<-mean(x)^2/var(x)   # set initial value
+    theta.mle<-optim(init,neg.loglike,method="L-BFGS-B", lower=init-6*(-loglike.
DD(init)^(-1/2))/sqrt(n), upper=init+6*(-loglike.DD(init)^(-1/2))/sqrt(n))$par
+
+    loglike.DD.mle <- loglike.DD(theta.mle) # second derivative at MLE
+
+    # approximation of the log-likelihood
+    loglike.est<-function(theta) loglike(theta.mle)+loglike.DD.mle*((theta-theta.
mle)^2)/2
+
+    # plot: the plotting limit of x-axis
+    tc<-theta.mle
+    rg<-6*((-loglike.DD.mle)^(-1/2) )/sqrt(n)   # half range
+
+    # plot the true log-likehood
+    plot(Vectorize(loglike),c(tc-rg,tc+rg),xlim=c(tc-rg,tc+rg),type="l",lty=1,
lwd=2,cex.lab=1.2,xlab=expression(theta),ylab=expression(paste("Log-likeli-
hood( ",theta,")")), main=paste0("n=",n))
+    # plot the approximation to the log-likehood
+    curve(loglike.est,from=tc-rg,to=tc+rg,type="l",lty=2,lwd=2,add=TRUE,col=
2)
+    lines(c(theta.mle,theta.mle), c(-1e+5,loglike(theta.mle)),lty=3)
+ }
>
```

It can be easily shown that the log-likelihood function $l(\theta)$ is highly peaked near the MLE $\hat{\theta}$, e.g., in the case of large samples. In such cases, the posterior density function $\Pr(\theta|X)$ is highly peaked about its maximum $\tilde{\theta}$, that is, the posterior mode ("generalized MLE"), at which the log posterior is maximized and has slope zero. Assume that $\tilde{\theta}$ exists and the prior $\pi(\theta)$ (positive), as well as the log-likelihood function $l(\theta)$, are three times differentiable near the posterior mode $\tilde{\theta}$. Then the posterior density $\Pr(\theta|X)$ for a large sample size n can be approximated by a normal distribution with mean $\tilde{\theta}$ and covariance matrix $\tilde{\Sigma} = (\mathbf{I}\tilde{l}(\tilde{\theta}))^{-1}$, where the "generalized" observed *Fisher information* matrix $\mathbf{I}\tilde{l}(\tilde{\theta}) = -\mathbf{H}\tilde{l}(\tilde{\theta})$, i.e., minus the *Hessian*

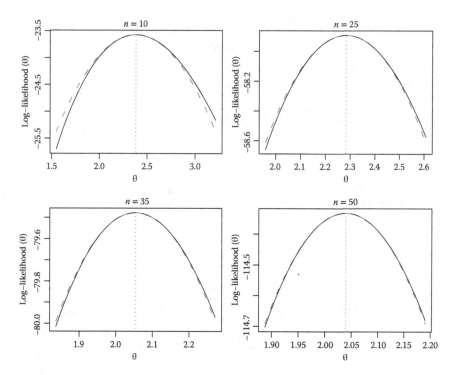

FIGURE 5.1

The plot of log-likelihood (solid line) and its quadratic approximation (dashed line) versus the shape parameter θ based on samples of sizes $n = 10, 25, 35, 50$ from a gamma distribution with the true shape parameter of $\theta = \theta_0 = 2$ and the known scale parameter 2.

matrix (second derivative matrix) of the log-posterior evaluated at $\tilde{\theta}$. Consequently, in such cases, for relatively large sample size n, the Bayes factor is approximately equivalent to the maximum likelihood ratio (for details, see the analysis shown below). In addition, the asymptotic distribution of the posterior mode depends on the Fisher information and not on the prior (Le Cam, 1986). Intuitively and consistent with the Bayesian concept, when the sample size n is relatively large, the impact of prior information has less effect on the form of the Bayes factor, i.e., large amounts of data minimize the weights of the prior knowledge in terms of the actual behavior of the likelihood function, since large data provide so much information that we do not need any prior knowledge.

For ease of exposition, and in an intuitive manner, we outline the proof of the normal approximation, considering a unidimensional case. Denote the log nonnormalized posterior

$$\tilde{l}(\theta) = \log(h(\theta)), \quad \text{where} \quad h(\theta) = \Pr(X \mid \theta, H)\pi(\theta \mid H).$$

Similar to the way of obtaining the approximation to the log-likelihood function, applying a Taylor expansion of $\tilde{l}(\theta)$ of second order at the posterior mode $\tilde{\theta}$, we have

$$\Pr(\theta \mid X) \propto \Pr(X \mid \theta, H)\pi(\theta \mid H) = \exp(\tilde{l}(\theta)) \approx \exp\{\tilde{l}(\tilde{\theta}) + \tilde{l}''(\tilde{\theta})(\theta - \tilde{\theta})^2/2\},$$

where $\propto$ represents "proportionality." Note that the posterior mode always lies between the peak of the prior and that of the likelihood, because it combines information from the prior density and the likelihood. This posterior density approximation technique is often referred to as the modal approximation because θ is estimated by the posterior mode.

For relatively large samples the choice of the prior density is generally not that relevant, and in fact the prior $\pi(\theta)$ might be ignored in the above derivation. Generally speaking, relatively large data provide so much information that we do not need any prior knowledge. In such cases, the posterior mode $\tilde{\theta}$ is replaced by the MLE $\hat{\theta}$ and the generalized observed Fisher information is replaced by the observed Fisher information $-l''(\hat{\theta})$. Then $\tilde{l}''(\tilde{\theta})(\theta - \tilde{\theta})^2 = \left\{n^{1/2}\left(\theta - \tilde{\theta}\right)\right\}^2 \tilde{l}''(\tilde{\theta})/n \approx \left\{n^{1/2}\left(\theta - \hat{\theta}\right)\right\}^2 l''(\theta)/n \sim \text{Normal}$, provided that θ is a true fixed value of the parameter (see Chapter 3). In this scenario, since $\tilde{\theta}$ maximizes $\tilde{l}(\theta)$, i.e., $\tilde{l}'(\tilde{\theta}) = 0$, the Taylor argument applied to $\tilde{l}'(\tilde{\theta})$ shows that

$$0 = \frac{d}{d\theta}\tilde{l}(\theta)\Big|_{\theta=\tilde{\theta}} = l'(\hat{\theta}) + \frac{d}{d}\{\log(\pi(\theta))\}\Big|_{\theta=\hat{\theta}} + \left(\tilde{\theta} - \hat{\theta}\right)\frac{d^2}{d\theta^2}\tilde{l}(\theta)\Big|_{\theta=\breve{\theta}}, \quad \text{with} \quad l'(\hat{\theta}) = 0$$

and then

$$\tilde{\theta} = \hat{\theta} - \left[\frac{d}{d}\{\log(\pi(\theta))\}\Big|_{\theta=\hat{\theta}}\right]\left\{\frac{d^2}{d\theta^2}\tilde{l}(\theta)\Big|_{\theta=\breve{\theta}}\right\}^{-1} = \hat{\theta} + o_p(1),$$

where $\breve{\theta} \in \left(\hat{\theta}, \tilde{\theta}\right)$ and $\frac{d^2}{d\theta^2}\tilde{l}(\theta)\Big|_{\theta=\breve{\theta}} = O_p(n)$ as a sum of random variables. This may also be considered a case where frequentist and Bayesian methods align in some regards.

It is interesting to note that asymptotic arguments similar to those shown above and in the forthcoming sections can also be employed to compare the Bayesian and *empirical Bayesian* concepts (Petrone et al., 2014).

The fact that some problems are of high dimension may also lead to intractable analytic evaluation of integrals. In this case Monte Carlo methods may be used, but these too need to be adapted to the statistical context. Bleistein and Handelsman (1975) as well as Evans and Swartz (1995) reviewed various numerical integration strategies for evaluating integral I. In this chapter we outline several techniques available to evaluate the Bayes factor, including the asymptotic approximation method, the simple Monte Carlo technique, importance sampling, and Gaussian quadrature strategies, as well as approaches based on generating samples from the posterior distributions. For general discussion and references, see, e.g., Kass and Raftery (1995) and Han and Carlin (2001).

5.3.1.1 Asymptotic Approximations

(1) Laplace's method. The Laplace approximation (De Bruijn, 1970; Tierney and Kadane, 1986) to the marginal density $I = \Pr(X \mid H) = \int \Pr(X \mid \theta, H)\pi(\theta \mid H)d\theta$ of the data is obtained by approximating the posterior with a normal distribution. It is assumed that the posterior density, which is proportional to the nonnormalized posterior $h(\theta) = \Pr(X \mid \theta, H)\pi(\theta \mid H)$, is highly peaked about its maximum $\tilde{\theta}$, the posterior mode. This assumption will usually be satisfied if the likelihood function $\Pr(X \mid \theta, H)$ is highly peaked near its maximum $\hat{\theta}$, e.g., in the case of large samples. Denote $\tilde{l}(\theta) = \log(h(\theta))$. Expanding $\tilde{l}(\theta)$ as a quadratic about $\tilde{\theta}$ and then exponentiating the resulting expansion yields an approximation to $h(\theta)$ that has the form of a normal density with mean $\tilde{\theta}$ and covariance matrix $\tilde{\Sigma} = (-\mathbf{H}\tilde{l}(\tilde{\theta}))^{-1}$, where $\mathbf{H}\tilde{l}(\tilde{\theta})$ is the Hessian matrix of second derivatives of the log-posterior evaluated at $\tilde{\theta}$. More specifically, component-wise, $\mathbf{H}\tilde{l}(\tilde{\theta})_{ij} = \left[\dfrac{\partial^2 \log \tilde{l}(\theta)}{\partial \theta_i \partial \theta_j} \right]_{\theta = \tilde{\theta}}$. Integrating the approximation to $h(\theta)$ with respect to θ yields

$$\hat{I}_L = (2\pi)^{d/2} \mid \tilde{\Sigma} \mid^{1/2} \Pr(X \mid \tilde{\theta}, H)\pi(\tilde{\theta} \mid H),$$

where d is the dimension of θ. Under conditions specified by Kass et al. (1990), it can be derived that $I = \hat{I}_L(1 + O(n^{-1}))$ as $n \to \infty$, that is, the relative error of Laplace's approximation to I is $O(n^{-1})$. Therefore when Laplace's method is applied to both the numerator and denominator of B_{10} in Equation 5.1, the resulting approximation leads to a relative error of order $O(n^{-1})$.

Laplace's method yields accurate approximations and is often computationally efficient. By employing Laplace's methods, one can show that the asymptotic properties of Bayes factor type procedures based on data are close to those based on *maximum-likelihood estimation* methods.

(2) Variants on Laplace's method. Laplace's method may be applied in alternative forms by omitting part of the integrand from the exponent when

performing the expansion. (For the general formulation, see Kass and Vaidyanathan (1992), which followed Tierney et al. (1989).) An important variant on the approximation $\hat{I}$ to I is

$$\hat{I}_{\text{MLE}} = (2\pi)^{d/2} \, |\hat{\Sigma}|^{1/2} \, \Pr(X \,|\, \hat{\theta}, H) \pi(\hat{\theta} \,|\, H),$$

where $\hat{\Sigma}^{-1}$ is the observed information matrix, that is, the negative Hessian matrix of the log-likelihood evaluated at the maximum likelihood estimator $\hat{\theta}$. This approximation again has relative error of order $O(n^{-1})$.

Define G to be the set of all possibilities that satisfy hypothesis H, and G' to be the set of all possibilities that satisfy hypothesis H'. We will call H' a *nested hypothesis* within H if $G' \subset G$.

Consider nested hypotheses, where there must be some parameterization under H_1 of the form $\theta = (\beta, \psi)^T$ such that H_0 is obtained from H_1 when $\psi = \psi_0$ for some ψ_0, with parameter (β, ψ) having prior $\pi(\beta, \psi)$ under H_1 and then $H_0 : \psi = \psi_0$ with prior $\pi(\beta \,|\, H_0)$. For instance, it is desired to check whether or not the collected data, denoted by X, could be described as a random sample from some normal distribution with mean μ_0, assuming that they may be described as a random sample from some normal distribution with unknown mean μ and unknown variance σ^2. In this case, notation-wise, $\psi_0 = \mu_0$, $\psi = \mu$, and $\beta = \sigma^2$.

Applying the approximation $\hat{I}_{\text{MLE}}$, one can show that

$$2 \log B_{10} \approx \Lambda + \log \pi(\hat{\beta}, \hat{\psi} \,|\, H_1) - \log \pi(\hat{\beta}^*, H_0) + (d_1 - d_0) \log(2\pi) + \log |\hat{\Sigma}_1| - \log |\hat{\Sigma}_0|,$$

where $\Lambda = 2 \left\{ \log \left(\Pr(X \,|\, (\hat{\beta}, \hat{\psi}), H_1) \right) - \log \left(\Pr(X \,|\, \hat{\beta}^*, H_0) \right) \right\}$ is the log-likelihood ratio statistic having approximately a chi-squared distribution with degrees of freedom $(d_1 - d_0)$, a difference between the numbers of the estimated parameters under H_1 and H_0, and $\hat{\beta}^*$ denotes the MLE under H_0. Here the covariance matrices $\hat{\Sigma}_k$ could be either observed or expected information, under which case the approximation of $2 \log B_{10}$ has relative error of order $O(n^{-1})$ or $O(n^{-1/2})$, respectively. For more information, we refer the reader to Kass and Raftery (1995).

Alternatively, we may consider the following MLE-based approach. We do not attempt a general proof but we instead provide an informal outline for the unidimensional case when regarding parameter θ we have the hypothesis $H_0 : \theta = \theta_0$ versus $H_1 : \theta \neq \theta_0$, where θ_0 is known. Note that in a Bayesian context, we are interested in testing for the model, where θ has a degenerate prior distribution with mass at θ_0 versus the model that states θ has a prior distribution $\pi(\theta)$. Recall that the log-likelihood ratio function $lr(\theta) = l(\theta) - l(\theta_0)$ attains its maximum at the MLE $\hat{\theta}$, satisfying $l'(\hat{\theta}) = 0$, and the likelihood function $l(\theta)$ increases up to the MLE $\hat{\theta}$ and decreases afterward. Define $\phi_n = c/n^{1/2-\gamma}$, where c is a constant and $\gamma < 1/6$. Then the marginal ratio (e.g., see the test statistic B_n defined in Section 5.2 when the observations are iid) can be divided into three components:

$$B_n = I / \exp(l(\theta_0)) = \int_{-\infty}^{\infty} \exp(lr(\theta))\pi(\theta)d\theta = I_1 + I_2 + \int_{\hat{\theta}-\phi_n}^{\hat{\theta}+\phi_n} \exp(lr(\theta))\pi(\theta)d\theta,$$

where $I_1 = \int_{-\infty}^{\hat{\theta}-\phi_n} \exp(lr(\theta))\pi(\theta)d\theta$ and $I_2 = \int_{\hat{\theta}+\phi_n}^{\infty} \exp(lr(\theta))\pi(\theta)d\theta$. We first consider the component I_1. Based on the fact that the log-likelihood ratio function $l(\theta)$ is a nondecreasing function of θ for $\theta \in (-\infty, \hat{\theta}-\phi_n)$ and that $lr(\hat{\theta}-\phi_n) \to -\infty$, under the null hypothesis, as $n \to \infty$, it can be derived that

$$I_1 \leq \exp(lr(\hat{\theta}-\phi_n)) \int_{-\infty}^{\infty} \pi(\theta)d\theta = \exp(lr(\hat{\theta}-\phi_n)) \to 0, \quad \text{as} \quad n \to \infty,$$

since the Taylor arguments can provide

$$lr(\hat{\theta}-\phi_n) \approx lr(\hat{\theta}) - \phi_n lr'(\hat{\theta}) + \phi_n^2 lr''(\hat{\theta})/2! = lr(\hat{\theta}) + \phi_n^2 lr''(\hat{\theta})/2$$

(here ϕ_n is considered around 0), where, under H_0, $2lr(\hat{\theta})$ has approximately a chi-squared distribution with one degree of freedom and

$$\phi_n^2 lr''(\hat{\theta}) = -n^{2\gamma}\left\{-lr''(\hat{\theta})\right\}/n \approx -n^{2\gamma}\left\{-lr''(\theta_0) - \left(\hat{\theta}-\theta_0\right)lr'''(\theta_0)\right\}/n$$

$$= -n^{2\gamma}|O_p(1)| \to -\infty$$

(here $\hat{\theta}$ is considered around θ_0) with $\left(\hat{\theta}-\theta\right) \to 0$ and $lr''(\theta_0) \sim n$, $lr'''(\theta_0) \sim n$; $lr''(\theta_0), lr'''(\theta_0)$ are sums of iid random variables.

This behavior is similar for the component I_2, since the log-likelihood function $l(\theta)$ is a non-increasing function of θ for $\theta \in (\hat{\theta}+\phi_n, \infty)$ and $lr(\hat{\theta}+\phi_n) \to -\infty$, under the null hypothesis, as $n \to \infty$, we have

$$I_2 \leq \exp(lr(\hat{\theta}+\phi_n)) \int_{-\infty}^{\infty} \pi(\theta)d\theta = \exp(lr(\hat{\theta}+\phi_n)) \to 0, \quad \text{as} \quad n \to \infty.$$

Therefore, we have that the Bayes factor $B_n = I / \exp(l(\theta_0))$ satisfies approximately

$$I / \exp(l(\theta_0)) \approx \int_{\hat{\theta}-\phi_n}^{\hat{\theta}+\phi_n} \exp(lr(\theta))\pi(\theta)d\theta, \quad \text{as} \quad n \to \infty.$$

In this approximation,

$$lr(\theta) = l(\theta) - l(\theta_0) = l(\hat{\theta}) - l(\theta_0) + (\theta - \hat{\theta})l'(\hat{\theta}) + (\theta - \hat{\theta})^2 l''(\hat{\theta}) / 2 + R(\theta)$$

$$= l(\hat{\theta}) - l(\theta_0) + (\theta - \hat{\theta})^2 l''(\hat{\theta}) / 2 + R(\theta),$$

where the remainder term $R(\theta) = (\theta - \hat{\theta})^3 l'''(\bar{\theta}) / 6$, $\bar{\theta} \in \left(\theta, \hat{\theta}\right)$ satisfies $R(\theta) = O_p(\phi_n^3)O_p(n)$, $R(\theta) = O_p(n^{-1/2+3\gamma}) = o_p(1)$, when $\theta \in \left[\hat{\theta}-\phi_n, \hat{\theta}+\phi_n\right]$, $\phi_n = c/n^{1/2-\gamma}$ and $\gamma < 1/6$. Then we conclude with

$$I / \exp(l(\theta_0)) \approx \int_{\hat{\theta}-\phi_n}^{\hat{\theta}+\phi_n} \exp(l(\hat{\theta}) - l(\theta_0) + (\theta - \hat{\theta})^2 l''(\hat{\theta}) / 2)\pi(\theta)d\theta$$

$$\approx \exp(l(\hat{\theta}) - l(\theta_0)) \int \exp(-(\theta - \hat{\theta})^2(-l''(\hat{\theta})) / 2)\pi(\theta)d\theta,$$

where $\int \exp(-(\theta - \hat{\theta})^2(-l''(\hat{\theta})) / 2)\pi(\theta)d\theta$ is a **Gaussian-type integral**. This result can be easily applied to control asymptotically the Type I error rate of the test statistic $B_n = I / \exp(l(\theta_0))$ in the frequentist manner.

In a more formal manner, Vexler et al. (2014) used the asymptotic principle shown above for constructing and evaluating nonparametric Bayesian procedures, where the empirical likelihood method was employed instead of the parametric likelihood. (Regarding the empirical likelihood approach, see Chapter 10.)

(3) The Schwarz criterion. It is possible to avoid the introduction of the prior densities $\pi_k(\theta_k | H_k)$ in Equation (5.1) by using

$$S = \left\{\log \Pr(X | \hat{\theta}_1, H_1) - \log \Pr(X | \hat{\theta}_0, H_0)\right\} - \frac{1}{2}(d_1 - d_0)\log(n),$$

where $\hat{\theta}_k$ is the MLE under H_k, d_k is the dimension of θ_k, $k = 0, 1$ and n is the sample size. The second term in S acts as a penalty term that corrects for differences in dimension between H_k, $k = 0, 1$. The quantity S is often called the **Schwarz criterion**. The **Bayesian information criterion** (BIC) can be defined as minus twice the Schwarz criterion; sometimes an arbitrary constant is added. The BIC is a criterion for ***model selection*** among a finite set of models. In this case, the model with the lowest BIC is preferred (e.g., Carlin and Louis, 2011). Schwarz (1978) showed that, under certain assumptions on the data distribution,

$$\frac{S - \log B_{10}}{\log B_{10}} \to 0, \quad \text{as} \quad n \to \infty.$$

Thus, the quantity exp(S) provides a rough approximation to the Bayes factor that is independent of the priors on the θ_k. Kass and Wasserman (1995) provided excellent discussion regarding the method mentioned above.

The benefits of asymptotic approximations in this context include the following: (1) numerical integration is replaced with numerical differentiation, which is computationally more stable; (2) asymptotic approximations do not involve random numbers, and consequently, two different analysts can produce a common answer based on the same dataset, model, and prior distribution; and (3) in order to investigate the sensitivity of the result to modest changes in the prior or the likelihood function, the computational complexity is greatly reduced; for more detail, we refer the reader to Carlin and Louis (2011). Among the asymptotic approximations described above, the Schwarz criterion is the easiest approximation to compute and requires no specification of prior distributions. In addition, as long as the number of degrees of freedom involved in the comparison is reasonably small relative to sample size, the analysis based on the Schwarz criterion will not mislead in a qualitative sense.

However, asymptotic approximations also have the following limitations: (1) in order to obtain a valid approximation, the posterior distribution must be unimodal, or at least nearly unimodal; (2) the size of the dataset must be fairly large, while it is hard to judge how large is large enough; (3) the accuracy of asymptotic approximations cannot be improved without collecting additional data; (4) the correct parameterization, on which the accuracy of the approximation depends, e.g., θ versus $\log(\theta)$, may be difficult to ascertain; (5) when the dimension of θ is moderate or high, say, greater than 10, Laplace's method becomes unstable, and numerical computation of the associated Hessian matrices will be prohibitively difficult; and (6) when the number of degrees of freedom involved in the comparison is large and the prior is very different from that for which the approximation is best, the asymptotic approximation based on the Schwarz criterion can be very poor; e.g., McCulloch and Rossi (1991) illustrated the poor approximation by the Schwarz criterion with an example of 115 degrees of freedom. For more details, we refer the reader to, e.g., Kass and Raftery (1995) as well as Carlin and Louis (2011). Therefore, in such cases, researchers may turn to alternative methods, e.g., Monte Carlo sampling, importance sampling, and Gaussian quadrature. These methods typically require longer runtimes, but can be programmed easily and can be applied in more general scenarios, which are the subject of the following section in this chapter.

5.3.1.2 Simple Monte Carlo, Importance Sampling, and Gaussian Quadrature

Dropping the notational dependence on the hypothesis indicator H_k, the integral I becomes $I = \Pr(X) = \int \Pr(X \mid \theta)\pi(\theta)d\theta$. The *simplest Monte Carlo integration* estimate of I is

$$\hat{\Pr}_1(X) = \frac{1}{m} \sum_{i=1}^{m} \Pr(X \mid \theta^{(i)}),$$

where $\{\theta^{(i)} : i = 1, \ldots, m\}$ is a sample from the prior distribution; this is the average of the likelihoods of the sampled parameter values, e.g., Hammersley and Handscomb (1964)

The precision of simple Monte Carlo integration can be improved by *importance sampling*. It involves generating a sample $\{\theta^{(i)} : i = 1, \ldots, m\}$ from a density $\pi^*(\theta)$. Under general conditions, a simulation-consistent estimate of I is

$$\hat{I}_{MC} = \frac{\sum_{i=1}^{m} w_i \Pr(X \mid \theta^{(i)})}{\sum_{i=1}^{m} w_i},$$

where $w_i = \pi(\theta^{(i)}) / \pi^*(\theta^{(i)})$, the function $\pi^*(\theta)$ is known as the importance sampling function. Then the approximation of Bayes factor can be computed accordingly; for general discussion, see Geweke (1989). Although the Monte Carlo integration and importance sampling methods are less precise and more computationally demanding, they may be the only applicable methods in complex models.

Genz and Kass (1997) demonstrated the evaluation of integrals that are peaked around a dominant mode and provided an adaptive Gaussian quadrature method. This method is efficient especially when the dimensionality of the parameter space is modest.

5.3.1.3 Generating Samples from the Posterior

Several methods can be applied to generate samples from posterior distributions, including direct simulation and rejection sampling for the simplest cases. In more complex cases, **Markov chain Monte Carlo** (MCMC) methods (e.g., Smith and Roberts, 1993) particularly the Metropolis–Hastings algorithm and the Gibbs sampler, as well as the weighted likelihood bootstrap, provide general schemes.

These methods provide a sample approximately drawn from the posterior density $\Pr(\theta \mid X) = \Pr(X \mid \theta)\pi(\theta) / \Pr(X)$. Substituting into $\hat{I}_{MC}$ defined in Section 5.3.1.2 yields as an estimate for $\Pr(X)$,

$$\hat{\Pr}_2(X) = \left\{ \frac{1}{m} \sum_{i=1}^{m} \Pr(X \mid \theta^{(i)})^{-1} \right\}^{-1},$$

which is the harmonic mean of the likelihood values (Newton and Raftery, 1994). This converges almost surely to the correct value, $\Pr(X)$, as $m \to \infty$, but it does not generally satisfy a Gaussian central limit theorem. See Kass and Raftery (1995) for additional modifications and discussion. Note that the MCMC methods have not yet been applied in many demanding problems and may require large numbers of likelihood function evaluations, resulting in difficulty in some cases.

5.3.1.4 Combining Simulation and Asymptotic Approximations

DiCiccio et al. (1997) provided a simulation based version of Laplace's method using generated observations from the posterior distributions by employing Markov chain Monte Carlo or other techniques. Following the previous notations of $\tilde{\theta}$ and $\tilde{\Sigma}$ described in Section 5.3.1.1 (Laplace's method), let $\tilde{\theta}$ be the posterior mode and let covariance matrix $\tilde{\Sigma}$ be minus the inverse of the Hessian of the log-posterior evaluated at $\tilde{\theta}$. If no analytical form can be obtained, then $\tilde{\theta}$ and $\tilde{\Sigma}$ can be estimated via simulation. The normal approximation to the posterior is $\varphi(\cdot) = \varphi(\cdot; \tilde{\theta}, \tilde{\Sigma})$, where $\varphi(\cdot; \mu, \Sigma)$ denotes a normal density with mean vector μ and covariance matrix Σ. Let $B = \left\{ \theta \in \Theta : \| (\theta - \tilde{\theta})^T \tilde{\Sigma}^{-1} (\theta - \tilde{\theta}) \|^2 < \delta^2 \right\}$, which has volume $\upsilon = \delta^p \pi^{p/2} \mid \tilde{\Sigma}^{1/2} \mid / \Gamma(p/2 + 1)$, where $\Gamma(u) = \int_0^\infty t^{u-1} \exp(-t) dt$ and $a^T = [a_1 \cdots a_k]$, for a vector $a = \begin{bmatrix} a_1 \\ \vdots \\ a_k \end{bmatrix}$. Define $\Pr(B) = \int_B \Pr(\theta \mid X) d\theta$ and $\alpha = \int_B \varphi(u; \tilde{\theta} \tilde{\Sigma}) du$.

A modification of Laplace's method can be obtained that simply estimates the unknown value of the posterior probability density at the mode using the simulated probability assigned to a small region around the mode divided by its area. Observing that

$$I = \frac{\Pr(X \mid \tilde{\theta})\pi(\tilde{\theta})}{\Pr(\tilde{\theta} \mid X)} = \frac{\Pr(X \mid \tilde{\theta})\pi(\tilde{\theta})}{\varphi(\tilde{\theta})} \frac{\varphi(\tilde{\theta})}{\Pr(\tilde{\theta} \mid X)} \approx \frac{\Pr(X \mid \tilde{\theta})\pi(\tilde{\theta})}{\varphi(\tilde{\theta})} \frac{\alpha}{\Pr(B)},$$

the volume-corrected estimator has the form

$$\hat{I}_L^* = \frac{\Pr(X \mid \tilde{\theta})\pi(\tilde{\theta})}{\varphi(\tilde{\theta})} \frac{\alpha}{\hat{P}},$$

where $\hat{P}$ is the Monte Carlo estimate of $\Pr(B)$, that is, a proportion of the sampled values inside B. DiCiccio et al. (1997) demonstrated that the simulated version of Laplace's method with a local volume correction approximates the Bayes factor accurately, which is especially useful in the case of costly likelihood function evaluations.

The importance of sampling techniques can be modified by restricting them to small regions about the mode. To improve the accuracy of approximations, Laplace's method can be combined with the simple bridge sampling technique proposed by Meng and Wong (1996). For detailed information, we refer the reader to DiCiccio et al. (1997).

5.3.2 The Choice of Prior Probability Distributions

Implementation of Bayes factor approaches requires the specification of priors, as is the case in all Bayesian analysis. In principle, priors formally represent available external information, providing a way to combine other information about the values of the target parameter with the data.

Typically, prior distributions are specified based on information accumulated from past studies or from the opinions of subject-area experts. The *elicited prior* is a means of drawing information from subject-area experts, who have a great deal of information about the substantive question but are not involved in the model construction process, with the goal of constructing a probability structure that quantifies their specific knowledge and experiential intuition about the studied effects.

In order to simplify the subsequent computational burden, e.g., make computation of the posterior distribution easier, experimenters often limit the choice of priors by restricting $\pi(\theta)$ to some familiar distributional family. In choosing a prior belonging to a specific distributional family, some choices may have more computational advantages than others. In particular, if the prior probability distribution $\pi(\theta)$ is in the same distributional family as the resulting posterior distribution $\Pr(\theta \mid X)$, then the prior and posterior are called *conjugate distributions*, and the prior is called a *conjugate prior* for the likelihood function. For example, the Gaussian family is conjugate to itself (or self-conjugate) with respect to a Gaussian likelihood function. That is, if the likelihood function is Gaussian, choosing a Gaussian prior over the mean will guarantee the Gaussian posterior distribution.

Often in practice, there is no reliable prior information regarding θ that exists, or it is desired to make an inference based solely on the data. In such cases, the *noninformative prior* plays a major role in Bayesian analyses.

A noninformative prior can be constructed by some formal rule that contains "no information" with respect to θ in the sense that no one θ value is favored over another, provided all values are logically possible. The simplest and oldest rule to determine a noninformative prior is the principle of indifference, which assigns equal probabilities to all possibilities. Noninformative priors can express objective information such as "the variable is within a certain range." For example, if we have a bounded continuous parameter space, say, $\Theta = [a,b]$, $-\infty < a < b < \infty$, then the uniform distribution $\pi(\theta) = I\{a \leq \theta \leq b\}/(b-a)$, where $I\{\cdot\}$ is the indicator function, is arguably noninformative for θ. If the parameter space is unbounded, i.e., $\Theta = (-\infty,\infty)$, then the appropriate uniform prior may be $\pi(\theta) = c$, $c > 0$. It is worth emphasizing that even if this distribution is improper in that $\int \pi(\theta)d\theta = \infty$, Bayesian inference is still possible provided that $\int \Pr(X \mid \theta)d\theta = K$, $K < \infty$. Then

$$\Pr(\theta \mid X) = \frac{\Pr(X \mid \theta)c}{\int \Pr(X \mid \theta)c\,d\theta} = \frac{\Pr(X \mid \theta)}{K}.$$

Since $\int \Pr(\theta \mid X)d\theta = 1$, the posterior density is indeed proper, and hence Bayesian inference may proceed as usual. Note that when employing improper priors, proper posteriors will not always result and extra care must be taken.

Krieger et al. (2003) have proposed several forms of a prior $\pi(\theta)$ and the corresponding distribution $H(\theta) = \int^{\theta} \pi(\theta)d\theta$ in the context of sequential change point detection (see Chapter 4). This method of choices of a prior can be adapted for the problem stated in this chapter. For example, if we suspect that the observations under the alternative hypothesis have a distribution that differs greatly from the distribution of the observations under the null, the prior distribution could be chosen as

$$H(\theta) = \left[\Phi\left(\frac{\mu}{\sigma}\right)\right]^{-1}\left(\Phi\left(\frac{\theta-\mu}{\sigma}\right) - \Phi\left(-\frac{\mu}{\sigma}\right)\right)^{+}, \tag{5.2}$$

where Φ is the standard normal distribution function and $a^{+} = aI(a \geq 0)$. A somewhat broader prior is

$$H(\theta) = \frac{1}{2}\left(\Phi\left(\frac{\theta-\mu}{\sigma}\right) + \Phi\left(\frac{\theta+\mu}{\sigma}\right)\right). \tag{5.3}$$

Note that the parameters μ and $\sigma > 0$ of the distributions $H(\theta)$ can be chosen arbitrarily. Krieger et al. (2003) recommended the specification of $\mu = 0$, and $\sigma = 1$ so that two forms of $H(\theta)$ specified above are simplified. In accordance with the rules shown in Marden (2000), where the author reviewed the Bayesian approach applied to hypothesis testing, the function H can be defined, e.g., for a fixed $\sigma > 0$, in the form

$$H \in \Psi = \left\{ \frac{1}{2}\left(\Phi\left(\frac{\theta-\mu}{\sigma}\right) + \Phi\left(\frac{\theta+\mu}{\sigma}\right) \right), \mu \in (\mu_{lower}, \mu_{upper}) \right\}. \tag{5.4}$$

Here Ψ is a set of distribution functions. The following R code shows the way to plot the distribution functions of priors specified in Equations (5.2) through (5.4) as shown in Figure 5.2.

```
> # The distribution function defined by Equation (5.2).
> H1<-function(theta,mu,sigma) {
+    tmp<-pnorm((theta-mu)/sigma)-pnorm(-mu/sigma)
+    H<-ifelse(tmp>0,tmp,0)/pnorm(mu/sigma)
+    return(H)
+ }
>
> # The distribution function defined by Equations (5.3) and (5.4).
> H2<-function(theta,mu,sigma) {
+    H<-(pnorm((theta-mu)/sigma)+pnorm((theta+mu)/sigma))/2
+    return(H)
+ }
> par(mfrow=c(1,2),mar=c(4,4,2,2))
> theta.seq<-seq(0,4,.1)
> H1.dist<-sapply(theta.seq,H1,mu=0,sigma=1)
> plot(theta.seq,H1.dist,type="l",xlim=c(-4,4),lty=1,lwd=2,xlab="theta",ylab=
"Probability")
>
> theta.seq2<-seq(-4,4,.1)
> H2.dist<-sapply(theta.seq2,H2,mu=0,sigma=1)
> lines(theta.seq2,H2.dist,lty=2,lwd=2)
>
> # fix sigma=1
> mu.seq<-seq(-5,5,1)
> H2.dist<-sapply(theta.seq2,H2,mu=mu.seq[1],sigma=1)
> plot(theta.seq2,H2.dist,lty=3,lwd=2,type="l",xlim=c(-4,4),ylim=c(0,1),xlab=
"theta",ylab="Probability")
> for (i in 2:length(mu.seq)){
+    H2.dist<-sapply(theta.seq2,H2,mu=mu.seq[i],sigma=1)
+    lines(theta.seq2,H2.dist,lty=i+2,lwd=2)
+ }
```

In Figure 5.2, the solid line and the dashed line in the left panel present $H(\theta)$ defined by (5.2) and (5.3) with $\mu = 0$ and $\sigma = 1$, respectively, and the right panel presents $H(\theta)$ defined by Equation (5.4) for μ changing from −5 to 5.

Example

As a specific example of the choice of the prior function, Gönen et al. (2005) provided a case study. Assuming the data points Y_{ir} ($i = 1, 2$, $r = 1, ..., n_i$) are independent and normally distributed with means μ_i and

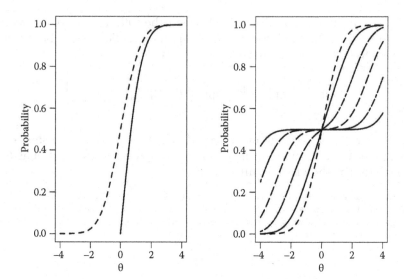

FIGURE 5.2
The cumulative distribution functions that correspond to the priors (5.2) through (5.4). The solid line and the dashed line in the left panel present $H(\theta)$ defined by (5.2) and (5.3) with $\mu = 0$ and $\sigma = 1$, respectively. The right panel presents $H(\theta)$ defined by (5.4), where $\mu = -5, ..., 5$.

a common variance σ^2, the goal is to test $H_0 : \delta = \mu_1 - \mu_2 = 0$ against $H_1 : \delta \neq 0$. In order to obtain the usual two-sample t statistic, prior knowledge is modeled for δ/σ instead of δ, which can be specified as $\delta/\sigma \,|\, \{\mu, \sigma^2, \delta/\sigma \neq 0\} \sim N(\lambda, \sigma_\delta^2)$. For sample size calculations, prior information to suggest the expected effect size λ is routinely used. The large-sample size calculation formula for two-sample tests is given by

$$n = \frac{2(z_{1-\alpha/2} + z_{1-\beta})^2}{(\delta/\sigma)^2} \quad \text{with} \quad \frac{1}{(2\pi)^{1/2}} \int_{-\infty}^{z_{1-\alpha/2}} e^{-u^2/2} du = 1 - \alpha/2$$

$$\text{and} \quad \frac{1}{(2\pi)^{1/2}} \int_{-\infty}^{z_{1-\beta}} e^{-u^2/2} du = 1 - \beta,$$

where $n = n_1 = n_2 = 2n_\delta$ is the sample size per group, δ/σ is the prespecified anticipated standardized effect size, and α, β are the Type I and Type II error probability, respectively. Note that the value σ_δ can be expressed as a function of the prior probability that the effect is in the wrong direction. For example, in the case of $\alpha = 0.05$, $\beta = 0.2$, $\lambda = (1.96 + 0.84)n_\delta^{-1/2} = 2.80n_\delta^{-1/2}$ and one thinks $Pr(\delta < 0 \,|\, \delta \neq 0) = 0.10$, one can obtain $\sigma_\delta = 2.19n_\delta^{-1/2}$ using normal distribution calculations.

These calculations involved the choice of zero for the tenth percentile of the prior on δ/σ. Note that other percentiles could have been selected as well. Another calibration would involve selection of σ_δ based on a prior assumed value for $Pr(\delta/\sigma > 2\lambda \,|\, \delta \neq 0) = 0.10$. In order to ensure consistency, it would be helpful to try several such values. The remaining parameter that needs to be specified is given in terms of the probability that H_0 is true, that is, $\pi_0 = \Pr(\delta = 0)$. Observing that it is unethical to randomize patients when the outcome is certain, the quantities $\Pr(\delta \le 0)$ and $\Pr(\delta > 0)$ should be roughly comparable. One may set $\pi_0 = 0.5$ as an "objective" value (Berger and Sellke, 1987), which, in conjunction with $\Pr(\delta < 0 \,|\, \delta \neq 0) = 0.10$, yields $\Pr(\delta \le 0) = 0.5 + 0.10 \times 0.5 = 0.55$. Alternatively, the prior π_0 can be assigned to reflect prior belief in the null; one may set $\Pr(\delta \le 0) = 0.5$, which implies $\pi_0 = 0.444$ in conjunction with $\Pr(\delta < 0 \,|\, \delta \neq 0) = 0.10$.

Note that a common criticism of Bayesian methods is that the priors may be chosen arbitrarily in some cases or subjective in a special way in other cases. Kass (1993) discussed that the value of a Bayes factor may be sensitive to the choice of priors on parameters in the competing models. A broad range of literature has discussed the selection of priors and various techniques for constructing priors, including Jeffrey's rules and their variants; see, e.g., Berger (1980, 1985), Kass and Wasserman (1996) and Sinharay and Stern (2002) for additional information.

5.3.3 Decision-Making Rules Based on the Bayes Factor

The Bayes factor is a summary of the evidence provided by the data in favor of one scientific theory, represented by a statistical model, as opposed to a competing model. Jeffreys (1961) provided a scale of interpretation for the Bayes factor in terms of evidence against the null hypothesis; see Table 5.1 for details. It is suggested to interpret B_{10} in half-units on the $\log_{10}$ scale.

It is interesting to note that in the frequentist manner of testing statistical hypotheses, mostly in the period before the Neyman–Pearson concept of setting the Type I error rates to be fixed was widely accepted, decisions based on the maximum likelihood ratio statistics were reported in a similar manner to those shown in Table 5.1 (e.g., Reid, 2000).

Probability itself provides a meaningful scale defined by betting, and so these categories are not a calibration of the Bayes factor, but rather a rough descriptive statement about standards of evidence in a scientific investigation; see Kass and Raftery (1995) for a detailed review.

TABLE 5.1

Bayes Factor as Evidence against the Null Hypothesis

$\log_{10}(B_{10})$	(B_{10})	Evidence against H_0
0–1/2	1–3.2	Weak
1/2–1	3.2–10	Substantial
1–2	10–100	Strong
>2	>100	Decisive

Asymptotic approximations to the Bayes factor are easy to compute using the output from standard packages that maximize likelihoods. Recall that we described the asymptotic behavior of the Bayes factor in Section 5.3.1.1, e.g., the Schwarz criterion, given as

$$S = \left\{ \log \Pr(X \mid \hat{\theta}_1, H_1) - \log \Pr(X \mid \hat{\theta}_0, H_0) \right\} - \frac{1}{2}(d_1 - d_0) \log(n),$$

which provides a rough approximation to the logarithm of the Bayes factor as $n \to \infty$. Note that $\Lambda = 2\left\{ \log \Pr(X \mid \hat{\theta}_1, H_1) - \log \Pr(X \mid \hat{\theta}_0, H_0) \right\}$ is the maximum log-likelihood ratio statistic, with approximately a $\chi^2_{d_1 - d_0}$ distribution. Consequently, Bayes factor type tests can be viewed as frequentist tests due to the asymptotic results, where corresponding critical values and powers can be obtained accordingly.

Example

Consider a straightforward but common example. Let $X = \{X_1, \ldots, X_n\}$ be a random sample from some normal distribution with mean μ and variance σ^2. It is desired to test the one-sided hypothesis $H_0 : \mu \leq \mu_{X0}$ versus $H_1 : \mu > \mu_{X0}$, where μ_{X0} is a prespecified number of interest. Let $\bar{X}$ denote the sample mean, $\bar{X} = n^{-1} \sum_{i=1}^{n} X_i$. We then consider two scenarios with known/unknown value of variance σ^2.

Scenario 1: *(The variance σ^2 is assumed to be known.)* Let the prior distribution function of μ be chosen in a conjugate manner to be normal, $N(\mu_0, \tau_0^2)$. Then the posterior density is

$$\Pr(\mu \mid X) \propto \pi(\mu) \Pr(X \mid \mu) \propto \exp\left(-\frac{1}{2} \left(\frac{(\mu - \mu_0)^2}{\tau_0^2} + \sum_{i=1}^{n} \frac{(X_i - \mu)^2}{\sigma^2} \right) \right),$$

which is associated with a normal density function with the mean and the variance as

$$\mu_n = \frac{\mu_0/\tau_0^2 + n\bar{X}/\sigma^2}{1/\tau_0^2 + n/\sigma^2}, \quad \tau_n^2 = \frac{1}{1/\tau_0^2 + n/\sigma^2},$$

respectively. Therefore, the posterior probability of H_0, denoted by q_0, is $\Pr(\mu \leq \mu_{X0} \mid X) = \Phi((\mu_{X0} - \mu_n)/\tau_n)$, where Φ is the standard normal distribution function. Denote the value of prior probability of H_0, $\Pr(\mu \leq \mu_{X0}) = \Phi((\mu_{X0} - \mu_0)/\tau_0)$, by p_0. Thus, the Bayes factor, the ratio of the posterior odds to the prior odds, has the form

$$B_{10} = \frac{\Pr(X \mid H_1)}{\Pr(X \mid H_0)} = \frac{\Pr(\mu > \mu_{X0} \mid X)}{\Pr(\mu \leq \mu_{X0} \mid X)} \bigg/ \frac{\Pr(\mu > \mu_{X0})}{\Pr(\mu \leq \mu_{X0})} = \frac{(1 - q_0)p_0}{(1 - p_0)q_0}.$$

Note that the prior precision, $1/\tau_0^2$, and the data precision, n/σ^2, play equivalent roles in the posterior distribution. Thus, for a large sample size n, the posterior distribution is largely determined by σ^2 and the sample mean $\bar{X}$; see Gelman et al. (2003) for detailed discussion.

Scenario 2: *(The variance σ^2 is assumed to be unknown.)* Let the conditional distribution of $^\mu$ given σ^2 be normal and the marginal distribution of σ^2 be scaled-inverse-χ^2 distribution, that is,

$$\mu \mid \sigma^2 \sim N(\mu_0, \sigma^2/\kappa_0), \quad \sigma^2 \sim \text{Inverse} - \chi^2(\nu_0, \sigma_0^2),$$

where the probability density function of the scaled-inverse-$\chi^2(\nu_0, \sigma_0^2)$ distribution is $f(y; \nu_0, \sigma_0^2) = \dfrac{(\sigma_0^2 \nu_0/2)^{\nu_0/2}}{\Gamma(\nu_0/2)} y^{-(1+\nu_0/2)} \exp\left(-\dfrac{\nu_0 \sigma_0^2}{2y}\right)$, $y > 0$. Then the joint prior density, a product form of $\Pr(\mu \mid \sigma^2)\Pr(\sigma^2)$, is

$$\Pr(\mu, \sigma^2) \propto \sigma^{-1}(\sigma^2)^{-(\nu_0/2+1)} \exp\left(-\dfrac{\nu_0 \sigma_0^2 + \kappa_0(\mu_0 - \mu)^2}{2\sigma^2}\right),$$

which is denoted as Normal-Inverse-$\chi^2(\mu_0, \sigma^2/\kappa_0 ; \nu_0, \sigma_0^2)$.

Let s^2 denote the sample variance, that is, $s^2 = (n-1)^{-1} \sum_{i=1}^{n} (X_i - \bar{X})^2$. Correspondingly, the joint posterior density is

$$\Pr(\mu, \sigma^2 \mid X) \propto \sigma^{-1}(\sigma^2)^{-(\nu_0/2+1)} \exp\left(-\dfrac{\nu_0 \sigma_0^2 + \kappa_0(\mu_0 - \mu)^2}{2\sigma^2}\right)(\sigma^2)^{-n/2} \exp\left(-\dfrac{(n-1)s^2 + n(\bar{X} - \mu)^2}{2\sigma^2}\right),$$

which is Normal-Inverse-$\chi^2(\mu_n, \sigma_n^2/\kappa_n ; \nu_n, \sigma_n^2)$, where

$$\mu_n = \dfrac{\kappa_0}{\kappa_0 + n}\mu_0 + \dfrac{n}{\kappa_0 + n}\bar{X}, \quad \kappa_n = \kappa_0 + n, \quad \nu_n = \nu_0 + n,$$

$$\nu_n \sigma_n^2 = \nu_0 \sigma_0^2 + (n-1)s^2 + \dfrac{\kappa_0 n}{\kappa_0 + n}(\bar{X} - \mu_0)^2.$$

To sample from the joint posterior distribution, we first draw σ^2 from its marginal posterior distribution Inverse-$\chi^2(\nu_n, \sigma_n^2)$, then draw μ from its normal conditional posterior distribution $N(\mu_n, \sigma^2/\kappa_n)$, using the generated value of σ^2.

The marginal posterior density of σ^2 is a scaled-inverse-χ^2 distribution, i.e.,

$$\sigma^2 \mid X \sim \text{Inverse} - \chi^2(\nu_n, \sigma_n^2).$$

The conditional posterior density of μ, given σ^2, is proportional to the joint posterior density in Scenario 1, where the value of σ^2 is assumed to be known, i.e.,

$$\mu \mid \sigma^2, X \sim N(\mu_n, \sigma^2/\kappa_n).$$

Integration of the joint posterior density with respect to σ^2 shows that the marginal posterior density for μ follows a nonstandardized Student's t distribution,

$$\Pr(\mu \mid X) \propto \left(1 + \frac{\kappa_n(\mu_n - \mu)^2}{v_n \sigma_n^2}\right)^{-(v_n/2+1)} = t_{v_n}(\mu_n, \sigma_n^2/\kappa_n),$$

where the probability density function of the nonstandardized Student's t distribution $t_v(\mu, \sigma)$ is $f(y; v, \mu, \sigma) = \dfrac{\Gamma((v+1)/2)}{\Gamma(v/2)\sqrt{\pi v}\sigma}\left(1 + \dfrac{1}{v}\left(\dfrac{y-\mu}{\sigma}\right)^2\right)^{-((v+1)/2)}$

with $\Gamma(u) = \displaystyle\int_0^\infty t^{u-1}\exp(-t)dt$. Denote the corresponding distribution function as $T(y; v, \mu, \sigma) = \displaystyle\int_{-\infty}^y f(t; v, \mu, \sigma)dt$. In this case, the posterior probability of H_0, denoted by q_0, is $\Pr(\mu \leq \mu_{X0} \mid X) = T(\mu_{X0}; v_n, \mu_n, \sigma_n^2/\kappa_n)$. The value of the prior probability of H_0, denoted by p_0, is $\Pr(\mu \leq \mu_{X0}) = \displaystyle\int_{-\infty}^{\mu_{X0}}\int_0^\infty \Pr(\mu, \sigma^2)d\mu d\sigma^2$, which can be computed based on previous derivation. Thus, the Bayes factor has the form of $B_{10} = \dfrac{(1-q_0)p_0}{(1-p_0)q_0}$.

The results based on the one-sample problem can be easily generalized to the two-sample case. A classic example would be to compare the means of two normal distributions with unknown variances. Let $X_1 = \{X_{11}, ..., X_{1m_1}\}$ and $X_2 = \{X_{21}, ..., X_{2m_2}\}$ be two independent random samples drawn from normal distributions $N(\mu_1, \sigma_1^2)$ and $N(\mu_2, \sigma_2^2)$, respectively, where μ_1, μ_2, σ_1^2 and σ_2^2 are unknown. We are interested in testing $H_0 : \mu_1 = \mu_2, \sigma_1^2 = \sigma_2^2$ versus $H_1 : \mu_1 \neq \mu_2, \sigma_1^2 \neq \sigma_2^2$.

As was mentioned above, Bayes factor type test statistics can be used in the context of traditional tests via a control of the corresponding Type I error rate, e.g., employing the asymptotic evaluations of the Bayes factor structures. We illustrate this principle in the following example.

Example

Let $X = \{X_1, ..., X_n\}$, $n = 30$, be a random sample drawn from $Y - 1$, where $Y \sim \exp(\lambda)$, i.e., $f(x; \lambda) = \lambda\exp(-\lambda(x+1))$, $\lambda > 0, x > -1$, is the density function of the observations. Denote the mean of X by θ ($\theta = 1/\lambda - 1$). Suppose it is of interest to test $H_0 : \theta = 0$ versus $H_1 : \theta \neq 0$. Under the alternative hypothesis, the prior function for θ is assumed to be the *Uniform*$[0,2]$-distribution function. In this case, based on the Schwarz criterion approximation, the relevant maximum likelihood ratio can be well approximation to $\log B_{10} + \log(n) / 2$, as $n \to \infty$. The corresponding maximum likelihood ratio has an asymptotic χ_1^2 distribution under the null hypothesis. Comparing $2\log B_{10} + \log(n)$ with the critical values related to χ_1^2 distribution one can provide an approach to make statistical decision rules from the traditional frequentist test perspective. Implementation of the testing procedure is presented in the following R code:

```
> n<-30
> lambda.true<-1/2
> 1/lambda.true-1 # theta.true
[1] 1
>
> set.seed(123456)
> x<-rexp(n,lambda.true)-1
> x
[1]  0.19113728  0.01426038  1.51633983  1.11874795  1.27664726  2.94610447
-0.86056815  4.24772281 -0.76769938
[10]  0.22111551 -0.72606026  1.06624316  0.10882527  2.32608560  3.73953110
1.89499414  2.52307509  1.35740018
[19] -0.76989244 -0.90812499 -0.83491881  0.29580491  3.72774643 -0.01274517
-0.57838195  2.79788529  0.74200029
[28] -0.93858993  1.18364253 -0.28730946
>
> theta0<-0 # EX under H_0
> lambda0<-(theta0+1)^(-1)
>
> neg.loglike<-function(x,theta){
+    length(x)*log(theta+1)+(sum(x)+length(x))/(theta+1)
+ }
>
> # Bayes factor
> # likelihood
> like<-function(x,theta){
+    exp(-(length(x)*log(theta+1)+(sum(x)+length(x))/(theta+1)))
+ }
>
> # prior
> ll<-0;uu<-2
> prior<-function(theta) 1/(uu-ll)*(theta<=uu)*(theta>=ll)
>
> integrand<-function(theta) like(theta,x=x) #*prior(theta)
> BF<-integrate(Vectorize(integrand), ll, uu)$value/like(theta0,x=x)
> log10(BF)
[1] 3.227941
> stat.est<-log(BF)+1/2*log(n)
> p.BF<-1-pchisq(2*stat.est,df=1)
> p.BF
[1] 1.920634e-05
> p.t<-t.test(x,mu=theta0)$p.val
> p.t
[1] 0.003940047
```

In this example, the value of $\log_{10}(B_{10})$ is 3.2279, greater than 2, suggesting a decisive evidence against H_0. From the traditional testing viewpoint, the approach based on the Bayes factor leads to a p-value far below 0.0001, suggesting the rejection of the null hypothesis, which is consistent with the result based on the *t*-test shown in the R code above.

The following points about Bayes factors should be emphasized: (1) Bayes factors provide a way to evaluate evidence in favor of a null hypothesis through the incorporation external information; (2) Bayes factor based decision-making procedures can be easily applied with respect to non-nested hypotheses (see Section 5.3.1.1 for the definition of nested hypotheses); (3) Technically, Bayes factors are simpler to compute as compared to deriving non-Bayesian significance tests based on "nonstandard" statistical models that do not satisfy common regularity conditions; (4) When estimation or prediction is of interest, Bayes factors can be converted to weights corresponding to various models so that a composite estimate or prediction may be obtained that takes into account structural or model uncertainty; (5) The use of Bayes factors allow us to feasibly assess the sensitivity of our conclusions relative to the choose of prior distribution; and (6) As shown in Section 5.2, Bayes factor type procedures can provide optimal decision rules as compared to other approaches. For more details, we refer the reader to Kass and Raftery (1995) as well as Vexler et al. (2010b).

5.3.4 A Data Example: Application of the Bayes Factor

In order to illustrate a use of the Bayes factor mechanism, we consider a study of survival among turtles where the question of comparing two nested models is of interest. In this study, 244 turtle eggs of the same age from 31 clutches (or families) were removed from their nests in a site in Illinois on the bank of the Mississippi River and taken to the laboratory where they were incubated and hatched (Janzen et al., 2000). Several days later, the baby turtles were released from the same place where the eggs were found. The turtles that traveled successfully to the water were marked as "survived." Five days after their release, turtles not identified as having survived were assumed dead. The birth weight of each turtle was collected as a covariate. The objective is to assess the effect of birth weight on survival and to determine whether there is any clutch effect on survival. Figure 5.3 shows a scatterplot of the birth-weight effect on survival status as well as the clutch effect on survival. The clutches are numbered from 1 through 31 in an increasing order of average birth weight of the turtles. Figure 5.3 suggests that the heaviest turtles tend to survive and the lightest ones tend to die. It also suggests some variability in survival rates across clutches. For example, in one clutch (with average birth weight 5.41), only 2 turtles out of 12 survived while in a second clutch (with average birth weight 7.50), 9 turtles out of 11 survived.

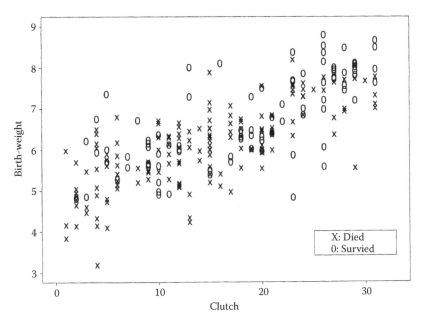

FIGURE 5.3
The snapshot from the paper by Sinharay and Stern (2002) regarding the scatterplot with the clutches sorted by average birth weight.

Let y_{ij} denote the response (survival status with 1 denoting survival) and x_{ij} the birth weight of the jth turtle in the ith clutch, $i = 1, 2...m = 31, j = 1, 2,...n_i$. The model we fit to the data is

$$y_{ij} \mid p_{ij} \sim \text{bern}(p_{ij}), \; i = 1, 2...m = 31, \; j = 1, 2,...n_i;$$

$$p_{ij} = \Phi(\alpha_0 + \alpha_1 x_{ij} + b_i), \; i = 1, 2...m = 31, \; j = 1, 2,...n_i;$$

$$b_i \mid \sigma^2 \overset{i.i.d.}{\sim} N(0, \sigma^2), \; i = 1, 2,...,m, \; \Phi(u) = \frac{1}{(2\pi)^{1/2}} \int_{-\infty}^{u} e^{-u^2/2} du,$$

where the b_i's are random effects for clutch (family). The clutch effects are assumed to be the same for all birth weights. To assess the importance of clutch effects, we compare our alternative model, the probit regression model with random effects, with the null model, a simple probit regression model with no random effects.

Suppose $p_0(\alpha)$ is the prior distribution for α under the null model, while the prior distribution for (α, θ) under the alternative model is $p(\alpha, \theta) = p(\sigma^2)p_1(\alpha \mid \sigma^2)$. Then, the Bayes factor for comparing the alternative model (M_1) against the null model (M_0) is $\text{BF}_{10} = p(y \mid M_1) / p(y \mid M_0)$, with

$$p(y \mid M_1) = \int p(y \mid \alpha, b) p(b \mid \sigma^2) p_1(\alpha \mid \sigma^2) p(\sigma^2) db d\alpha d\sigma^2,$$

$$p(y \mid M_0) = \int p(y \mid \alpha, b = 0) p_0(\alpha) d\alpha.$$

For this example,

$$p(y \mid a, b) = \prod_{i=1}^{m} \prod_{j=1}^{n_i} \{\Phi(a_0 + a_1 x_{ij} + b_i)\}^{y_{ij}} \{1 - \Phi(a_0 + a_1 x_{ij} + b_i)\}^{1 - y_{ij}},$$

$$p(y \mid \alpha, b = 0) = \prod_{i=1}^{m} \prod_{j=1}^{n_i} \{\Phi(a_0 + a_1 x_{ij})\}^{y_{ij}} \{1 - \Phi(a_0 + a_1 x_{ij})\}^{1 - y_{ij}},$$

$$p(b \mid \sigma^2) \propto (\sigma^2)^{-m/2} \exp\left\{-\sum_{i=1}^{m} b_i^2 / (2\sigma^2)\right\}.$$

Furthermore, we use a proper vague prior distribution on α, a bivariate normal distribution with mean 0 and variance 20.1 under both models.

The approximated value of the Bayes factor, obtained using the importance sampling method, with an importance sample size of 5,000 under both models, is 0.31 with an estimated standard deviation of 0.01. The value of the Bayes factor indicates some evidence in favor of the null model.

We then investigate the sensitivity of the Bayes factor to the choice of prior distributions. The prior distributions on α under the two models do not affect the Bayes factor much because there are 244 data points in the dataset. However, the prior distribution for the variance component σ^2 is influential on any posterior inference because our ability to learn about σ^2 is determined by the number of clutches rather than the number of animals. Furthermore, there is little prior information available for σ^2 because very few studies like the turtle study have been performed. To study the effect of the choice of the prior distribution for σ^2 on the Bayes factor, let BF_{10,σ^2} denote the "point mass prior Bayes factor" comparing the probit regression model with random effects, where the variance component is fixed at σ^2, against the simple probit regression model without any variance component. For grid values of σ^2, the approximated values of the Bayes factor, $\hat{BF}_{10,\sigma^2}$, obtained by the importance sampling method are computed. Figure 5.4 presents a plot of $\hat{BF}_{10,\sigma^2}$ against σ^2. The figure demonstrates that $\hat{BF}_{10,\sigma^2} = 1$ when $\sigma^2 = 0$, implying that the two models are identical at that value. The estimated Bayes factor then increases with increase in σ^2 until it reaches its maximum value of about 4.55 at around $\sigma^2 = 0.09$. This is sensible because the restricted maximum likelihood estimate (REML) of σ^2 is 0.091. Also, when it comes to choosing between a small hypothesized value (by small here we mean less than 0.3) of σ^2 and σ^2

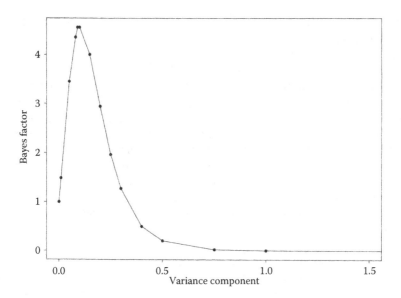

FIGURE 5.4
The snapshot from the paper by Sinharay and Stern (2002) regarding the plot of $\hat{BF}_{10,\sigma^2}$ against σ^2.

equal to zero, the approximated Bayes factor favors the small positive value of σ^2. However, when it comes to choosing between a large value of σ^2 and σ^2 equal to zero, the approximated Bayes factor favors the σ^2 equal to zero; we refer the reader to Sinharay and Stern (2002) for more details.

5.4 Remarks

The Bayes factor, the ratio of the posterior odds (not probability) of a hypothesis to the prior odds, is equal to a likelihood ratio in the simplest case (and only then); see Good (1992) for details. It can be described as a multiplicative weight of evidence. In the frequentist setting of testing statistical hypotheses, problems may arise when inference about the truth or believability of the null hypothesis is based on the classical formulation of a p-value (see forthcoming material in this book regarding p-values). In this context, it should be noted that the p-value is not the probability that the null hypothesis is true. Unfortunately, many practitioners and students have tried to use the p-value to measure the evidence of the null hypothesis as the probability that the null hypothesis is true. This is the wrong concept, since, in general, p-values are random variables. Formal arguments about incorrect interpretations of p-values are provided in Chapter 9. We also remark again (as in Chapter 4) that almost no null hypothesis is exactly true in practice. Consequently, when sample sizes are large enough, almost any null hypothesis will have a tiny p-value, and hence will be rejected at conventional levels. As alternatives to the classical formulation of p-values for testing hypotheses, Bayes factors have been suggested as a measure of the extent to which the observed data align with a given hypothesis by incorporating prior information about the parameter of interest. The use of the p-value should not be discarded all together. A small p-value does not necessarily mean that we should reject the null hypothesis and leave it at that. Rather, it is a red flag indicating that something is up; the null hypothesis may be false, possibly in a substantively uninteresting way, or maybe we got unlucky. On the other hand, a large p-value does mean that there is not much evidence against the null. For example, in many settings the Bayes factor is bounded above by $1/p$-value. Even Bayesian analyses can benefit from classical testing at the model-checking stage (see Box (1980) or the Bayesian p-values in Gelman et al. (2013)). In this context, for more details, we refer the reader to Marden (2000).

Warning: Assume the parameter of interest is θ. In the frequentist manner, the meaning of testing statistical hypotheses, say $H_0 : \theta = \theta_0$ versus $H_1 : \theta = \theta_1 \neq \theta_0$, is clear. In the Bayesian setting, we believe that θ is random. Then it is possible that the statement $\Pr(\theta = \theta_0) = \Pr(\theta = \theta_1) = 0$ has a sense. If your statistical world is completely Bayesian, you compare the model $H_0 : \theta \sim \pi_0$ with the model $H_1 : \theta \sim \pi_1$, where π_0 and π_1 are prior density functions of θ. In this case, we can still write $H_0 : \theta = \theta_0$, assuming that π_0 is an appropriate degenerated density function (e.g., Berger, 1985; Vexler et al., 2010b). Let us consider briefly the following simple scenario, in which using the Bayes factor procedure we would like to compare the following models: $M_0 : q \sim \pi_0 = Unif[0,1]$ versus $M_1 : q \sim \pi_1 = Unif[1,1.5]$, where q is a quintile that satisfies $F(q) = \alpha \equiv 0.1$ for the independent and identically F-distributed data points $X_1, ..., X_n$. Let $X_1, ..., X_n$ be exponentially distributed with the density function $f(x \mid \lambda_q)$, where $\lambda_q : \int_0^q f(u \mid \lambda_q)du = \alpha = 0.1$. Then the Bayes factor statistic is

$$BF = \frac{\displaystyle\int_1^{1.5} \prod_{i=1}^n f(X_i \mid \lambda_q)dq}{\displaystyle\int_0^1 \prod_{i=1}^n f(X_i \mid \lambda_q)dq}.$$

For illustrative purposes, we can simulate 5,000 times the scenario mentioned above under the model M_0 with $n = 25$ using the following R code:

```
alpha<-0.1
n<-25
MC<-5000
```

```
BF<-array()
for(mc in 1:MC)
{
a0<-0
b0<-1
a1<-b0
b1<-b0+0.5
q<-runif(1,a0,b0) # model M0
#q<-runif(1,a1,b1)# model M1
QQ<-function(u) pexp(q,u)-alpha
lambda<-uniroot(QQ,c(0,1000000))$root # to find lambda corresponding to the q's value
x<-rexp(n,lambda)
Intr <-function(uu){
        fix<-uu
        QQ1<-function(u) pexp(fix,u)-alpha
        QQ1V<-Vectorize(QQ1)
        lambda1<-uniroot(QQ1V,c(0,100000000))$root
        S<-sum(log(dexp(x,lambda1)))
        return(exp(S))
        }
```

Intr(uu) is the function $\prod_{i=1}^{n} f(X_i|\lambda_q)$, where λ_q corresponds to the argument uu

```
Inegr<-Vectorize(Intr)
Num<-integrate(Inegr,a1,b1)[[1]]
Den<-integrate(Inegr,a0,b0,stop.on.error = FALSE)[[1]]

BF[mc]<-Num/Den

print(length(BF[BF<1]))
print(length(BF[(BF>=1)&(BF<10^0.5)]))
print(length(BF[(BF>=10^0.5)&(BF<10^1)]))
print(length(BF[(BF>=10^1)&(BF<10^1.5)]))
}
```

We would like to invite the reader to run the code above and obtain the results, evaluating them with respect to Table 5.1.

Note again that, in the frequent perspective, the approaches mentioned in this chapter show that Bayes factor type procedures can provide very efficient decision-making mechanisms.

6

A Brief Review of Sequential Methods

6.1 Introduction

Retrospective studies are generally derived from already existing databases or combining existing pieces of data, e.g., using electronic health records to examine risk or protection factors in relation to a clinical outcome, where the outcome may have already occurred prior to the start of the analysis. The investigator collects data from past records, with no or minimal patient follow-up, as is the case with a prospective study. Many valuable studies, such as the first major case-control study published by Lane-Claypon (1926), investigating risk factors for breast cancer, were retrospective investigations. Prospective studies may be analyzed similar to retrospective studies or they may have a *sequential* element to them, which we will describe below, that is, data may be analyzed continuously or in stages during the course of study.

In retrospective studies it is common to have sources of error due to confounding and various biases such as selection bias, e.g., bias due to missing data elements, misclassification, or information bias. In addition, the inferential decision procedures for retrospective studies are based on data sets, where the corresponding samples sizes are fixed in advance and can oftentimes be quite large. It is possible in these settings to have underpowered or overpowered designs. For example medical claims data may lead to an overpowered design, i.e., a study that will detect small differences from the null hypothesis that may not be scientifically interesting. Consequently, retrospective studies may induce unnecessarily high financial and/or human cost or statistically significant results that are not necessarily meaningful. Armitage (1981) stated that

> The classical theory of experimental design deals predominantly with experiments of predetermined size, presumably because the pioneers of the subject, particularly R.A. Fisher, worked in agricultural research, where the outcome of a field trial is not available until long after the experiment has been designed and started.

In fact, in an experiment in which data accumulate steadily over a period of time, it is natural to monitor results as they occur, with a view toward taking action such as certain modifications or early termination of the study. For example, a disease prevention trial or an epidemiological cohort study of occupational exposure may run on a time scale of tens of years. It is not uncommon for phase III cancer clinical trials, where the primary objective is final confirmation of safety and efficacy, with a survival endpoint, to run 10 years.

From a logistical and cost-effectiveness point of view it is natural to employ sequential statistical procedures. *Sequential analysis* will be performed as "a method allowing hypothesis tests to be conducted on a number of occasions as data accumulate through the course of a trial. A trial monitored in this way is usually called a sequential trial" (Everitt and Palmer, 2010). In fully sequential approaches statistical conclusions are conducted after the collection of every observation. In *group sequential testing*, tests are conducted after batches of data are observed. Both approaches allow one to draw decisions during the data collection and possibly reach a final conclusion at a much earlier stage as is the case in classical hypothesis testing. In classical retrospective hypothesis testing where the sample size is fixed at the beginning of the experiment and the data collection is conducted without considering the data and/or the analysis, the sample size in sequential analysis is a random variable (see Chapters 2 and 4 for several examples).

The sequential analysis methodology possesses many advantages, including economic savings in sample size, time and cost. It also has advantages in terms of ethical considerations and monitoring, e.g., a clinical trial might be stopped early if a new treatment is more efficacious than originally assumed. Sequential analysis methods have different operating characteristics as compared to corresponding fixed sample size procedures. Given the potential cost savings and the interesting theoretical properties of sequential tests, many corresponding variations have become well established and thoroughly investigated. There are formal guidelines for use of sequential statistical procedures in many research areas (DeGroot, 2005; Dmitrienko et al., 2005). For example, in terms of government regulated trials in the United States there are formal published requirements pertaining to interim analyses and the reporting of the corresponding statistical results. It is stated in a Food and Drug Administration Guideline (1988) that

> *The process of examining and analyzing data accumulating in a clinical trial, either formally or informally, can introduce bias. Therefore all interim analyses, formal or informal, by any study participant, sponsor staff member, or data monitoring group should be described in full even if treatment groups were not identified. The need for statistical adjustment because of such analyses should be addressed. Minutes of meetings of the data monitoring group may be useful (and may be requested by the review division).*

Armitage (1975, 1991) argued that ethical considerations demand a trial be stopped as soon as possible when there is clear evidence of the preference for one or more treatments over the standard of care or placebo, which logically leads to the use of a sequential trial. In his publications cited above, Armitage described a number of sequential testing methods and their application to trials comparing two alternative treatments.

Sequential methods are well suited for use in clinical trials with short-term outcomes, e.g., a one-month follow-up value. When dealing with human subjects, regular examinations of accumulating results and early termination of the study are ethically desirable (Armitage, 1975). Sequential methods touch much of modern statistical practice and hence we cannot possibly include all relevant theory and examples. In this chapter, we will outline several of the more well-applied sequential testing procedures, including two-stage designs, the sequential probability ratio test, group sequential tests, and adaptive sequential designs.

Warning: (1) Note that the scheme of sequential testing may result in very complicated estimation issues in the post-sequential analyses of the data. Investigators should be careful applying standard estimation techniques to data obtained via a sequential data collection procedure. For example, estimation of the sample mean and variance of the data can be very problematic in terms of obtaining unbiased estimates (Liu and Hall, 1999). (2) In the retrospective setting, one can pretest parametric assumptions regarding underlying data and implement a parametric statistical procedure, e.g., estimation, adjusting its results with respect to the pretest. Oftentimes, parametric sequential procedures suppose parametric distribution assumptions even before the data is observed. (3) Common statistical sequential schemes stop at random times with lengths that depend on observations. Thus, in general, data obtained after sequential analyses cannot be evaluated for goodness-of-fit using the classical tests developed for retrospective testing. For example, the Shapiro–Wilk test for normality (e.g., Vexler et al., 2016a) has a Type I error rate that does not depend on the data distribution. This property is not held if the number of observations is random with a distribution that depends on underlying data characteristics.

In Sections 6.2, 6.5, 6.6, and 6.7 we introduce two-stage sequential procedures, concepts of group sequential tests, adaptive sequential designs and futility analysis. The classical sequential probability ratio test is detailed in Section 6.3. In Section 6.4 we show a technique that can be applied to evaluate asymptotic properties of stopping times used in statistical sequential schemes. In Section 6.8 we provide some remarks regarding post-sequential procedures data evaluations.

6.2 Two-Stage Designs

The rudiments of sequential analysis can be traced to the works of Huyghens, Bernoulli, DeMoivre, and Laplace with respect to the gambler's ruin problem (Lai, 2001). The formal applications of sequential procedures started in the late 1920s in the area of statistical quality control in manufacturing production. The early two-stage designs, which can be extended to multi-stage designs, were proposed for industrial acceptance sampling of a production lot where the decision was that the lot met specification or the lot was defective. In a two-stage acceptance sampling plan, there are six parameters: the sample sizes for each stage (n_1 and n_2), acceptance numbers (c_1 and c_2), and rejection numbers (d_1 and d_2), where $d_1 > c_1 + 1$ and $d_2 = c_2 + 1$. To implement the plan, one first takes an initial sample of n_1 items, and if this contains c_1 defective items or fewer, the lot is accepted; but if d_1 defective items or more are found, the lot is rejected. Otherwise, the decision is deferred until a second sample of size n_2 is inspected. The lot is then accepted if the total cumulative number of defective items is less than or equal to c_2 and rejected if this number is greater than or equal to d_2; see Dodge and Romig (1929) for more details. The two-stage sequential testing idea can be generalized to a multistage sampling plan where up to K stages are permitted (see Bartky, 1943, for details). This approach was subsequently developed by Freeman et al. (1948) to form the basis of the U.S. military standards for acceptance sampling.

A similar problem arises in the early stages of drug screening and in Phase II clinical trials, where the primary objective is to determine whether a new drug or regimen has minimal level of therapeutic efficacy, i.e., sufficient biological activity against the disease under study, to warrant more extensive development. Such trials are often conducted in a multi-institution setting where designs of more than two stages are difficult to manage. Simon (1989) proposed an optimal two-stage design, which has the goal to "minimize the expected sample size if the new drug or regimen has low activity subject to constraints upon the size of the Type I error rate (α) and the Type II error rate (β)." These types of interim stopping rules are often termed a futility analysis; we will discuss futility analysis in detail in Section 6.7.

Simon's two-stage designs are based on testing for the true response probability p that $H_0 : p \leq p_0$ versus $H_1 : p \geq p_1$, for some desirable target levels p_0 and p_1. Each Simon's two-stage design is indexed by four numbers n_1, n_2, r_1, and r, where n_1 and n_2 denote the numbers of patients studied in the first and second stage, and r_1 and r denote the stopping boundaries in the first and second stage, respectively. Let the total sample size be $n = n_1 + n_2$. The study is terminated at the end of the first stage and the drug is rejected for further investigation if r_1 or fewer responses out of n_1 participants are observed; otherwise, the study proceeds to the second stage, with a total sample size n, and the drug is rejected for further development if r or fewer responses are observed at the end of the second stage, i.e., at the end of the study. A Type I error occurs when there are more than r_1 responses at the end of the first stage and more than r responses at the end of the study when $p \leq p_0$. A Type II error occurs if there are r_1 or fewer responses in the first stage or there are r or fewer responses at the end of the study when $p \geq p_1$. The values of $n_1, n_2, r_1,$

and r are found for fixed values of p_0, p_1, α (the Type I error rate), and β (the Type II error rate), and are determined as follows.

The decision of whether or not to terminate after the first or the second stage is based on the number of responses observed. The number of responses X, given a true response rate p and a sample size m, follows a binomial distribution, that is, $\Pr(X = x) = b(x; p, m)$ and $\Pr(X \leq x) = B(x; p, m)$, where b and B denote the binomial probability mass function, and the binomial cumulative distribution function, respectively. Therefore, the total sample size is random. The probability of early termination, and the expected sample size depend on the true probability of response p. By using exact binomial probabilities, the probability of early termination after the first stage, denoted as $\text{PET}(p)$, has the form $B(r_1; p, n_2)$, and the expected sample size based a true response probability p for this design can be defined as $E(N \mid p) = n_1 + \{1 - \text{PET}(p)\} n_2$. The probability of rejecting a drug with a true response probability p, denoted as $\bar{R}(p)$, is

$$\bar{R}(p) = B(r_1; p, n_2) + \sum_{x=r_1+1}^{\min\{n_1, r\}} b(x; p, n_1) B(r - x; p, n_2).$$

For pre-specified values of the parameters p_0, p_1, α and β, if the null hypothesis is true, then we require that the probability that the drug should be accepted for further study in other clinical trials should be less than α, i.e., concluding that the drug is sufficiently promising. We also require that the probability of rejecting the drug for further study should be less than β under the alternative. That is, an acceptable design is one that satisfies the error probability constraints $\bar{R}(p_0) \geq 1 - \alpha$ and $\bar{R}(p_1) \geq 1 - \beta$. Let Ω be the set of all such designs. A grid search is used to go through every combination of n_1, n_2, r_1 and r, with an upper limit for the total sample size n, usually between 0.85 and 1.5 times the sample size for a single stage design (Lin and Shih, 2004). The optimal design under H_0 is the one in Ω that has the smallest expected sample size $E(N \mid p_0)$. For more details, we refer the reader to Simon (1989). Extensions of this design for testing both efficacy and/or futility after the first set of subjects has enrolled are well developed, e.g., see Kepner and Chang (2003).

6.3 Sequential Probability Ratio Test

The modern theory of sequential analysis originates from the research of Barnard (1946) and Wald (1947). In particular, the method of the *sequential probability ratio test* (**SPRT**) has been the predominant influence of the subsequent developments in the area. Inspired by the Neyman–Pearson lemma (Chapter 3), Wald (1947) proposed the SPRT, which provides a method of constructing efficient sequential statistical schemes.

The intuitive idea is this: while testing statistical hypotheses in many situations the decision-making procedures produce outcomes with respect to conclusions of the form to reject or not to reject the corresponding null hypothesis. Assume we have $n = 100$ observations and the appropriate likelihood ratio test statistic based on first 35 data points is relatively too small. Then we will have a very rare chance to reject the null hypotheses using the full data. In this case we do not need to observe 100 data points to make the test decision. Similarly, we can consider situations when the likelihood ratio has relatively large values. Thus, one can terminate the testing procedure when the likelihood ratio is greater or smaller than presumed threshold values instead of calculating the test statistic based upon $n = 100$ observations.

Let $X_1, X_2, \ldots$ be a sequence of data points with joint probability density function f. Consider a basic form for testing a simple null hypothesis $H_0 : f = f_0$ against a simple alternative hypothesis $H_1 : f = f_1$, where f_0 and f_1 are known. Recall that the likelihood ratio has the form

$$LR_n = \frac{f_1(X_1, \ldots, X_n)}{f_0(X_1, \ldots, X_n)}.$$

The goal of the SPRT is to inform a decision as to which hypothesis is more likely as soon as possible relative to the desired Type I and Type II error rates. To accomplish this goal, observations are collected sequentially one at a time; when a new observation has been made, a decision rule has to be made among the following options: (1) not to reject the null hypothesis and stop sampling; (2) reject the null hypothesis and stop sampling; or (3) collect another observation as a piece of information and repeat (1) and (2). Towards this end, we specify boundaries (thresholds) for the decision process given as $0 < A < 1 < B < \infty$, and sample $X_1, X_2, \ldots$ sequentially until the random time N, where

$$N = N_{A,B} = \inf\{n \geq 1 : LR_n \notin (A, B)\}.$$

In other words, we stop sampling at time N and decide not to reject H_0 if $LR_N \leq A$ or decide to reject H_0 if $LR_N \geq B$; see Figure 6.1 for an illustration. The determination of A and B is given below.

Graphically we plot the likelihood value as a function of the sample size and examine the time series process as to whether it crossed either the A or B boundary. The R code for producing the plot is:

```
> # For any pre-specified A and B (0<A<1<B). For example, A=.11, B=0.
> A=.11
> B=9
```

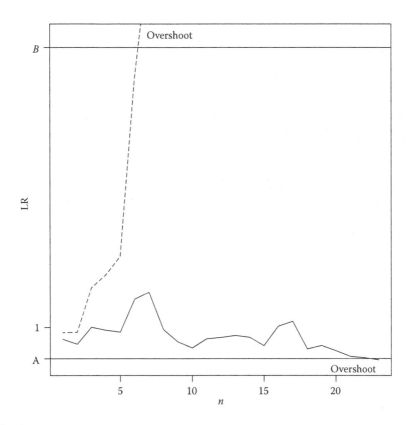

FIGURE 6.1

The sampling process via the SPRT; the solid line shows the case where the sampling process stops when $LR_N \leq A$ and that leads to the decision not to reject H_0, and the dashed line represents the case where the sampling process stops when $LR_N \geq B$ and we decide to reject H_0. The shown overshoots have the values of $LR_N - A$ or $LR_N - B$, respectively.

```
> muX0<-0 # A simple example where X~i.i.d. N(0,1) under H0
> muX1<-0.5 # A simple example where X~i.i.d. N(0.5,1) under H1
> L<-1
> n<-0
> L.seq.A<-c()
> while(L>A & L<B){
+    x<-rnorm(1,muX0,1)
+    L<-L*exp((muX1-muX0)*x+(muX0^2-muX1^2)/2) #dnorm(x,muX1,1)/dnorm(x,muX0,
1)
+    L.seq.A<-c(L.seq.A,L)
+    n<-n+1
+ }
>
> L<-1
> n<-0
> L.seq.B<-c()
> while(L>A & L<B){
```

```
+    x<-rnorm(1,muX1,1)
+    L<-L*exp((muX1-muX0)*x+(muX0^2-muX1^2)/2)
+    L.seq.B<-c(L.seq.B,L)
+    n<-n+1
+ }
> # to plot
> par(mar=c(4,4,2,2))
> plot(L.seq.A,type="l",lty=1,ylim=c(0,9.3),yaxt="n",xlab="n",ylab="L")
> lines(L.seq.B,type="l",lty=2)
> abline(h=c(A,B))
> axis(2,c(A,1,B),label=c("A","1","B"),las=2)
```

The SPRT stopping boundaries: The thresholds A and B are chosen so that the Type I error and Type II error probabilities are approximately equal (bounded appropriately) to the prespecified values α and β, respectively, and formally defined as

$$\alpha = \Pr_{H_0}(LR_N \geq B) \leq B^{-1}(1-\beta) \quad \text{and} \quad \beta = \Pr_{H_1}(LR_N \leq A) \leq A(1-\alpha).$$

Proof. We have

$$
\begin{aligned}
\alpha &= \Pr_{H_0}(LR_N \geq B) = \sum_{n=1}^{\infty} \Pr_{H_0}(LR_n \geq B, N=n) \\
&= \sum_{n=1}^{\infty} E_{H_0}\{I(LR_n \geq B, N=n)\} = \sum_{n=1}^{\infty} \int I(LR_n \geq B, N=n) f_0(x_1,...,x_n)dx_1...dx_n \\
&= \sum_{n=1}^{\infty} \int I(LR_n \geq B, N=n) \frac{f_0(x_1,...,x_n)}{f_1(x_1,...,x_n)} f_1(x_1,...,x_n)dx_1...dx_n \\
&= \sum_{n=1}^{\infty} \int I(LR_n \geq B, N=n) \frac{f_1(x_1,...,x_n)}{LR_n} dx_1...dx_n \\
&\leq B^{-1} \sum_{n=1}^{\infty} \int I(LR_n \geq B, N=n) f_1(x_1,...,x_n)dx_1...dx_n = B^{-1} \sum_{n=1}^{\infty} E_{H_1}\{I(LR_n \geq B, N=n)\} \\
&= B^{-1} \Pr_{H_1}(LR_N \geq B) = B^{-1}(1-\beta).
\end{aligned}
$$

Similarly, it can be derived that $\beta = \Pr_{H_1}(LR_N \leq A) \leq A\Pr_{H_0}(LR_N \leq A) = A(1-\Pr_{H_0}(LR_N \geq B)) = A(1-\alpha)$. The proof is complete.

Note that the inequalities shown above account for values of the likelihood ratio that may "overshoot" the boundary at any given decision point; e.g., see Figure 6.1. Treating the above inequalities as approximate equalities and solving for α and β leads to the useful error rate approximations

$$\alpha \approx \frac{1-A}{B-A} \quad \text{and} \quad \beta \approx \frac{A(B-1)}{B-A};$$

or equivalently, solving for A and B leads to the approximations of the threshold values

$$A \approx \frac{\beta}{1-\alpha} \quad \text{and} \quad B \approx \frac{1-\beta}{\alpha},$$

where the symbol "$\approx$" means that the overshoot values are disregarded.

The Wald approximation to the average sample number (ASN): The expected stopping time $E(N)$ is often called the *average sample number* (*ASN*). Being able to calculate the ASN is practically relevant in terms of the logistics of planning a given study. To study the ASN and the asymptotic properties of the stopping time N, we consider the following reformulation and make an additional assumption that the observations $X_i, i \geq 1$, are iid. Therefore, the log-likelihood ratio $\log(LR_n)$ is a sum of iid random variables $Z_i = \log\{f_1(X_i)/f_0(X_i)\}$, i.e., $\log(LR_n) = \sum_{i=1}^{n} Z_i = S_n$, where we define $\log(LR_n)$ as S_n for simplicity. Then the stopping time can be rewritten as

$$N = N_{c_1,c_2} = \inf\{n \geq 1 : S_n \leq -c_1 \text{ or } S_n \geq c_2\},$$

where $c_1 = -\log(A)$ and $c_2 = \log(B)$ are positive thresholds.

Denote $\mu_{Zi} = E_i(Z_1) = \int \log\{f_1(x)/f_0(x)\} f_i(x)dx$ and $\sigma_{Zi}^2 = E_i(Z_1 - \mu_{Zi})^2$, under the hypothesis $H_i, i = 0,1$. By Wald's fundamental identity (see Proposition 4.3.2 in Chapter 4 as well as Wald, 1947), the Wald approximation to the expected sample size can be expressed in the form

$$E_0 N \cong \mu_{Z0}^{-1}\left\{\alpha \log\left(\frac{1-\beta}{\alpha}\right) + (1-\alpha)\log\left(\frac{\beta}{1-\alpha}\right)\right\}, \text{ under } H_0$$

and

$$E_1 N \cong \mu_{Z1}^{-1}\left\{(1-\beta)\log\left(\frac{1-\beta}{\alpha}\right) + \beta \log\left(\frac{\beta}{1-\alpha}\right)\right\}, \text{ under } H_1,$$

where $\mu_{Zk} \neq 0, k = 0, 1$. These approximations are obtained using Proposition 4.3.2, which provides

$$E_k\{\log(LR_N)\} = E_k\left\{\sum_{i=1}^{N} Z_i\right\} = E_k(N)\mu_{Zk}, k = 0, 1,$$

where, ignoring values of the overshoots, we can approximate

$$\log(LR_N) \approx \log(B)I(LR_N \geq B) + \log(A)I(LR_N \leq A),$$

$$E_k\left\{\log(LR_N)\right\} \approx \log(B)\Pr_{H_k}(LR_N \geq B) + \log(A)\Pr_{H_k}(LR_N \leq A), k = 0,1,$$

$$\alpha = \Pr_{H_0}(LR_N \geq B) = 1 - \Pr_{H_0}(LR_N \leq A), \beta = \Pr_{H_1}(LR_N \leq A) = 1 - \Pr_{H_1}(LR_N \geq B),$$

since LR_N can take only values that satisfy $LR_N \geq B$, $LR_N \approx B$, or $LR_N \leq A$, $LR_N \approx A$ with $A \approx \beta(1-\alpha)^{-1}$ and $B \approx (1-\beta)\alpha^{-1}$.

Note that the Wald approximation to $E_k(N), k = 0,1$ underestimates the true ASN. The accuracy of the Wald approximation to $E(N)$ is mostly determined by the amount that S_N will tend to overshoot $-c_1$ or c_2. If this overshoot tends to be small, the approximations will be quite good; otherwise, the approximation can be poor (Berger, 1985).

Asymptotic properties of the stopping time N: Define $c = \min(c_1,c_2)$ and suppose that $E(Z_1) = \mu \neq 0$, where c_1 and c_2 are defined above. It is clear that, under H_0, $\mu = \mu_{Z0} = E_0(Z_1) = \int \log\{f_1(x)/f_0(x)\}f_0(x)dx < 0$, whereas, under H_1, $\mu = \mu_{Z1} = E_1(Z_1) = \int \log\{f_1(x)/f_0(x)\}f_1(x)dx > 0$ (see Section 3.2 for details). Based on the central limit theorem result shown by Siegmund (1968), it is easy to check that for $\mu > 0$,

$$(c_2/\mu)^{-1/2}[N - (c_2/\mu)] \xrightarrow{d} N(0,\sigma^2/\mu^2), \quad \text{as} \quad c \to \infty.$$

Similarly, if $\mu < 0$, then $(c_1/|\mu|)^{-1/2}[N - (c_1/|\mu|)] \xrightarrow{d} N(0,\sigma^2/\mu^2)$ as $c \to \infty$. See Martinsek (1981) as well as the next section for more detail. Additionally, Martinsek (1981) presented the following result:

Theorem 6.3.1.

Let $Z_1, Z_2,\ldots$ be iid with $E(Z_1) = \mu \neq 0$, $\mathrm{var}(Z_1) = \sigma^2 \in (0,\infty)$, and assume $E|Z_1|^p < \infty$, where $p \geq 2$. Then

(1) If $\mu > 0$ and $c_2 = o(c_1)$ as $c \to \infty$, then $\{c_2^{-p/2} | N - (c_2/\mu)|^p : c \geq 1\}$ is uniformly integrable and hence $E|N - (c_2/\mu)|^r \sim (c_2/\mu)^{r/2}(\sigma/\mu)^r E|N(0,1)|^r$ as $c \to \infty$, for $0 < r \leq p$;

(2) If $\mu < 0$ and $c_1 = o(c_2)$ as $c \to \infty$, then $\{c_1^{-p/2} | N - (c_1/|\mu|)|^p : c \geq 1\}$ is uniformly integrable and hence $E|N - (c_1/|\mu|)|^r \sim (c_1/|\mu|)^{r/2}(\sigma/|\mu|)^r E|N(0,1)|^r$ as $c \to \infty$, for $0 < r \leq p$. (Here the notation $N(0,1)$ presents a normally (0,1) distributed random variable.)

When $p = 2$, the asymptotic behavior of $\mathrm{var}(N)$ is shown in the following corollary (Martinsek, 1981):

Corollary 6.3.1. Let $Z_1, Z_2, \ldots$ be iid with $E(Z_1) = \mu \neq 0$, $\text{var}(Z_1) = \sigma^2 \in (0, \infty)$. Then

(1) If $\mu > 0$ and $c_2 = o(c_1)$ as $c \to \infty$, then $\text{var}(N) \sim c_2 \sigma^2 / \mu^3$ as $c \to \infty$;

(2) If $\mu < 0$ and $c_2 = o(c_1)$ as $c \to \infty$, then $\text{var}(N) \sim c_1 \sigma^2 / |\mu|^3$ as $c \to \infty$, where $c = \min(c_1, c_2)$.

Example:

As a typical example of the SPRT, we consider the situation where $X \sim N(\mu, \sigma^2)$, $\sigma^2 = 1$, and it is desired to test $H_0 : \mu = \mu_0$ versus $H_1 : \mu = \mu_1$ with $\alpha = 0.05$ and $\beta = 0.2$, where $\mu_0 = -1/2$ and $\mu_1 = 1/2$. For purpose of the comparison of the required sample size, in addition to the SPRT, we also considered the nonsequential likelihood ratio test (LRT), that is, the fixed sample size test. Define $\bar{X}_n = n^{-1} \sum_{i=1}^{n} X_i$. In this case, it is clear that the likelihood ratio is

$$LR_n = \exp\left(n(\mu_1 - \mu_0)\bar{X}_n + n(\mu_0^2 - \mu_1^2)/2\right),$$

and

$$\alpha = \Pr(LR_n > C_\alpha \mid H_0) = \Pr(\bar{X}_n > \log(C_\alpha)/(n(\mu_1 - \mu_0)) + (\mu_1 + \mu_0)/2 \mid H_0),$$

$$\beta = 1 - \Pr(LR_n > C_\alpha \mid H_1) = 1 - \Pr(\bar{X}_n > \log(C_\alpha)/(n(\mu_1 - \mu_0)) + (\mu_1 + \mu_0)/2 \mid H_1).$$

Therefore, since $\bar{X}_n \sim N(\mu, \sigma^2/n)$, one can easily obtain that $\log(C_\alpha)/(n(\mu_1 - \mu_0)) + (\mu_1 + \mu_0)/2 = \Phi^{-1}_{(\mu_0, \sigma^2/n)}(1 - \alpha)$, where $\Phi^{-1}_{(\mu_0, \sigma^2/n)}(1 - \alpha)$ denotes the $(1 - \alpha)$th quantile of a normal distribution with a mean of μ_0 and a variance of σ^2/n. As a consequence, $\beta = \Pr(\bar{X}_n < \Phi^{-1}_{(\mu_0, \sigma^2/n)}(1 - \alpha) \mid H_1)$, and hence the fixed sample size n in the nonsequential LRT test can be obtained by solving $\Phi^{-1}_{(\mu_1, \sigma^2/n)}(\beta) = \Phi^{-1}_{(\mu_0, \sigma^2/n)}(1 - \alpha)$. In this example, assuming $\alpha = 0.05$ and $\beta = 0.2$, the nonsequential LRT test requires a sample size that is approximately 6.1826 (6.1826 corresponds to how much sample information is required to achieve the desired error probabilities). Here we use the *uniroot* function in R to estimate the sample size. The R code to obtain the results is shown below:

```
## set up parameters
> alpha <- 0.05 # the significance level
> beta <- 0.2  # power=1-beta=0.8
> muX0 <- -1/2
> muX1 <- 1/2
>
```

```
> ### Likelihood ratio test
> # power as a function of the number of observations n
> get.power <- function(n){
+    right.part <- qnorm(1-alpha,mean=muX0,sd=1/sqrt(n))
+    pnorm(right.part,mean=muX1,sd=1/sqrt(n))
+ }
> power <- 1-beta
> n.LR <- uniroot(function(n) get.power(n)-beta, c(0, 10000))$root
> n.LR
[1] 6.182566
```

For the sequential test, it can be easily obtained that the stopping boundaries of the SPRT are $A \approx 4/19$ and $B \approx 16$ based on $\alpha = 0.05$ and $\beta = 0.2$. Note first by simple calculation that $\mu_{Zi} = \mu_i$ and $\sigma_{Zi}^2 = 1$, $i = 0,1$, and thus the Wald approximation to the ASN is 2.6832 and 3.8129 under the H_0 and H_1, respectively. The ASNs obtained via the Monte Carlo simulations (we refer the reader to Chapter 2 for more details related to Monte Carlo studies) are 4.1963 and 5.6990 under the null and the alternative, respectively. This proves that the Wald approximations are indeed underestimates of the ASN (however, considerably smaller than the sample size required in the nonsequential LRT test). The R code to obtain the results is shown below:

```
> ##### the function to get the ASN via Monte Carlo simulations ######
> # case: "H0" for the null hypothesis; "H1" or "Ha" for the alternative
> # alpha: the type I error rate, i.e., presumed significance level
> # beta: the type II error rate, where the power is 1-beta
> # muX0: the mean specified under the null hypothesis
> # muX1: the mean specified under the alternative hypothesis
> # MC: the number of Monte Carlo repetitions
>
> get.n<-function(case="H0",alpha=0.05,beta=0.2,muX0=-1/2,muX1=1/2,MC=5000){
+    if (missing(alpha)|missing(beta)) stop("missing alpha value or beta value
")
+    if (missing(muX0)|missing(muX1)) stop("missing mean value under H_0 or H_
1") else {
+       if (case=="H0") mu<-muX0 else if (case=="H1"|case=="Ha") mu<-muX1 else
stop("wrong specification of case")
+    }
+    if (!missing(alpha) & !missing(beta) & !missing(muX0) & !missing(muX1) &
case%in%c("H0","H1","Ha")){
+       if (missing(MC)) MC<-5000
+       A<-beta/(1-alpha)
+       B<-(1-beta)/alpha
+       n.seq<-c()
+       for (i in 1:MC){
+          L<-1
+          n<-0
+          while(L>A & L<B){
+             x<-rnorm(1,mu,1)
+             L<-L*exp(-(2*(muX0-muX1)*x+muX1^2-muX0^2)/2)
+             n<-n+1
+          }
+          n.seq[i]<-n
```

```
+       }
+       return(n.seq)
+     }
+ }
>
> ## SPRT under H_0
>
n.seq.0<-get.n(case="H0",alpha=0.05,beta=0.2,muX0=-1/2,muX1=1/2,MC=50000)
> mean(n.seq.0)
[1] 4.1963
> var(n.seq.0)
[1] 11.2889
>
> ## SPRT under H_1
>
n.seq.1<-get.n(case="H1",alpha=0.05,beta=0.2,muX0=-1/2,muX1=1/2,MC=50000)
> mean(n.seq.1)
[1] 5.6990
> var(n.seq.1)
[1] 13.5441
```

The SPRT is very simple to apply in practice and this procedure typically leads to lower sample sizes on average than fixed sample size tests given fixed α and β.

For this example the asymptotic ASN calculated based on Theorem 6.3.1 under H_0 and H_1 is 3.1163 and 5.5452, respectively. The result is closer to the ASN obtained via the Monte Carlo simulations as compared to the Wald approximation to the ASN. The asymptotic var (N) calculated based on Corollary 6.3.1 under H_0 and H_1 is 12.4652 and 22.1807, respectively, whereas the one obtained via the Monte Carlo simulations is 11.2889 and 13.5441, respectively.

In conclusion, there are a variety of fully sequential tests. The SPRT is theoretically optimal in the sense that it attains the smallest possible expected sample size before a decision is made as compared to all sequential tests that do not have larger error probabilities than the SPRT (Wald and Wolfowitz, 1948). However, it should be noted that the SPRT is an open scheme with an unbounded sample size; as a consequence, the non-asymptotic distribution of sample size can be skewed with a large variance. For more detail, we refer the reader to Martinsek (1981) and Jennison and Turnbull (2000).

6.4 The Central Limit Theorem for a Stopping Time

In Chapter 2 we considered the stopping time

$$N(H) = \min\left\{ n \geq 1 : \sum_{i=1}^{n} X_i \geq H \right\},$$

where $X_i > 0, i = 1, 2, \ldots$, are iid random variables. The random process $N(H)$ has not only a central role in **renewal theory**, but also is widely applied in statistical sequential schemes. Evaluations of $N(H)$ can demonstrate several basic principles that can be adapted to analyze various stopping rules used in sequential procedures.

In Chapter 2 we obtained the result $E\{N(H)\} \sim H / E(X_1)$ as $H \to \infty$. In order to derive an asymptotic distribution of $N(H)$, we define $\mu = E(X_1), \sigma^2 = \mathrm{var}(X_1)$ and provide the central limit theorem for the variable $\zeta(H) = (N(H) - H / a)(H\sigma^2 / a^3)^{-1/2}$ in the following proposition.

Proposition 6.4.1. If $\sigma^2 < \infty$, then the distribution function of $\zeta(H)$ converges to the $N(0,1)$ distribution as $H \to \infty$.

Proof. Following previous material of this book, we know how to deal with sums of iid random variables. Therefore we are interested in associating the distribution function of $\zeta(H)$ with that of a sum of iid random variables. To this end, we note that

$$\Pr\{N(H) \geq k\} = \Pr\left\{\sum_{i=1}^{k} X_i \leq H\right\} = \Pr\left\{\frac{\sum_{i=1}^{k}(X_i - a)}{\sigma(k)^{1/2}} \leq \frac{H - ak}{\sigma(k)^{1/2}}\right\}.$$

It is clear that when we use $k \to \infty$ and $H \to \infty$ restricted to hold $(H - ak)(\sigma^2 k)^{-1/2} = u$, where u is a fixed variable, the central limit theorem (Chapter 2) provides

$$\Pr\{N(H) \geq k\} = \Pr\left\{\sum_{i=1}^{k} X_i \leq H\right\} = \Pr\left\{\frac{\sum_{i=1}^{k}(X_i - a)}{\sigma(k)^{1/2}} \leq u\right\} \to \Phi(u),$$

where $\Phi(u)$ is the standard normal distribution function. Then let us solve $(H - ak)(\sigma^2 k)^{-1/2} = u$ with respect to k:

$$k = \frac{H}{a} + \frac{u\sigma\left\{u\sigma \pm 2(aH)^{1/2}\left(1 + u^2\sigma^2 / (4Ha)\right)^{1/2}\right\}}{2a^2} = \frac{H}{a} \pm \frac{u\sigma}{a^2}(aH)^{1/2}\left\{1 + O\left(H^{-1/2}\right)\right\}.$$

Thus, since $\zeta(H) = (N(H) - H/a)(H\sigma^2/a^3)^{-1/2}$, we have

$$\Pr\{N(H) \geq k\} = \Pr\{\zeta(H) \geq \pm u + O(H^{-1/2})\} \to \Phi(u).$$

Since the function $\Phi(u)$ increases when its argument increases, we should choose $\Pr\{N(H) \geq k\} = \Pr\{\zeta(H) \geq -u + O(H^{-1/2})\}$ to satisfy $\Pr\{\zeta(H) \geq -u\} \nearrow$ when $u \nearrow$. Therefore, we have $\Pr\{\zeta(H) \geq -u\} \to \Phi(u)$ as $H \to \infty$.

Since $\Phi(u)$ is a symmetric distribution function, we can rewrite

$$\Pr\{\zeta(H) \geq -u\} \to \Phi(u) = 1 - \Phi(-u) \quad \text{or} \quad 1 - \Pr\{\zeta(H) \leq -u\} \to 1 - \Phi(-u).$$

Defining $v = -u$, we conclude with $\Pr\{\zeta(H) \leq v\} \to \Phi(v)$. This completes the proof of Proposition 6.4.1.

6.5 Group Sequential Tests

In practice, especially in the context of clinical trials, it is convenient to analyze the data after collecting groups of observations, as opposed to a fully sequential test in which the collection of a single observation at a time and continuous data monitoring can be a serious practical burden.

The introduction of group sequential tests has led to a wide use of sequential methods and has achieved the most efficient gains as compared with fully sequential tests. The group sequential designs and corresponding methods of analysis are particularly useful in clinical trials, where it is standard practice that monitoring committees meet at regular intervals to assess the progress of a study and to add formal interim analyses of the primary patient response. Group sequential tests address the ethical and efficiency concerns in clinical trials. They can be conducted conveniently with most of the benefits of fully sequential tests in terms of lower expected sample sizes and shorter average study lengths (Jennison and Turnbull, 2000).

In this section, we introduce the general idea of group sequential tests. In group sequential designs, subjects are allocated in up to K groups of an equal group size m, according to a constrained randomization scheme, which ensures m subjects receive each treatment in every group and the accumulating data are analyzed after each group of $2m$ responses. The experiment can stop early to reject the null hypothesis if the observed difference is sufficiently large. For each $k = 1,...,K$, assume that S_k is the test statistic computed from the first k groups of observations, C_k is the corresponding threshold, and the decision rule is to reject H_0 when $S_k > C_k$; the test terminates if H_0 is rejected, i.e., $S_k > C_k$. If the test continues to the Kth analysis and $S_K < C_K$, it stops at that point and H_0 is not rejected.

The problem in which many authors are interested in the field of sequential analysis is the calculation of the sequence of critical values, $\{C_1,...,C_K\}$, to give an overall Type I error rate. Various different types of group sequential test give rise to different sequences. In choosing the appropriate number of groups K and the group size m there may be external influences such as a predetermined cost or length of trial to fix mK or a natural interval between analyses to fix m. However, it is useful to evaluate the statistical power constraint by the possible designs under consideration. Note that when significance tests at a fixed level are repeated at stages during the accumulation of data, the probability of obtaining a significant result rises above the nominal significance level in the case that the null hypothesis is true. Therefore, repeated significance testing of the accumulated data is applied after each group is evaluated, with critical boundaries adjusted for multiple testing (e.g., Dmitrienko et al., 2010). For more details, we refer the reader to, e.g., Jennison and Turnbull (2000).

As a specific example, consider a clinical trial with two treatments, A and B, where the response variable for each patient to treatment A or B is normally distributed with known variance, σ^2, and unknown mean, μ_A or μ_B, respectively. The group sequential procedure for testing $H_0 : \mu_A = \mu$ versus $H_1 : \mu_A \neq \mu_B$ is specified by the maximum number of stages, K, the number of patients, m, to be accrued on A and B at each stage (assume equal sample sizes for each stage and for A and B), and decision boundaries $a_1,...,a_K$. The sequential procedure is as follows: upon completion of each stage k of sampling ($1 \leq k \leq K$), compute the test statistic

$$S_k = \sqrt{m}\sum_{i=1}^{k}\left(\bar{X}_{Ai} - \bar{X}_{Bi}\right)/\left(\sqrt{2}\sigma\right),$$

where $\bar{X}_{Ai}$ and $\bar{X}_{Bi}$ denote the sample mean to treatments A and B at the ith stage of m patients, respectively. If $|S_k| < a_k$ and $k < K$, continue to the stage $k+1$; if $|S_k| \geq a_k$ or $k = K$, stop sampling. Let M denote the stopping stage. The null hypothesis is accepted if $|S_M| < a_M$ or rejected if $|S_M| \geq a_M$. Note that $S_1, S_2 - S_1,...,S_k - S_{k-1}$ are independent and identically distributed normal random variables with mean $\mu = \sqrt{n}(\mu_A - \mu_B)/(\sqrt{2}\sigma)$ and variance one. Pocock (1977) proposed the boundaries $a_k = ak^{1/2}$, $k = 1,2,...,K$, where the constant a satisfies

$$\alpha = 1 - \text{Pr}(\,|S_1| < a, |S_2| < a2^{1/2},...,|S_k| < ak^{1/2}\,|\mu = 0).$$

This group sequential design can sometimes be statistically superior to standard sequential designs. And the results based on a normal response can be easily adapted to other types of response data. For more details and discussion regarding other types of response data, we refer the reader to Pocock (1977).

The assumption of equal numbers of observations in each group can be relaxed and then more flexible methods for handling unequal and unpredictable group sizes have been developed (Jennison and Turnbull, 2000).

6.6 Adaptive Sequential Designs

In recent years, there has been a great deal of interest in the work of adaptive sequential designs, an alternative and somewhat dissimilar methodology to the sequential approaches described above. Adaptive designs allow the modification of the design and the sample size after a portion of the data has been collected. This can be done using sequentially observed and estimated treatment effects at interim analyses to modify the maximal statistical information to be collected or re-examine the variance assumptions about the original design based on estimates.

For each $k = 1,...,K$, assume that S_k is the test statistic computed from the first k groups of observations. Essentially, the technique of the adaptive design is based on the assumption of multivariate normality for $S_1,...,S_K$ and was first described by Bauer and Kohne (1994). The authors focused on a two-stage design and assumed that the data from each stage are independent of those from the previous stage. We outline the basic idea with a simple two-arm parallel clinical trial as follows: suppose that it is desired to test the null hypothesis $H_0 : \theta = 0$, where θ represents the treatment difference between the experimental and control groups. Based on the data obtained from each of the two stages, two p-values, p_1 and p_2, can be obtained. Using Fisher's combination method, Bauer and Kohne (1994) showed that $-2\log(p_1 p_2)$ follows a chi-square distribution on four degrees of freedom under the null hypothesis, giving the ability to combine the data from the two stages in a single test. The approach only assumes the independence of data from the two stages, leading to great flexibility in the design and analysis of trials without inflating the Type I error rate. The adaption methodology can be extended to trials with greater numbers of stages. The adaptations can be based on unblinded data collected in a trial, as well as external information. In addition, the adaptation rules need not be specified in advance.

Note that the adaptive design approach makes use of a test statistic, which is not a sufficient statistic for the treatment difference, resulting in a lack of power for the test. However, the enhanced flexibility of the adaptive design makes it extremely attractive and important.

6.7 Futility Analysis

We introduced Simon's two-stage designs in Section 6.2, which provide a simple futility rule for an early stop in clinical trials. The term futility refers to the inability to achieve its objectives in a clinical trial. Futility analyses involve the decision-making process to terminate a trial prior to completion conditional on the data accumulated so far when the interim results suggest that it is unlikely to achieve statistical significance. It can save resources that could be used on more promising research. One can combine the sequential testing concept with futility analysis.

Stochastic curtailment is one approach to futility analysis. It refers to a decision to terminate the trial based on an assessment of the conditional power, where conditional power is the probability that the final result will be statistically significant conditional on the data observed thus far and a specific assumption about the pattern of the data to be observed in the remainder of the study. Common assumptions include the original design effect, or the effect estimated from the current data, or under the null hypothesis. While a conditional power computation could be used as the basis for terminating a trial when a positive effect emerges, a group sequential procedure is usually employed for such decisions. A conditional power assessment is usually used to assess the futility of continuing a trial when there is little evidence of a beneficial effect. In some studies such monitoring for conditional power is done in an ad hoc manner, whereas in others a futility-stopping criterion is specified.

There are other approaches proposed to assess futility, such as group sequential methods described in Section 6.5, predictive power, and predictive probability. For more details, we refer the reader to, e.g., Snapinn et al. (2006).

6.8 Post-Sequential Analysis

In the previous sections, we discussed the advantages of sequential procedures. However, in the framework of sequential experiments, once data have been collected, the hypothesis testing paradigm may no longer be the directly useful one for the following statistical analysis; see, e.g., the discussion in Cutler et al. (1966). In practice, medical studies usually require a more complete analysis rather than the simple "accept" or "reject" decision of a hypothesis test. Once a sequential procedure is executed, generally speaking, we will meet the disadvantages of post-sequential analysis. The problem is that all simple statistical approaches based on retrospectively collected data should be completely modified when data is collected via sequential schemes.

Moreover, analyzing the data arising from sequential experiments commonly require very complicated adjustments.

The probability properties of the statistics obtained in a trial that is stopped early at only n samples are different from those attained in a similar trial that is run for a predetermined number of trials, even if they end up collecting the same number of samples. Because the sampling procedure stops randomly during a sequential study, classical methods related to the fixed sample size test do not work for the sequential designs, in many situations. If these issues are not accounted for in the interpretation of the sequential trial, the results of analysis of data collected via sequential procedures will be biased. For a simple example, we assume N is a stopping time based on sequentially obtained iid observations $X_1, X_2, ..., X_n$, then $\sum_{i=1}^{N} X_i / N$ may not be an unbiased estimator of $E(X_1)$, that is, $E\left(\sum_{i=1}^{N} X_i / N\right) \neq E(X_1)$. Piantadosi (2005) argued that the estimate of a treatment effect will be biased when a trial is terminated at an early stage: the earlier the decision, the larger the bias. Whitehead (1986) investigated the bias of maximum likelihood estimates calculated at the end of a sequential procedure. Liu and Hall (1999) showed that in a group sequential test about the drift θ of a Brownian motion $X(t)$ stopped at time T, the sufficient statistic $S = (T, X(T))$ is not complete for θ. In addition, there exist infinitely many unbiased estimators of θ and none has uniformly minimum variance.

Furthermore, most sequential analyses involve parametric approaches, especially in the group sequential designs. In contrast with the analysis of data obtained retrospectively, the parametric assumptions are posed before data points are observed. Even if we have strong reasons to assume parametric forms of the data distribution, it will be extremely hard, for example, to test for the goodness of fit of data distributions after the execution of sequential procedures. In this case, perhaps, e.g., the known Shapiro–Wilk test for normality will not be exact and its critical value will depend on the underlying data distribution.

Therefore, it is important that proper methodology is followed in order to avoid invalid conclusions based on sequential data. For more information about the analysis following a sequential test, we refer the reader to Jennison and Turnbull (2000).

7

A Brief Review of Receiver Operating Characteristic Curve Analyses

7.1 Introduction

Receiver operating characteristic (ROC) curve analysis is a popular tool for visualizing, organizing, and selecting classifiers based on their classification accuracy. The ROC curve methodology was originally developed during World War II to analyze classification accuracy in differentiating signal from noise in radar detection (Lusted, 1971). Recently, the ROC methodology has been extensively adapted to medical areas heavily dependent on screening and diagnostic tests (Lloyd, 1998; Zhou and Mcclish, 2002; Pepe, 2000, 2003), in particular, radiology (Obuchowski, 2003; Eng, 2005), bioinformatics (Lasko et al., 2005), epidemiology (Green and Swets, 1966; Shapiro, 1999), and laboratory testing (Campbell, 1994). For example, in laboratory diagnostic tests, which are central in the practice of modern medicine, common uses of ROC-based methods include screening a specific population for evidence of disease and confirming or ruling out a tentative diagnosis in an individual patient, where the interpretation of a diagnostic test result depends on the ability of the test to distinguish between diseased and non-diseased subjects. In cardiology, diagnostic testing and ROC curve analysis plays a fundamental role in clinical practice, e.g., using serum markers to predict myocardial necrosis and using cardiac imaging tests to diagnose heart disease. ROC curves are increasingly used in the machine-learning field, due in part to the realization that simple classification accuracy is often a poor standard for measuring performance (Provost and Fawcett, 1997). In addition to being a generally useful graphical method for visualizing classification accuracy, ROC curves have properties that make them especially useful for domains with skewed discriminating distributions and/or unequal classification error costs. These characteristics have become increasingly important as research continues into the areas of cost-sensitive learning and learning in the presence of unbalanced classes (Fawcett, 2006).

ROC curve analysis can also be applied generally for evaluating the accuracy of goodness-of-fit tests of statistical models (e.g., logistic regression) that classify subjects into two categories such as diseased or non-diseased (e.g., in the context of a linear discriminant analysis). For example, in cardiovascular research, predictive modeling to evaluate expected outcomes, such as mortality or adverse cardiac events, as functions of patient risk characteristics is common. In this setting, ROC curve analysis is very useful in terms of sorting out important risk factors from less important risk factors.

The ROC curve technique has been widely used in disease classification with low-dimensional biomarkers because (1) it accommodates case-control designs and (2) it allows treating discriminatory accuracy of a biomarker (diagnostic test) for distinguishing between two populations in an efficient and relatively simple manner.

This chapter will outline the following ROC curve topics: ROC Curve Inference, Area under the ROC Curve, ROC curve Analysis and Logistic Regression, Best Combinations Based on Values of Multiple Biomarkers. These themes are considered in the contexts of definitions, parametric/nonparametric estimation/testing and the relevant literature in the field of the ROC curve analyses.

7.2 ROC Curve Inference

In this chapter we assume, without loss of generality, that $X_1, \ldots, X_n$ and $Y_1, \ldots, Y_m$ are iid observations from diseased and non-diseased populations, respectively and let F and G denote the corresponding continuous distribution functions of X and Y. The ROC curve $R(t)$ is defined as $R(t) = 1 - F(G^{-1}(1-t))$, where $t \in [0, 1]$ and the function G^{-1} defines the inverse function of G, i.e., $G^{-1}(t): G(G^{-1}(t)) = t$ (e.g., Pepe, 2003). The ROC curve is a plot of sensitivity (true positive rate, $1 - F(t)$) against one minus specificity (true negative rate, $1 - G(t)$) for different values of the threshold t. Note that the ROC curve is a special case of a probability-probability plot (P-P plot) (e.g., Vexler et al., 2016a). As an example, we consider three biomarkers with their corresponding ROC curves presented in Figure 7.1, whose underlying distributions are $F_1 \sim N(0,1)$, $G_1 \sim N(0,1)$ for biomarker A (the diagonal line), $F_2 \sim N(1,1)$, $G_2 \sim N(0,1)$ for biomarker B (in a dashed line), and $F_3 \sim N(10,1)$, $G_3 \sim N(0,1)$ for biomarker C (in a dotted line), respectively.

The following R code is used to plot the ROC curves shown in Figure 7.1:

```
> t<-seq(0,1,0.001)
> R1<-1-pnorm(qnorm(1-t,0,1),0,1)   # biomarker A
> R2<-1-pnorm(qnorm(1-t,1,1),0,1)   # biomarker B
> R3<-1-pnorm(qnorm(1-t,10,1),0,1)  # biomarker C
> plot(R1,t,type="l",lwd=1.5,lty=1,cex.lab=1.1,ylab="Sensitivity",xlab="1-Spe
cificity")
> lines(R2,t,lwd=1.5,lty=2)
> lines(R3,t,lwd=1.5,lty=3)
```

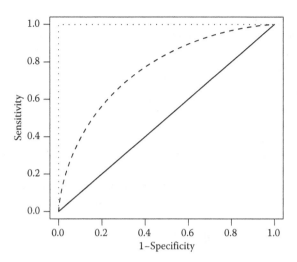

FIGURE 7.1
The ROC curves related to the biomarkers. The solid diagonal line corresponds to the ROC curve of biomarker A, where $F_1 \sim N(0,1)$ and $G_1 \sim N(0,1)$. The dashed line displays the ROC curve of biomarker B, where $F_2 \sim N(1,1)$ and $G_2 \sim N(0,1)$. The dotted line close to the upper left corner plots the ROC curve for biomarker C, where $F_3 \sim N(10,1)$ and $G_3 \sim N(0,1)$.

It can be seen that the farther apart the two distributions F and G are in terms of location, the more the ROC curve shifts to the top left corner. A near perfect biomarker would have an ROC curve coming close to the top left corner, and a biomarker without any discriminability would result in an ROC curve that is a diagonal line from the points (0,0) to (1,1).

The ROC curve displays a distance between two distribution functions. The ROC curve is a well-accepted statistical tool for evaluating the discriminatory ability of biomarkers (e.g., Shapiro, 1999). It is a convenient way to compare diagnostic biomarkers because the ROC curve places tests (biomarkers values) on the same scale where they can be compared for accuracy.

There exists extensive research on estimating ROC curves from the parametric and nonparametric perspectives (e.g., Pepe, 2003; Hsieh and Turnbull, 1996; Wieand et al., 1989). For example, assuming that both the diseased and non-diseased populations are normally distributed, that is, $F \sim N(\mu_1, \sigma_1^2)$ and $G \sim N(\mu_2, \sigma_2^2)$, the corresponding ROC curve can be expressed as

$$R(t) = \Phi(a + b\Phi^{-1}(t)),$$

where $a = (\mu_1 - \mu_2)/\sigma_1$, $b = \sigma_2/\sigma_1$, and Φ is the standard normal cumulative distribution function. This is oftentimes referred to as the bi-normal ROC curve. The estimated ROC curve is obtained by substituting the maximum likelihood estimators (MLE) of the parameters μ_1, μ_2, σ_1, and σ_2 into the formula above. The nonparametric estimation of the ROC curve incorporates empirical distribution functions in place of their parametric counterparts. Toward this end we define the empirical distribution function of F based on iid observations $X_1,...,X_n$ from F as

$$\hat{F}_n(t) = \frac{1}{n}\sum_{i=1}^{n} I\{X_i \le t\},$$

where $I\{\cdot\}$ denotes the indicator function. The empirical distribution function $\hat{G}_m$ of G can be defined similarly, using iid observations $Y_1,...,Y_m$ from G. Estimating F and G by their corresponding empirical estimates $\hat{F}_n$ and $\hat{G}_m$, respectively, gives the empirical estimator of the ROC curve in the form

$$\hat{R}(t) = 1 - \hat{F}_n(\hat{G}_m^{-1}(1-t)),$$

which can be shown to converge to $R(t)$ for large sample sizes n and m. Figure 7.2 presents the nonparametric estimators of the ROC curves based on data related to generated values ($n = m = 1000$) of the three biomarkers described with respect to Figure 7.1, i.e., $F_1 \sim N(0,1)$, $G_1 \sim N(0,1)$ for biomarker A (the diagonal line), $F_2 \sim N(1,1)$, $G_2 \sim N(0,1)$ for biomarker B (in a

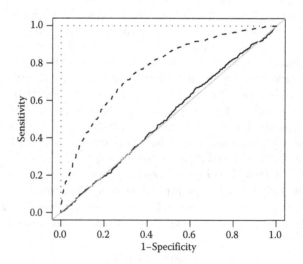

FIGURE 7.2
The nonparametric estimators of the ROC curves related to three different biomarkers based on $n = 1000$ and $m = 1000$ data points. The solid diagonal line corresponds to the nonparametric estimator of the ROC curve of biomarker A, where $F_1 \sim N(0,1)$ and $G_1 \sim N(0,1)$. The dashed line displays the nonparametric estimator of the ROC curve of biomarker B, where $F_2 \sim N(1,1)$ and $G_2 \sim N(0,1)$. The dotted line close to the upper left corner plots the nonparametric estimator of the ROC curve for biomarker C, where $F_3 \sim N(0,1)$ and $G_3 \sim N(10,1)$.

dashed line), and $F_3 \sim N(10, 1)$, $G_3 \sim N(0, 1)$ for biomarker C (in a dotted line), respectively, using the following R code:

```
> if(!("pROC" %in% rownames(installed.packages()))) install.packages("pROC")
> library(pROC)
> n<-1000
> set.seed(123)   # set the seed
> # Simulate data from the normal distribution
> X1<-rnorm(n,1,1)
> Y1<-rnorm(n,0,1)
> group<-cbind(rep(1,n),rep(0,n))
> measures<-c(X1,Y1)
> roc1<-roc(group, measures)
> plot(1-roc1$specificities,roc1$sensitivities,type="l",ylab="Sensitivity",x
lab="1-Specificity")
> abline(a=0,b=1,col="grey")   # add the diagonal line for reference
```

It should be noted that for large sample sizes, the ROC curves are well approximated by the nonparametric estimators.

In health-related studies, the ROC curve methodology is commonly related to *case-control studies*. As a type of observational study, case-control studies differentiate and compare two existing groups differing in outcome on the basis of some supposed causal attributes. For example, based on factors that may contribute to a medical condition, subjects can be grouped as cases (subjects with a condition/disease) and controls (subjects without the condition/disease), e.g., cases could be subjects with breast cancer and controls may be health subjects. For independent populations, e.g., cases and controls, various parametric and nonparametric approaches have been proposed to evaluate the performance of biomarkers (e.g., Pepe, 1997; Hsieh and Turnbull, 1996; Wieand et al., 1989; Pepe and Thompson, 2000; McIntosh and Pepe, 2002; Bamber, 1975; Metz et al., 1998).

7.3 Area under the ROC Curve

A rough idea of the performance of a set of biomarkers, in terms of their diagnostic accuracy, can be obtained through visual examination of the corresponding ROC curves. However, judgments based solely on visual inspection of the ROC curve are far from enough to precisely describe the diagnostic accuracy of biomarkers. The *area under the ROC curve (AUC)* is a common summary index of the diagnostic accuracy of a binary biomarker. The AUC measures the ability of the marker to discriminate between the case and control groups (Pepe and Thompson, 2000; McIntosh and Pepe, 2002).

Bamber (1975) noted that the AUC is equal to $\Pr(X > Y)$.

Proof. By the definition of the ROC curve, $R(t) = 1 - F(G^{-1}(1-t))$, where $t \in [0, 1]$ and F and G are distribution functions of X and Y, respectively, the AUC can be expressed as

$$\int_0^1 R(t)dt = \int_0^1 (1 - F(G^{-1}(1-t)))dt = \int_{-\infty}^{\infty} (1 - F(w))dG(w)$$

$$= 1 - \int_{-\infty}^{\infty} F(w)dG(w) = 1 - \Pr(X \leq Y) = \Pr(X > Y).$$

The proof is complete.

Values of the AUC can range from 0.5, in the case of no differentiation between the case and control distributions, to 1, where the case and control distributions are perfectly separated. For more details, see Kotz et al. (2003), for wide discussions regarding evaluations of the AUC-type objectives.

7.3.1 Parametric Approach

Under binormal assumptions, where for the diseased population $X \sim N(\mu_1, \sigma_1^2)$ and for the non-diseased population $Y \sim N(\mu_2, \sigma_2^2)$, a closed form of the AUC is presented as

$$A = \Phi\left(\frac{\mu_1 - \mu_2}{\sqrt{\sigma_1^2 + \sigma_2^2}}\right), \quad \Phi(u) = \frac{1}{\sqrt{2\pi}} \int_{-\infty}^{u} \exp\left(-\frac{z^2}{2}\right) dz.$$

Noting that X and Y are independent, we obtain that

$$A = \Pr(X > Y) = \Pr(X - Y > 0) = 1 - \Pr\left\{\frac{(X - Y) - (\mu_1 - \mu_2)}{\sqrt{\sigma_1^2 + \sigma_2^2}} \leq -\frac{\mu_1 - \mu_2}{\sqrt{\sigma_1^2 + \sigma_2^2}}\right\}$$

$$= 1 - \Phi\left(-\frac{\mu_1 - \mu_2}{\sqrt{\sigma_1^2 + \sigma_2^2}}\right) = \Phi\left(\frac{\mu_1 - \mu_2}{\sqrt{\sigma_1^2 + \sigma_2^2}}\right).$$

The index $A \geq 0.5$, when $\mu_1 \geq \mu_2$. By substituting maximum likelihood estimators for μ_i and σ_i^2, $i = 1, 2$ into the above formula, the maximum likelihood estimator of the AUC can be obtained directly. Given the estimator of the AUC under binormal distributional assumptions, one can easily construct large-sample confidence interval-based tests for the AUC using the *delta method* (we outline this method below). For nonnormal data a transformation of observations to normality may first be applied, e.g., the Box–Cox transformation (Box and Cox, 1964), prior to the parametric ROC curve approach being applied. In general, when data distributions are assumed to have parametric forms different than the normal distribution function for F and G, the AUC can be expressed as $\Pr(X > Y) = \int G(x)dF(x)$, in a similar manner to the technique shown above (Kotz et al., 2003).

When parametric forms of the distribution functions F and G are specified in nonnormal shapes, methods for evaluating the AUC can be proposed in a similar manner to those shown above. The maximum likelihood estimation of $A = \Pr(X > Y) = \int G(x)dF(x)$ can be provided by expressing one of parameters of F and G as a function of A. For example, the following approach can be easily extended to be appropriate for different parametric forms of F and G: when $A = \Phi\left(\dfrac{\mu_1 - \mu_2}{\sqrt{\sigma_1^2 + \sigma_2^2}}\right)$, we have $\mu_1 = \left(\sqrt{\sigma_1^2 + \sigma_2^2}\right)\Phi^{-1}(A) + \mu_2$, where $\Phi\left(\Phi^{-1}(u)\right) = u$, and then using the likelihood function based on observations from $X \sim N\left(\left(\sqrt{\sigma_1^2 + \sigma_2^2}\right)\Phi^{-1}(A) + \mu_2, \sigma_1^2\right)$ and $Y \sim N(\mu_2, \sigma_2^2)$, the maximum likelihood estimator of A can be calculated maximizing the corresponding likelihood with respect to $A \in (0,1), \mu_2, \sigma_1 > 0$ and $\sigma_2 > 0$. It is clear the properties of the maximum likelihood estimator of A can be obtained via the material of Chapter 3 (see, e.g., Vexler et al., 2008a as well as Vexler et al., 2008b, for more details). Note that, statistical software packages such as R, SAS, or SPlus allow us to numerically perform the maximization of the corresponding log-likelihood functions without using closed forms of the estimators of the unknown parameters. The basic procedure *"optim"* in R (R Development Core Team, 2014) can be carried out with respect to minimizing the negative log-likelihoods and the procedure *"multiroot"* can help finding these minimizations.

The ***delta method*** for evaluating estimators of the AUC, e.g., in terms of their asymptotic variances and distributions, can be employed similarly to the following scheme: when $X \sim N(\mu_1, \sigma_1^2)$ and $Y \sim N(\mu_2, \sigma_2^2)$, one can estimate the parameters $\mu_1, \sigma_1^2, \mu_2, \sigma_2^2$ as $\hat{\mu}_1, \hat{\sigma}_1^2, \hat{\mu}_2, \hat{\sigma}_2^2$, obtaining the estimators $\hat{\delta} = \dfrac{\hat{\mu}_1 - \hat{\mu}_2}{\sqrt{\hat{\sigma}_1^2 + \hat{\sigma}_2^2}}$ of $\delta = \dfrac{\mu_1 - \mu_2}{\sqrt{\sigma_1^2 + \sigma_2^2}}$ and $\hat{A} = \Phi(\hat{\delta})$ of A. Then Taylor's theorem yields the approximation

$$\hat{A} \approx \Phi(\delta) + (\hat{\delta} - \delta)\Phi'(\delta) = A + (\hat{\delta} - \delta)\Phi'(\delta);$$

see, e.g., Kotz et al. (2003) for details.

Example:

Assume that biomarker levels were measured from diseased and healthy populations, with iid observations $X_1 = 0.39$, $X_2 = 1.97$, $X_3 = 1.03$, and $X_4 = 0.16$, which are assumed to be from a normal distribution $N(\mu_1, \sigma_1^2)$, and iid observations $Y_1 = 0.42$, $Y_2 = 0.29$, $Y_3 = 0.56$, $Y_4 = -0.68$, and $Y_5 = -0.54$, which are assumed to be from a normal distribution $N(\mu_2, \sigma_2^2)$, respectively. In this case, the maximum likelihood estimators of the parameters are $\hat{\mu}_1 = 0.8875$, $\hat{\mu}_2 = 0.01$, $\hat{\sigma}_1^2 = 0.4922$, and $\hat{\sigma}_2^2 = 0.2655$. Based on the definition described in Section 7.2, $\hat{a} = (\hat{\mu}_1 - \hat{\mu}_2)/\hat{\sigma}_1 = 1.251$ and $\hat{b} = \hat{\sigma}_2/\hat{\sigma}_1 = 0.734$, and therefore the ROC curve can be estimated as $\hat{R}(t) = \Phi(\hat{a} + \hat{b}\Phi^{-1}(t)) = \Phi(1.251 + 0.734\Phi^{-1}(t))$. The AUC can be estimated as $\hat{A} = \Phi\left((\hat{\mu}_1 - \hat{\mu}_2)/\sqrt{\hat{\sigma}_1^2 + \hat{\sigma}_2^2}\right) = 0.8433$, which summarizes the discriminating ability of the biomarker with respect to the disease. The interpretation of the AUC is that this particular marker accurately predicts a case to be a case and a control to be control 84% of the time and that 16% of the time the marker will misclassify the groupings.

7.3.2 Nonparametric Approach

Conversely, a nonparametric estimator for the AUC can be obtained as

$$\hat{A} = \frac{1}{mn} \sum_{i=1}^{m} \sum_{j=1}^{n} I(X_i > Y_j),$$

where $X_i, i = 1, \ldots, m$ and $Y_j, j = 1, \ldots, n$ are the observations for diseased and non-diseased populations, respectively (Zhou et al., 2011). It is equivalent to the well-known Mann–Whitney statistic, and the variance of this empirical estimator can be obtained using U-statistic theory (Serfling, 2002). Replacing the indicator function by a **kernel function**, one can obtain a smoothed ROC curve (Zou et al., 1997). For details regarding nonparametric evaluations and comparisons of ROC curves and AUCs we refer the reader to Vexler et al. (2016a).

Example:

Biomarker levels were measured from diseased and healthy populations, providing iid observations $X_1 = 0.39$, $X_2 = 1.97$, $X_3 = 1.03$, and $X_4 = 0.16$, which are assumed to be from a continuous distribution, and iid observations $Y_1 = 0.42$, $Y_2 = 0.29$, $Y_3 = 0.56$, $Y_4 = -0.68$, and $Y_5 = -0.54$, which are also assumed to be from a continuous distribution, respectively. In this case, the empirical estimates of the distribution functions F and G have the forms $\hat{F}_4(t) = \frac{1}{4} \sum_{i=1}^{4} I(X_i < t)$ and $\hat{G}_5(t) = \frac{1}{5} \sum_{j=1}^{5} I(Y_j < t)$, respectively, and the empirical estimate of the ROC curve is $\hat{R}(t) = 1 - \hat{F}_4(\hat{G}_5^{-1}(1-t))$. The AUC can be estimated as $\hat{A} = \frac{1}{4 \times 5} \sum_{i=1}^{4} \sum_{j=1}^{5} I(X_i > Y_j) = 0.75$, suggesting a moderate discriminating ability of the biomarker with respect to discriminating the disease population from the health population. Note that in this case, the non-parametric estimator of the AUC is smaller than the estimator of the

AUC under the normal assumption (Section 7.3.1). For such a small data-set used in our examples the difference in AUC estimates is likely due more to the discreteness of the nonparametric method than any real difference between the approaches.

7.4 ROC Curve Analysis and Logistic Regression: Comparison and Overestimation

In general, the discriminant ability of a continuous covariate, e.g., biomarker measurements, can be considered based on logistic regression or the ROC curve methodology (Pepe, 2003). Logistic regression has been proposed as a mean of modeling the probability of disease given several test results (e.g., Richards et al., 1996). It is often used to find a combination of covariates that discriminates between two groups or populations, for example, diseased and non-diseased populations. Suppose we have a data set consisting of a binary outcome, $q \in \{0,1\}$, which indicates the membership of the individual, and m components in covariate vector z. Table 7.1 illustrates the connection between the ROC curve and logistic regression with a case-control study. Let X and Y represent the measurements of the biomarker in the case and control group, respectively. Individuals in the case group ($q = 1$) have values of z given $q = 1$, that is, $X = z \mid q = 1$, while individuals in the control group ($q = 0$) have values of z given $q = 0$, that is, $Y = z \mid q = 0$.

The logistic regression models

$$\Pr(q = 1 \mid z) = \frac{e^{\beta^T z}}{1 + e^{\beta^T z}},$$

where the covariate vector z can include a component with the value of 1 to present an intercept coefficient of the model and the vector β consists of the parameters of the regression, the operator ^{T} denotes the transpose.

Logistic regression relies only on an assumption about the form of the conditional probability for disease given the covariate vector z and does not

TABLE 7.1

The outcome levels and the biomarker values z, where X and Y represent values of measurements of the biomarker in the case and control group, respectively

Class	z (Biomarker values)
Case ($q = 1$)	$X = z \mid q = 1$ (values of z given $q = 1$)
Control ($q = 0$)	$Y = z \mid q = 0$ (values of z given $q = 0$)

require specification of the much more complex joint distribution of the covariate vector z.

It can be emphasized that logistic regression focuses on $\Pr(q = 1 \mid z)$ and the covariant z is assumed to be not a random variable, whereas the ROC curve methodology attends to $\Pr(z \mid q)$ and z is assumed to be a random variable.

In this section, we present the fact that using the same data to fit both the discriminant score and to estimate its ROC curve leads to an overly optimistic estimate of the accuracy of the test as compared to how the model would perform on samples of future cases (Copas and Corbett, 2002). In general, for large studies data are split into *training samples* and *validation samples*. The training sample is used to fit the model and the validation sample is used to assess the performance of the model fit relative to how it would function on a future set of patients. This is discussed further below.

The ROC curve is a standard way of illustrating and evaluating the performance of a discriminant score or screening marker. Let s be such a score, e.g., $s = \beta^T z$, where z is the covariate vector. And we have two groups or populations indexed by the binary outcome $q \in \{0,1\}$, e.g., which represents the membership of the diseased or non-diseased populations. Then threshold u gives the *false positive rate*

$$F_0(u) = \Pr(s \geq u \mid q = 0)$$

and the *true positive rate*

$$F_1(u) = \Pr(s \geq u \mid q = 1).$$

The ROC curve, R, is the graph of $F_1(u)$ against $F_0(u)$ as u ranges over all possible values,

$$R = \{(F_1(u), F_0(u)), -\infty < u < +\infty\}.$$

It is important to recognize that an empirical ROC curve, such as that shown in Figure 7.2, is a retrospective calculation, using the same data to estimate the score and to assess its performance. What we really want to know is how well this particular score would perform if it were to be adopted in practice. This would involve a prospective assessment of how well the score discriminates between future and independent cases with $q = 1$ and $q = 0$. Thus we distinguish between the retrospective (training set) ROC, $\hat{R}(\hat{\beta})$, the curve with $s = \hat{\beta}^T z$ and with F_0 and F_1 taken as the empirical distributions of s in the sample, and the prospective (validation set) ROC, $R(\hat{\beta})$, the curve with the same score $s = \hat{\beta}^T z$ but with F_0 and F_1 taken as the true population distributions of s. The term *overestimation* in the title of this section refers to the difference

$$\hat{R}(\hat{\beta}) - R(\hat{\beta}),$$

where the difference between two curves denotes the curve of differences in vertical coordinates graphed against common values for the horizontal coordinate. In other words, this is the difference in true positive rates having chosen the thresholds to match the false positive rates. Typically, the term overestimation is positive, that is, the retrospective ROC gives an inflated assessment of the true performance of the score.

Consider the classifier $\hat{q} = 1$, if $\hat{\beta}^T z \geq u$, and $\hat{q} = 0$, if $\hat{\beta}^T z < u$. Then it is well known that the retrospective error rate, namely the proportion of cases in the sample for which $\hat{q} \neq q$, is a downward biased estimate of the true prospective error rate, which would be obtained if the classifier $\hat{q}$ were to be applied to the whole population. Efron (1986) derives an asymptotic approximation to the expected bias. Efron's formula is consistent with the approximation based on the ROC curve methodology, which we will present in the following subsection.

7.4.1 Retrospective and Prospective ROC

Suppose we have a total sample size of n individuals with data (z_i, q_i), where q denotes the group membership as before and there are m components in covariate vector z, including the intercept term $z_1 = 1$. We assume throughout that the data fit well to the logistic regression model

$$\Pr(q = 1 | z) = \frac{e^{\beta^T z}}{1 + e^{\beta^T z}}.$$

Let $\hat{\beta}$ be the maximum likelihood estimator of β. Then, if we apply the scores $\hat{u} = \hat{\beta}^T z_i$ to the data against a threshold u, the observed proportions of false and true positives are

$$\hat{F}_0(u) = \frac{1}{n(1-\bar{q})} \sum_i H(\hat{u}_i - u)(1 - q_i), \quad \hat{F}_1(u) = \frac{1}{n\bar{q}} \sum_i H(\hat{u}_i - u) q_i,$$

respectively, where $\bar{q} = \sum q_i / n$ and H is the Heaviside function: $H(z) = 1$ if $z \geq 0$, and $H(z) = 0$ if $z < 0$. The sums in these and subsequent expressions run from 1 to n. The ROC curve $\hat{R} = \hat{R}(\hat{\beta})$ is then the graph of $\hat{F}_1(u)$ against $\hat{F}_0(u)$.

For the prospective ROC fit, suppose the random q's in these data are replicated a large number of times. Then, at each x_i, we expect a proportion p_i of replicated cases to have $q = 1$, where

$$p_i = \frac{e^{u_i}}{1+e^{u_i}}, \ u_i = \beta^T z_i.$$

If the scores $\hat{u}_i$ are applied to the replicated data against a threshold v, the future proportions of false and true positives are

$$F_0(v) = \frac{1}{n(1-\bar{p})} \sum_i H(\hat{u}_i - v)(1-p_i), \ F_1(v) = \frac{1}{n\bar{p}} \sum_i H(\hat{u}_i - v)p_i,$$

where $\bar{p} = \sum p_i / n$. Then $R = R(\hat{\beta})$ is the graph of $F_1(v)$ and $F_0(v)$.

7.4.2 Expected Bias of the ROC Curve and Overestimation of the AUC

To simplify the notation, let $\varepsilon_i = q_i - p_i$, $H_i = H(\hat{u}_i - u)$, and $H_i^* = H(\hat{u}_i - v)$. Then we can obtain

$$\bar{q} = \bar{p} + \bar{\varepsilon},$$

and

$$n\{\hat{F}_0(u) - F_0(v)\} = \sum_i H_i \left(\frac{1-p_i-\varepsilon_i}{1-\bar{p}-\bar{\varepsilon}} - \frac{1-p_i}{1-\bar{p}} \right) - \frac{1}{1-\bar{p}} \sum_i (H_i^* - H_i)(1-p_i).$$

For large n, values of p_i will be close to p_u, which is the true value of $\Pr(y=1 \mid \beta^T z = u)$. Hence

$$n\{\hat{F}_0(u) - F_0(v)\} \approx \sum_i H_i \left(\frac{1-p_i-\varepsilon_i}{1-\bar{p}-\bar{\varepsilon}} - \frac{1-p_i}{1-\bar{p}} \right) - \frac{1-p_u}{1-\bar{p}} \sum_i (H_i^* - H_i).$$

Similarly, we can obtain

$$n\{\hat{F}_1(u) - F_1(v)\} \approx \sum_i H_i \left(\frac{p_i+\varepsilon_i}{\bar{p}+\bar{\varepsilon}} - \frac{p_i}{\bar{p}} \right) - \frac{p_u}{\bar{p}} \sum_i (H_i^* - H_i).$$

Define v_u to be the value of v such that $n\{\hat{F}_0(u) - F_0(v)\} = 0$. We have

$$\hat{F}_1(u) - F_1(v_u) \approx n^{-1} \sum_i H_i A(i,u),$$

where $A(i,u) = \left(\dfrac{p_i+\varepsilon_i}{\bar{p}+\bar{\varepsilon}} - \dfrac{p_i}{\bar{p}} \right) - \dfrac{(1-\bar{p})p_u}{\bar{p}(1-p_u)} \left(\dfrac{1-p_i-\varepsilon_i}{1-\bar{p}-\bar{\varepsilon}} - \dfrac{1-p_i}{1-\bar{p}} \right).$

Note that $\bar{\varepsilon} = O_p(n^{-1/2})$. Let $\Omega = n^{-1}\sum_i p_i(1-p_i)z_iz_i^T$ and $d_i^2 = z_i^T\Omega^{-1}z_i$, then we can obtain

$$S(u) = E\{\hat{F}_1(u) - F_1(v_u)\} = \frac{p_u}{n^{3/2}\bar{p}}\sum_i\left\{d_i - \frac{1}{\bar{p}(1-\bar{p})d_i}\right\}\varphi\left(\frac{n^{1/2}(u_i - u)}{d_i}\right),$$

$$\varphi(u) = (2\pi)^{-1/2}\exp(-u^2/2).$$

The terms p_u and u_i in the right-hand side are functions of the true parameter vector β, and the terms d_i and $\bar{p}$ depend on p_i and hence are also functions of β. Estimating these in the obvious way using $\hat{\beta}$ gives the corresponding estimator $\hat{S}(u)$. The corrected ROC curve

$$R^* = \{\hat{F}_1(u) - \hat{S}(u), \hat{F}_0(u)\}$$

is an estimator of the ROC curve that would be obtained if the fitted score $\hat{\beta}^Tz$ were to be validated on a large replicated sample. As expected, this indicates that this score discriminates between the two populations noticeably less well than the retrospective analysis seems to suggest.

The estimated AUC is

$$\int\hat{F}_1(u)d\hat{F}_0(u) = \frac{1}{n(1-\bar{q})}\sum_j(1-q_j)\hat{F}_1(\hat{u}_j).$$

Similar to the overestimation in the ROC curve described above, the overestimation in the AUC is

$$\int\{\hat{F}_1(u) - F_1(u_v)\}d\hat{F}_0(u) = \frac{1}{n(1-\bar{q})}\sum_j(1-q_j)\{\hat{F}_1(\hat{u}_j) - F_1(v_{\hat{u}_j})\}$$

$$= \frac{1}{n^2(1-\bar{q})}\sum_{i,j}H(\hat{u}_i - \hat{u}_j)(1-q_i)A(i,\hat{u}_j) \approx \frac{1}{2n^{5/2}\bar{p}(1-\bar{p})}\sum_{i\neq j}p_i(1-p_i)b_{ij}\varphi\left\{\frac{n^{1/2}(u_j - u_i)}{b_{ij}}\right\},$$

where $a_{ij} = (z_j - z_i)^T\Omega^{-1}z_i$, $b_{ij}^2 = a_{ij} + a_{ji} = (z_i - z_j)^T\Omega^{-1}(z_i - z_j)$. Therefore, the overestimation in the AUC is approximately

$$\frac{1}{n\bar{p}(1-\bar{p})}\bar{E}[p_v(1-p_v)f(u)\text{tr}\{\Omega^{-1}\,\bar{\text{var}}(z\,|\,U)\}],$$

where $U = \beta^Tz$ has probability density function $f(u)$, $\bar{E}(.)$ and $\bar{\text{var}}(.)$ denote the empirical expectation and variance over the empirical distribution of the sample covariate vectors $z_1,...,z_n$. Note that the overestimation is again of the order $O(n^{-1})$. For more details see Copas and Corbett (2002).

7.4.3 Example

Let $X_1, ..., X_m$ and $Y_1, ..., Y_n$ denote biomarker measurements from non-diseased and diseased populations, respectively. Assume that we would like to examine the discriminant ability of the biomarker based on the AUC, that is, testing for $H_0: AUC = 1/2$ versus $H_1: AUC \neq 1/2$ as well as based on the logistic regression, i.e., testing for the coefficient, β, $H_0: \beta = 0$ versus $H_1: \beta \neq 0$.

As described in Section 7.3.2, a nonparametric estimator of the AUC is equivalent to the well-known Mann–Whitney statistic, which follows an asymptotic normal distribution, and the variance of this empirical estimator can be obtained using U-statistic theory (Serfling, 2002). Then the nonparametric estimator of the AUC is $\hat{A} = \dfrac{1}{mn} \sum_{i=1}^{m} \sum_{j=1}^{n} I(X_i > Y_j)$. Let R_i be the rank of X_i's (the ith ordered value among X_i's) in the combined sample of X_i's and Y_j's, and S_j be the rank of Y_j's (the jth ordered value among Y_j's) in the combined sample of X_i's and Y_j's. Define

$$S_{10}^2 = \frac{1}{(m-1)n^2} \left[\sum_{i=1}^{m}(R_i - i)^2 - m\left(\frac{1}{m}\sum_{i=1}^{m} R_i - \frac{m+1}{2} \right)^2 \right],$$

$$S_{01}^2 = \frac{1}{(n-1)m^2} \left[\sum_{j=1}^{n}(S_j - j)^2 - n\left(\frac{1}{n}\sum_{j=1}^{n} S_j - \frac{n+1}{2} \right)^2 \right].$$

Then the estimated variance of this empirical estimator of the AUC is

$$S^2 = \left(\frac{mS_{01}^2 + nS_{10}^2}{m+n} \right) \bigg/ \left(\frac{mn}{m+n} \right).$$

Based on the asymptotic normal distribution of the empirical estimator of the AUC, the corresponding p-value can be easily obtained and the 95% confidence interval of the AUC is $[\hat{A} - 1.96 \times S, \hat{A} + 1.96 \times S]$.

The test for $H_0: \beta = 0$ versus $H_1: \beta \neq 0$ is based on the asymptotic distribution of the estimated coefficient β from the logistic regression fit (Hosmer and Lemeshow, 2004). It should be noted that the test $H_0: \beta = 0$ versus $H_1: \beta \neq 0$ is a test of association, which is a less stringent measure than prediction.

In order to evaluate the test procedures described above, we conducted 10,000 Monte Carlo generations of $X_1, ..., X_m$ and $Y_1, ..., Y_n$. In the simulation setting, we assume that both the case group X and the control group Y follow a log-normal distribution $\log N(\mu, \sigma^2)$ with different μ's and a common σ^2, where $E(Y) = 3$, $E(X) = 3 + \delta$, and δ ranges from 0 to 2.

Figure 7.3 demonstrates the experimental comparison of the Monte Carlo powers between the test for $H_0: AUC = 1/2$ versus $H_1: AUC \neq 1/2$ (upper curves) and the test based on the logistic regression $H_0: \beta = 0$ versus $H_1: \beta \neq 0$

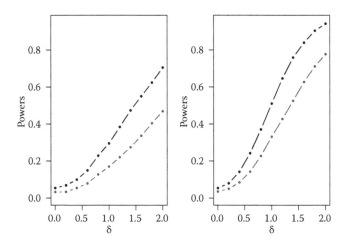

FIGURE 7.3

The experimental comparisons based on the Monte Carlo powers related to the test for $H_0 : AUC = 1/2$ versus $H_1 : AUC \neq 1/2$ (upper curves) and the test for $H_0 : \beta = 0$ versus $H_1 : \beta \neq 0$ (lower curves). The tests were performed in order to detect the discriminant ability of the biomarker at the 0.05 significance level. The left and the right panels correspond to the sample sizes $n = m = 50$ and $n = m = 100$, respectively.

(lower curves) to detect the discriminant ability of the biomarker at the 0.05 significance level, where the left and the right panel corresponds to the sample sizes $n = m = 50$ and $n = m = 100$, respectively. In these cases, the test based on the AUC concept demonstrates better discriminant ability of the biomarker compared to the test based on the logistic regression.

The R code to implement the procedures is presented below:

```
> # empirical AUC (Mann-Whitney stat), returns p-value for H_0: AUC=1/2
versus H_1: AUC!=1/2
> AUC.pval<-function(x,y) {
+    m<-length(x)
+    n<-length(y)
+    x<-sort(x)
+    y<-sort(y)
+    rankall<-rank(c(x,y))
+    R<-rankall[1:m]
+    S<-rankall[-c(1:m)] # ranks of y
+
+    S10<-1/((m-1)*n^2)*(sum((R-1:m)^2)-m*(mean(R)-(m+1)/2)^2)
+    S01<-1/((n-1)*m^2)*(sum((S-1:n)^2)-n*(mean(S)-(n+1)/2)^2)
+    S2<-(m*S10+n*S01)/(m+n)
+
+    a<-wilcox.test(y,x)$statistic/(n*m)
+    AUC<-as.numeric(ifelse(a>=0.5,a,1-a))  # empirical AUC
+    pval<- 2*(1-pnorm(abs(AUC-0.5)/sqrt(S2/(m*n/(m+n)))))
+    return(pval)
+ }
>
```

```
> # logistic regression
> logistic.pval<-function(x,y){
+   if (!is.null(ncol(x))) {
+     Z<-rbind(x,y)
+     m<-nrow(x)
+     n<-nrow(y)
+   } else{
+     Z<-c(x,y)
+     m<-length(x)
+     n<-length(y)
+   }
+   q<-c(rep(0,m),rep(1,n))
+   newdata<-data.frame(cbind(q,Z))
+   glm.out = glm(q ~Z, family=binomial(logit), data=newdata)
+   return(summary(glm.out)$coef[-1,c(1,4)])
+ }
>
> MC<-10000
> alpha<-0.05
>
> Ex=3
> sigma2.x<-sigma2.y<-1
> delta.seq<-seq(0,2,.2)
> n.seq<-c(50,100)
>
> powers.all<-lapply(n.seq,function(n){
+   m<-n
+   powers<-sapply(delta.seq,function(delta){
+     Ey=Ex+delta
+     ux<-log(Ex)-0.5*sigma2.x
+     uy<-log(Ey)-0.5*sigma2.y
+     tmp<-sapply(1:MC,function(b){
+       x<-exp(rnorm(m,ux,sqrt(sigma2.x))) #x is lognormal
+       y<-exp(rnorm(n,uy,sqrt(sigma2.y))) #y is lognormal
+       pvals<-c(logistic.pval(x,y)[2]<alpha,AUC.pval(x,y)<alpha)
+       names(pvals)<-c("logistic","AUC")
+       return(pvals)
+     })
+     pow.delta<-apply(tmp,1,mean)
+     return(pow.delta)
+   })
+   colnames(powers)<-delta.seq
+   return(powers)
+ })
>
> names(powers.all)<-paste0("m=n=",n.seq)
> powers.all
$`m=n=50`
```

	0	0.2	0.4	0.6	0.8	1	1.2	1.4	1.6	1.8	2
logistic	0.0326	0.0332	0.0548	0.0796	0.1273	0.1695	0.2208	0.2743	0.3371	0.4046	0.4692
AUC	0.0540	0.0687	0.0998	0.1494	0.2286	0.2955	0.3845	0.4738	0.5499	0.6237	0.7055

```
$`m=n=100`
```

	0	0.2	0.4	0.6	0.8	1	1.2	1.4	1.6	1.8	2
logistic	0.0350	0.0501	0.0850	0.1423	0.2272	0.3317	0.4277	0.5252	0.6270	0.7122	0.7781
AUC	0.0538	0.0796	0.1414	0.2419	0.3710	0.5107	0.6464	0.7595	0.8397	0.9042	0.9422

Note that in the case where both the case group X and the control group Y follow a log-normal distribution $\log N(\mu, \sigma^2)$ with a common value for μ and we vary the values for σ^2 between the case group and the control group, the AUC does not allow us to detect any significant difference between the two groups. This is because a simple log transformation of observed data points shows that the AUC is equal to 0.5 in this case. We refer the reader to Section 7.3.1 for the computation of the AUC under normal assumptions.

7.5 Best Combinations Based on Values of Multiple Biomarkers

In practice, different biomarker levels are usually associated with disease in various magnitudes and in different directions. For example, low levels of high-density lipoprotein (HDL) cholesterol and high levels of thiobarbuturic acid reacting substances (TBARS), biomarkers of oxidative stress and anti-oxidant status, are indicators of coronary heart disease (Schisterman et al., 2001a). When multiple biomarkers are available, it is of great interest to seek a combination of biomarkers to improve diagnostic accuracy (e.g., Liu et al., 2011). Due to the simplicity in practical applications, we will attend to the best linear combination (BLC) of biomarkers, such that the combined score achieves the maximum AUC or the maximum treatment effect over all possible linear combinations. We refer the reader to Pepe (2003) and Pepe and Thompson (2000) for information regarding general methods related to best combinations of biomarkers that improve diagnostic accuracy.

Warning: Note that the implementation of logistic regression based on several biomarkers does not aim to maximize the AUC, its objective is to maximize the likelihood function. However, we motivate the reader, e.g., via the Monte Carlo simulations, to compare the AUC based on BLC described in this section with the AUC based on the linear combinations of biomarkers obtained from logistic regression.

Consider a study with d continuous-scale biomarkers yielding measurements $\mathbf{X}_i = (X_{1i}, ..., X_{di})^T$, $i = 1, ..., n$, on n diseased patients, and measurements $\mathbf{Y}_j = (Y_{1j}, ..., Y_{dj})^T$, $j = 1, ..., m$, on m non-diseased patients, respectively, where ^{T} denotes the transpose. It is of interest to construct effective one-dimensional combined scores of biomarker measurements, i.e., $X(\mathbf{a}) = \mathbf{a}^T\mathbf{X}$ and $Y(\mathbf{a}) = \mathbf{a}^T\mathbf{Y}$, such that the AUC based on these scores is maximized over all possible linear combinations of biomarkers. Define $A(\mathbf{a}) = \Pr(X(\mathbf{a}) > Y(\mathbf{a}))$; the statistical problem is to estimate the maximum AUC defined as $A = A(\mathbf{a}_0)$, where the vector $\mathbf{a}_0$ consists of the BLC coefficients satisfying $\mathbf{a}_0 = \arg\max_{\mathbf{a}} A(\mathbf{a})$. For simplicity, we assume that the first component of the vector $\mathbf{a}$ equals 1. For example, in the case of two biomarkers, i.e., $d = 2$, the AUC can be defined as $A(a) = \Pr(X_1 + aX_2 > Y_1 + aY_2)$.

7.5.1 Parametric Method

Assuming $\mathbf{X}_i \sim N(\mu_X, \Sigma_X)$, $i = 1, \ldots, n$ and $\mathbf{Y}_j \sim N(\mu_Y, \Sigma_Y)$, $j = 1, \ldots, m$, Su and Liu (1993) derived the BLC coefficients $\mathbf{a}_0 \propto \Sigma_C^{-1}\mu$ and the corresponding optimal AUC as $\Phi(\omega^{1/2})$, where $\mu = \mu_X - \mu_Y$, $\Sigma_C = \Sigma_X + \Sigma_Y$, $\omega = \mu^T \Sigma_C^{-1}\mu$, and Φ is the standard normal cumulative distribution function.

Based on Su and Liu's point estimator, we can derive the confidence interval estimation for the BLC-based AUC under multivariate normality assumptions (e.g., Reiser and Faraggi, 1997).

7.5.2 Nonparametric Method

In the nonparametric context, the BLC-based maximum AUC can be evaluated using different nonparametric schemes to estimate the probability $\Pr(X(\mathbf{a}) > Y(\mathbf{a}))$ as a function of the vector $\mathbf{a}$ (e.g., Vexler et al., 2006; Chen et al., 2015).

7.6 Remarks

Medical diagnoses usually involve the classification of patients into two or more categories. When subjects are categorized in a binary manner, i.e., non-diseased and diseased, the ROC curve methodology is an important statistical tool for evaluating the accuracy of continuous diagnostic tests, and the AUC is one of the common indices used for overall diagnostic accuracy. In many situations, the diagnostic decision is not limited to a binary choice. For example, a clinical assessment, NPZ-8, of the presence of HIV-related cognitive dysfunction (AIDS Dementia Complex [ADC]) would discriminate between patients exhibiting clinical symptoms of ADC (combined stages 1–3), subjects exhibiting minor neurological symptoms (ADC stage 0.5) and neurologically unimpaired individuals (ADC stage 0) (Nakas and Yiannoutsos, 2004). For such disease processes with three stages, binary statistical tools such as the ROC curve and AUC need to be extended. In this case of three ordinal diagnostic categories, the ROC surface and the volume under the surface can be applied to assess the accuracy of tests. For details, we refer the reader to, for example, Nakas and Yiannoutsos (2004). In contrast, logistic regression can be easily generalized, e.g., to multinomial logistic regression, in order to deal with multiclass problems.

There are several measurements that are often used in conjunction with the ROC curve technique. For example: (1) the **Youden index** is a summary measure of the ROC curve. It both measures the effectiveness of a diagnostic marker and enables the selection of an optimal threshold value (cutoff point) for the biomarker. The Youden index, J, is the point on the ROC curve that is farthest from line of equality (diagonal line), that is, using the definitions applied in Section 7.2, one can show that $J = \max_{-\infty < c < \infty}\{\Pr(X \geq c) + \Pr(Y \leq c) - 1\}$ (e.g., Fluss et al., 2005; Schisterman et al., 2005). (2) The *partial AUC (pAUC)* has been proposed as an alternative measure to the full AUC. When using the partial AUC, one considers only those regions of the ROC space where data have been observed, or which correspond to clinically relevant values of test sensitivity or specificity, that is, $pAUC = \int_a^b R(t)dt$ for prespecified $0 \leq a < b \leq 1$. Assume, for example, random variables Y_D and $Y_{\bar{D}}$ are from the distribution functions F_{Y_D} and $F_{Y_{\bar{D}}}$ that correspond to biomarker's measurements from diseased (D) and non-diseased ($\bar{D}$) subjects, respectively. The partial area under the ROC curve is the area under a portion of the ROC curve, oftentimes defined as the area between two false positive rates (FPRs). For example, the pAUC with two fixed *a priori* values for FPRs t_0 and t_1 is

$$pAUC = \int_{t_0}^{t_1} R(t)dt = \Pr\left\{Y_D > Y_{\bar{D}}, Y_{\bar{D}} \in \left(S_{Y_{\bar{D}}}^{-1}(t_1), S_{Y_{\bar{D}}}^{-1}(t_0)\right)\right\},$$

where S_{Y_D} and $S_{Y_{\bar{D}}}$ are the survival functions of the diseased and healthy group, respectively. To simplify this notation, we denote $q_0 = S_{Y_{\bar{D}}}^{-1}(t_0)$ and $q_1 = S_{Y_{\bar{D}}}^{-1}(t_1)$. Then

$$pAUC = \Pr\{Y_D > Y_{\bar{D}}, Y_{\bar{D}} \in (q_0, q_1)\}.$$

8

The Ville and Wald Inequality: Extensions and Applications

8.1 Introduction

The purpose of this chapter is twofold with respect to: (1) Our desire to introduce a very powerful theoretical scheme for constructing statistical procedures, and (2) We would like to show again arguments against statistical stereotypes. For example, one generally can state that if a statistical test has a reasonable fixed Type I error rate then the test cannot be of power one. In this chapter, a test with power one is presented.

In previous chapters we employed *the law of large numbers* and *the central limit theorem* to propose and examine statistical tools. In this chapter we apply *the law of the iterated logarithm.* The material presented in this chapter may seem overly technical, however we encourage the reader to study the methodological technique introduced below in order to obtain beneficial skills in developing advanced statistical procedures.

The Ville and Wald inequality: In Chapter 4, Doob's inequality was introduced with a focus on developing a bound for the distribution of a statistic, which can be anticipated to be increasing when the sample size n increases. In this case, we concluded that Doob's inequality can be expected to be very accurate in terms of such a bound. The right side of Doob's inequality (the bound) does not depend on n. In the asymptotic framework this result begs the following question: Can we apply the symbolic expression "$\lim_{n\to\infty} \Pr(.) = \Pr(\lim_{n\to\infty}) \leq$ The Bound" with respect to Doob's inequality?

In general, since the probability can be written as $\Pr(.) = E\{I(.)\} = \int I(.)$, where $I(.)$ denotes the indicator function, the action "$\lim_{n\to\infty} \Pr(.) = \Pr(\lim_{n\to\infty})$" corresponds to complicated issues related to possibly plugging the operator $\lim_{n\to\infty}$ into the integral. In this context, the Fatou–Lebesgue theorem (Titchmarsh, 1976) can justify the operation "$\lim_{n\to\infty} \Pr(.) = \Pr(\lim_{n\to\infty})$", provided that the conditions of the theorem are satisfied. In this chapter, when $n = \infty$, we introduce a simple extension of Doob's inequality that is entitled **the *Ville and Wald inequality.*** This result was presented by Ville in 1939 as well as by Wald in 1947 (Ville, 1939; Wald, 1947). As mentioned above the Ville and Wald inequality can be assumed to be extremely accurate. We will target to formulate the inequality in terms of sums of iid random variables, offering general opportunities to construct various powerful statistical procedures (see also Section 2.4.5.2 in this context) including, e.g., tests with power one.

The law of the iterated logarithm: In Section 2.4.5.2 we stated a question regarding the asymptotic behavior of the statistic S_n/b_n, where $S_n = \sum_{i=1}^{n} X_i$ is a sum of n iid random variables with zero expectation and a deterministic sequence $b_n \to \infty$ as $n \to \infty$, "in between" the law of large numbers ($b_n = n$) and the central limit theorem ($b_n = n^{1/2}$). *The law of the iterated logarithm,*

$$\Pr\left\{\limsup_{n \to \infty} \frac{S_n}{\left(2n \operatorname{var}(X_1) \log\left(\log(n)\right)\right)^{1/2}} = 1\right\} = 1 \quad (\log(e) = 1),$$

precisely assesses the asymptotic behavior of S_n/b_n. Thus we need to "press" on S_n a "little bit" more than $b_n = n^{1/2}$ to force S_n/b_n to not be considered as a random variable even with respect to its maximum values as $n \to \infty$. Note that, *in the statistical context and in many scenarios, the quality of a statistical tool depends on its possibility for predicting deterministically bounds of the random variable S_n.* In this context we have the following scheme: (1) having the rule to control S_n/n, one can provide several statistical procedures, e.g., consistent estimation; (2) having the rule to control $S_n/n^{1/2}$, one can evaluate properties of statistical procedures at Item (1) above and develop efficient tests (see previous chapters in this book); and (3) the law of the iterated logarithm detects very accurately deterministic bounds for S_n, providing extremely efficient statistical algorithms (e.g., a test with power one we will show in this chapter) based on an anticipated deterministic (data-free) forecasting related to S_n's values. It turns out that the sequence $\left(2n \operatorname{var}(X_1) \log\left(\log(n)\right)\right)^{1/2}$ increases about as slowly as is possible for sums of iid random variables with mean 0,

$$\Pr\left\{\max_{1 \le n}\left(S_n - \left(2n \operatorname{var}(X_1) \log\left(\log(n)\right)\right)^{1/2}\right) \ge 0\right\}$$

$$= \Pr\left\{S_n \ge \left(2n \operatorname{var}(X_1) \log\left(\log(n)\right)\right)^{1/2} \text{ for some } n \ge 1\right\} < 1.$$

For example, when $X_1, \ldots, X_n$ are iid data points it is reasonable to reject the hypothesis $E(X_1) = 0$, if S_n does not follow the law of the iterated logarithm related to the case with $E(X_1) = 0$. For illustrative purposes, we generated 5,000

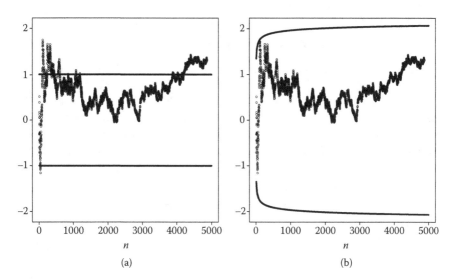

FIGURE 8.1

Values of $S_n/n^{1/2}$ (ooo) plotted against $n = 12, \ldots, 5000$. Panel (a) represents the bounds ± 1 and panel (b) represents the bounds $\pm\left(2\log\left(\log\left(n\right)\right)\right)^{1/2}$.

iid random variables $X_i = \xi_i - 1 \geq -1$ with $\Pr(\xi_1 < u) = 1 - \exp(-u)$ and computed the sequence of $S_1 = X_1$, $S_2 = (X_1 + X_2)/2^{1/2}$, $S_3 = (X_1 + X_2 + X_3)/3^{1/2}, \ldots$ Values of $S_n/n^{1/2}$ are depicted in Figure 8.1 against $n = 12, \ldots, 5000$ using "o" symbols. In this figure, panel (a) represents the bounds ± 1 (the central limit theorem) and panel (b) represents the bounds $\pm\left(2\log\left(\log\left(n\right)\right)\right)^{1/2}$ (the law of the iterated logarithm).

It is clear that, in terms of the Type I error rate control, the law of the iterated logarithm could insure the use of a test procedure based on $S_n/n^{1/2}$ in a better manner than the use of the central limit theorem. And the "payment" for this improvement is only $\left(2\log\left(\log\left(n\right)\right)\right)^{1/2}$, which clearly cannot significantly impact the power of the test when $S_n \sim nE(X_1)$ with $E(X_1) \neq 0$.

In this chapter we will apply the law of the iterated logarithm to judge the proposed techniques.

The reader has all ingredients, including those provided in this book, to prove the law of the iterated logarithm. However, in actuality the proof is quite technical and thus we omit it, referring the reader to Petrov (1975). We suggest that the reader who is interested in more details regarding this chapter's material consult the fundamental publications of Professor Herbert Robbins (e.g., Robbins, 1970).

In Section 8.2 we consider the Ville and Wald inequality. This inequality is extended and rewritten in terms of sums of iid random variables in Section 8.3. The statistical significance of the obtained results is introduces in Section 8.4.

8.2 The Ville and Wald inequality

Consider two assumptions H and H'. Under H the random variables (not necessary iid) $X_1,...,X_n$ with a specified joint distribution function P have a density function $g_n(x_1,...,x_n)$, whereas under H' for each $n \geq 1$ the sequence $X_1,...,X_n$ is from P', any other joint probability distribution, with a density function $g'_n(x_1,...,x_n)$. In this case, the likelihood ratio is $LR_n = g'_n(X_1,...,X_n)/g_n(X_1,...,X_n)$ when $g_n(X_1,...,X_n) > 0$. Then, under H, for any $\varepsilon > 0$,

$$\Pr_H\left(LR_n \geq \varepsilon \text{ for some } n \geq 1\right) \leq 1/\varepsilon.$$

Proof. Define the stopping rule $N = \inf\{n \geq 1: LR_n \geq \varepsilon\}$ with $N = \infty$ if no such $n: LR_n \geq \varepsilon$. Thus, we have

$$\Pr_H\left(LR_n \geq \varepsilon \text{ for some } n \geq 1\right)$$

$$= \Pr_H\left(N < \infty\right) = \sum_{j=1}^{\infty} \Pr_H\left(N = j\right) = \sum_{j=1}^{\infty} E_H\left\{I(N = j)\right\}$$

$$= \sum_{j=1}^{\infty} \int I(N = j) g_j(x_1,...,x_j) dx_1...dx_j$$

$$= \sum_{j=1}^{\infty} \int I\left(\max_{1 \leq k < j} LR_k < \varepsilon, LR_j \geq \varepsilon\right) \frac{g_j(x_1,...,x_j)}{g'_j(x_1,...,x_j)} g'_j(x_1,...,x_j) dx_1...dx_j$$

$$= \sum_{j=1}^{\infty} \int I\left(\max_{1 \leq k < j} LR_k < \varepsilon, LR_j \geq \varepsilon\right) \frac{1}{LR_j} g'_j(x_1,...,x_j) dx_1...dx_j$$

$$\leq \sum_{j=1}^{\infty} \int I\left(\max_{1 \leq k < j} LR_k < \varepsilon, LR_j \geq \varepsilon\right) \frac{1}{\varepsilon} g'_j(x_1,...,x_j) dx_1...dx_j$$

$$= \frac{1}{\varepsilon} \sum_{j=1}^{\infty} \int I(N = j) g'_j(x_1,...,x_j) dx_1...dx_j = \frac{1}{\varepsilon} \Pr_{H'}\left(N < \infty\right) \leq \frac{1}{\varepsilon}.$$

This completes the proof.

Note that $\Pr_H\left(LR_n \geq \varepsilon \text{ for some } n \geq 1\right) = \Pr_H\left(\max_{1 \leq k \leq \infty} LR_k \geq \varepsilon\right)$ and LR_n with the sigma algebra based on $(X_1,...,X_n)$ is an H-martingale. This supports our conclusion presented in Chapter 4 that statistics with martingale properties can provide efficient decision-making schemes. It turns out that even maximum values of the likelihood ratio are in control over all $n \geq 1$.

8.3 The Ville and Wald Inequality Modified in Terms of Sums of iid Observations

As discussed in Section 8.1, it is reasonable to study several techniques presented as examples of reformulations of the Ville and Wald inequality in terms of sums of iid observations. Towards this end, we will employ an approach that can be associated with the material presented in Chapter 5 when the likelihood function is proposed to be integrated over different values of the parameter. Let the observations $X_1, ..., X_n$ be iid $N(0,1)$, under H. In this case, $g_n(x_1, ..., x_n) = \prod_{i=1}^{n} \phi(x_i)$ with $\phi(x) = (2\pi)^{-1/2} \exp(-x^2/2)$. Assume that H' corresponds to a mixture of distribution functions P_θ, where P_θ denotes that $X_1, ..., X_n$ are iid $N(\theta, 1)$, defining $g_n'(x_1, ..., x_n) = \int_{-\infty}^{\infty} \prod_{i=1}^{n} \phi(x_i - \theta) dF(\theta)$, for an arbitrary distribution function F. Thus we obtain the likelihood ratio

$$LR_n = g_n'(X_1, ..., X_n)/g_n(X_1, ..., X_n) = \int_{-\infty}^{\infty} \exp(\theta S_n - n\theta^2/2) dF(\theta), \quad S_n = \sum_{i=1}^{n} X_i.$$

This likelihood ratio can be interpreted in the contexts shown in Chapter 5. Section 5.2 provides to the reader a necessary proof scheme to extend the Ville and Wald inequality to be appropriate for the **Bayes factor**, when the null hypothesis H states that the parameter equals to zero. For reasons which will become apparent in the next sections related to applications of the presented method, we replace $F(\theta)$ by $F(\theta m^{1/2})$, where m is an arbitrary positive constant, since F is an arbitrary distribution function. Then we rewrite

$$LR_n = \int_{-\infty}^{\infty} \exp(\theta S_n - n\theta^2/2) dF(\theta m^{1/2}).$$

Define the function

$$f(x,t) = \int_{-\infty}^{\infty} \exp(yx - ty^2/2) dF(y).$$

Then

$$LR_n = \int_{-\infty}^{\infty} \exp(\theta S_n - n\theta^2/2) dF(\theta m^{1/2})$$

$$= \int_{-\infty}^{\infty} \exp(yS_n m^{-1/2} - ny^2(2m)^{-1}) dF(y) = f(S_n m^{-1/2}, n/m).$$

Thus the Ville and Wald inequality states

$$\Pr\nolimits_H \left\{ f\left(S_n m^{-1/2}, n / m\right) \geq \varepsilon \text{ for some } n \geq 1\right\} =$$

$$\Pr\nolimits_{\theta=0}\left\{ f\left(S_n m^{-1/2}, n / m\right) \geq \varepsilon \text{ for some } n \geq 1\right\} \leq 1 / \varepsilon \ (m > 0, \varepsilon > 0).$$

The following examples illustrate the significance of the result above, considering particular choices of F.

Example 1. Suppose the distribution function F corresponds to random variables having support over $(0, \infty)$. Then $f(x, t) = \int_0^\infty \exp\left(yx - ty^2 / 2\right) dF(y)$ is an increasing function of x. This concludes with

$$f(x, t) \geq \varepsilon \text{ if and only if } x \geq A(t, \varepsilon), \text{ for all } t > 0,$$

where $A(t, \varepsilon)$ is the positive solution x of the equation $f(x, t) = \varepsilon$, i.e., $f(x = A(t, \varepsilon), t) = \varepsilon$. In this case, the Ville and Wald inequality shows that

$$\Pr\nolimits_H \left\{ S_n \geq m^{1/2} A(n / m, \varepsilon) \text{ for some } n \geq 1\right\}$$

$$= \Pr\nolimits_{\theta=0}\left\{ S_n \geq m^{1/2} A(n / m, \varepsilon) \text{ for some } n \geq 1\right\} \leq 1 / \varepsilon.$$

This result remains valid if instead of being iid $N(\theta, 1)$ the observations are any iid random variables that satisfy $E\{\exp(uX_1)\} < \infty$ for all $0 < u < \infty$ (Robbins, 1970). This comment is applicable regarding the following examples too.

Example 2. Suppose the distribution function F is degenerate with mass one assigned to the point $2a > 0$. This scenario can be associated with the hypothesis $H : \theta = 0$ versus $H' : \theta = 2a$. As in Example 1 above, we have

$$f(x, t) = \exp\left(2ax - 2a^2 t\right) \geq \varepsilon \text{ if and only if } x \geq at + \{\log(\varepsilon)\} / (2a),$$

$$\text{for all } t > 0.$$

Thus

$$\Pr\nolimits_H \left\{ S_n \geq an / m^{1/2} + dm^{1/2} \text{ for some } n \geq 1\right\}$$

$$= \Pr\nolimits_{\theta=0}\left\{ S_n \geq an / m^{1/2} + dm^{1/2} \text{ for some } n \geq 1\right\} \leq e^{-2ad},$$

where $d = \log(\varepsilon) / (2a) > 0$, $a > 0$ and $m > 0$.

Example 3. Suppose the distribution function F is defined by

$$F(y) = I(y > 0) \left(\frac{2}{\pi} \right)^{1/2} \int_0^y e^{-u^2/2} \, du. \text{ Then for } t > -1 \text{ we have}$$

$$f(x,t) = \left(\frac{2}{\pi} \right)^{1/2} \int_0^\infty e^{-yx - (t+1)y^2/2} \, dy$$

$$= \frac{2 \exp\left\{ \frac{1}{2} x^2 / (t+1) \right\}}{(t+1)^{1/2}} \Phi\left(\frac{x}{(t+1)^{1/2}} \right), \quad \Phi(u) = \frac{1}{(2\pi)^{1/2}} \int_{-\infty}^u e^{-y^2/2} \, dy.$$

Defining $h^{-1}(u)$ as the inverse function to $h(u) = u^2 + 2\log(\Phi(u))$, one can obtain $A(t,\varepsilon) = (t+1)^{1/2} h^{-1} \left(2\log(\varepsilon/2) + \log(t+1) \right)$, which yields

$$\Pr_{\theta=0}\left\{ S_n \geq (m+n)^{1/2} h^{-1}\left(h(a) + \log\left(\frac{n}{m} + 1 \right) \right) \text{ for some } n \geq 1 \right\}$$

$$\leq \frac{1}{2\Phi(a)} e^{-a^2/2},$$

where $0 < a$ satisfies $0 < \varepsilon = 2\Phi(a)e^{a^2}$, $m > 0$ and it is known that $h(u) \sim u^2$, $h^{-1}(u) \sim u^{1/2}$ as $u \to \infty$.

Example 4. Omitting technical details, one can show that the choice of

$$F(y) = I\left(0 < y < e^{-e} \right) \delta \int_0^y \frac{1}{u \log(1/u) \{\log(\log(1/u))\}^{1+\delta}} \, du \text{ for all } \delta > 0$$

provides that

$$\Pr_H \{ S_n \geq c_n \text{ for some } n \geq 1 \} = \Pr_{\theta=0}\{ S_n \geq c_n \text{ for some } n \geq 1 \} \leq 1/\varepsilon, \, c_n = m^{1/2} A(n/m, \varepsilon)$$

with $c_n \sim \left(2n \log(\log(n)) \right)^{1/2}$ as $n \to \infty$ (Robbins and Siegmund, 1970).

Example 5. Define the distribution function F to be **symmetric** $(F(-u) = 1 - F(u), u \in (-\infty, \infty))$. Then $f(x,t) \geq \varepsilon$ if and only if $|x| \geq A(t,\varepsilon)$, for all $t > 0$. For example, if $F(u) = \Phi(u)$ we obtain

$$\Pr_{\theta=0}\left\{ |S_n| \geq (m+n)^{1/2}\left(a^2 + \log\left(\frac{n}{m} + 1 \right) \right)^{1/2} \text{ for some } n \geq 1 \right\} \leq e^{-a^2/2},$$

where $a > 0$ and $m > 0$. As a one-sided version of this inequality, noting that for all $t > 1$ $\left(a^2 + \log(t) \right)^{1/2} > h^{-1}\left(h(a) + \log(t) \right)$ (the reader can simply plot the functions $\left(a^2 + \log(t)\right)^{1/2}$ and $h^{-1}\left(h(a) + \log(t)\right)$ against $t > 1$, where h and h^{-1} are defined in Example 3 above), we can use the output of Example 3 to obtain

$$\mathrm{Pr}_{\theta=0}\left\{S_n \ge (m+n)^{1/2}\left(a^2 + \log\left(\frac{n}{m}+1\right)\right)^{1/2} \text{ for some } n \ge 1\right\} \le e^{-a^2/2}/(2\Phi(a)).$$

In a similar manner to that shown above, Robbins (1970) and Robbins and Siegmund (1970) concluded with

$$\mathrm{Pr}_{\theta=0}\left\{|S_n| \ge (n)^{1/2}\left(a^2 + \log\left(\frac{n}{m}\right)\right)^{1/2} \text{ for some } n \ge m\right\} \le 2\left(1 - \Phi(a) + a\phi(a)\right),\ \phi(u) = (2\pi)^{-1/2} e^{-u^2/2}.$$

Actually, in the above inequality we can see the role of $m > 0$, when it is stated that "for some $n \ge m$." The integer m can define a pre-sample size of observations after which we analyze $\max_{m \le n < \infty}|S_n|$.

The preceding examples show how to transform the Ville and Wald inequality to the form $\mathrm{Pr}_H\{S_n \ge c_n \text{ for some } n\} \le 1/\varepsilon$ or $\mathrm{Pr}_H\{|S_n| \ge c_n \text{ for some } n\} \le 1/\varepsilon$, where c_n depends on $\varepsilon > 0$. Example 2 derives $c_n = an/m^{1/2} + dm^{1/2} \sim an/m^{1/2}$, Example 3 derives $c_n = (m+n)^{1/2}h^{-1}\left(h(a) + \log\left(\frac{n}{m}+1\right)\right) \sim (n\log(n))^{1/2}$ and Example 4 concludes with $c_n \sim \left(2n\log\left(\log(n)\right)\right)^{1/2}$ as $n \to \infty$. Let us focus again on the law of the iterated logarithm. The sequence $c_n \sim \left(2n\log\left(\log(n)\right)\right)^{1/2}$ increases about as slowly as is possible for sums of iid random variables with mean 0 and variance 1, $\mathrm{Pr}_H\{S_n \ge c_n \text{ for some } n \ge 1\} < 1$. Assume, for example, a researcher attempts to improve upon $c_n \sim \left(2n\log\left(\log(n)\right)\right)^{1/2}$, with the aim of providing a limit to the expression $\mathrm{Pr}_H\left\{S_n \ge c_n \left(\log(\log(\log(n)))\right)^{1/2} / \left(\log(\log(n))\right)^{1/2} \text{ for some } n\right\}$. In this case, the law of the iterated logarithm implies that this approach would be invalid given that

$$\mathrm{Pr}_H\left\{S_n \ge c_n \log(\log(\log(n)))^{1/2}/\log(\log(n))^{1/2} \text{ for some } n\right\} = 1.$$

In order to demonstrate this point, we generated 10,000 iid random variables $X_i \sim N(0,1)$ and computed the sequence of $S_1 = X_1, S_2 = (X_1 + X_2)$, $S_3 = (X_1 + X_2 + X_3), \dots$ Values of S_n are plotted in Figure 8.2 against $n = 150, \dots, 10000$ using "o" symbols. In this figure, we present the bounds $\pm\left(2n\log\left(\log(n)\right)\right)^{1/2}$ (curves —) and $\pm\left(2n\log\left(\log(\log(n))\right)\right)^{1/2}$ (curves - - - -).

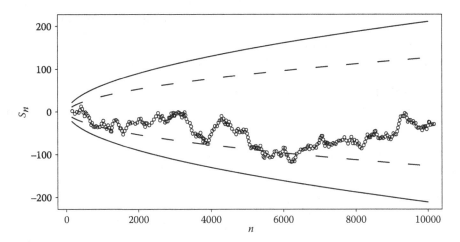

FIGURE 8.2

Values of S_n (ooo) plotted against $n = 150, ..., 10000$. The figure presents the bounds $\pm \left(2n \log \left(\log \left(n\right)\right)\right)^{1/2}$ (curves —) and $\pm \left(2n \log \left(\log \left(\log(n)\right)\right)\right)^{1/2}$ (curves - - - -).

8.4 Applications to Statistical Procedures

Consider the statistical significance of the results mentioned in Section 8.3.

8.4.1 Confidence Sequences and Tests with Uniformly Small Error Probability for the Mean of a Normal Distribution with Known Variance

Let the observations $X_1, ..., X_n, X_{n+1}, ...$ be independent and identically $N(\theta, 1)$ distributed, where θ is an unknown parameter, $-\infty < \theta < \infty$. We are interested in obtaining the intervals $I_n = ((S_n - c_n)/n, (S_n + c_n)/n)$, where $n \geq 1$, $S_n = X_1 + ... + X_n$ and c_n is a sequence of positive constants, such that we can control the cover probability $\text{Pr}_\theta(\theta \in I_n$ for every $n \geq 1)$.

It is clear that

$$\text{Pr}_\theta(\theta \in I_n \text{ for every } n \geq 1) = \text{Pr}_\theta\left(S_n - c_n < \theta n < S_n + c_n \text{ for every } n \geq 1\right)$$

$$= \text{Pr}_\theta\left(S_n - c_n < \theta n, S_n + c_n > \theta n \text{ for every } n \geq 1\right)$$

$$= \text{Pr}_\theta\left(S_n - \theta n < c_n, S_n - \theta n > -c_n \text{ for every } n \geq 1\right)$$

$$= \text{Pr}_\theta\left(\left|\sum_{i=1}^{n}(X_i - \theta)\right| < c_n \text{ for every } n \geq 1\right)$$

$$= \text{Pr}_{\theta=0}\left(\left|S_n\right| < c_n \text{ for every } n \geq 1\right).$$

Note that, in the equation above, we changed the measure Pr_θ to be $\text{Pr}_{\theta=0}$, since, under the assumption $X_i \sim N(\theta, 1)$, the expression $\dfrac{S_n - c_n}{n} < \theta < \dfrac{S_n + c_n}{n}$ is equivalent to $|S_n| < c_n$, when $X_i \sim N(0, 1)$. Thus

$$\text{Pr}_\theta(\theta \in I_n \text{ for every } n \geq 1) = \text{Pr}_0(|S_n| < c_n \text{ for every } n \geq 1)$$

$$= 1 - \text{Pr}_0(|S_n| \geq c_n \text{ for some } n \geq 1).$$

Define $c_n = [(n+m)(a^2 + \log(n/m+1))]^{1/2}$, with $0 < c_n/n \to 0$ as $n \to \infty$. In this case, Example 5 in Section 8.3 provides

$$\text{Pr}_0(|S_n| \geq c_n \text{ for some } n \geq 1) \leq e^{-a^2/2}.$$

Hence

$$\text{Pr}_\theta(\theta \in I_n \text{ for every } n \geq 1) = \text{Pr}_0\left(\theta \in \bigcap_{i=1}^{\infty} I_i\right) \geq 1 - e^{-a^2/2},$$

which can be made near 1 by choosing a sufficiently large, e.g., $a^2 = 6$ yields $1 - \exp(-a^2/2) \cong 0.95$. Thus for $a^2 = 6$ and any $m > 0$, the sequence I_n with c_n defined above forms a 95% confidence sequence for an unknown θ with coverage probability ≥ 0.95.

Following the conventional concept of confidence interval constructions (see Chapter 9 in this context), one can use the fact $S_n = X_1 + \ldots + X_n \sim N(\theta n, n)$ to propose, for any *fixed* n,

$$\text{Pr}_\theta\{(S_n - 1.96n^{1/2})/n < \theta < (S_n + 1.96n^{1/2})/n\} = \text{Pr}_\theta\{\theta < (S_n + 1.96n^{1/2})/n\}$$

$$-\text{Pr}_\theta\{\theta < (S_n - 1.96n^{1/2})/n\} = 1 - \text{Pr}_\theta\{(S_n - \theta n)/n \leq -1.96n^{1/2}\}$$

$$-1 + \text{Pr}_\theta\{(S_n - \theta n)/n \leq 1.96n^{-1/2}\} = \Phi(1.96) - \Phi(-1.96) \cong 0.95.$$

However, by virtue of the law of the iterated logarithm, we conclude with

$$\text{Pr}_\theta\{(S_n - 1.96n^{1/2})/n < \theta < (S_n + 1.96n^{1/2})/n \text{ for every } n \geq 1\} = 0.$$

The advantage of the confidence sequence I_n as compared to a fixed sample size confidence interval is that it allows us to "follow" the unknown parameter throughout the whole sequence $X_1, \ldots$ with an interval I_n whose length shrinks to 0 as the sample size increases, in such a way that with probability ≥ 0.95 the interval I_n contains the parameter at every stage. This advantage costs us a widening of the intervals $\left((S_n - 1.96n^{1/2})/n, (S_n + 1.96n^{1/2})/n\right)$ to $\left((S_n - c_n)/n, (S_n + c_n)/n\right)$ with respect to an asymptotic order of $O\left([\log(n)]^{1/2}/n\right)$ as $n \to \infty$.

8.4.2 Confidence Sequences for the Median

Let $Z_1, Z_2, \ldots$ be iid data points with median M that satisfy $\Pr(Z_1 \leq M) = 0.5$. The usual *confidence interval* for M, provided that the sample size n is relatively large, is

$$\Pr\{Z_{a_1}^{(n)} \leq M \leq Z_{a_2}^{(n)}\} \cong 2\Phi(a) - 1,$$

where $Z_1^{(n)} \leq \ldots \leq Z_n^{(n)}$ denote the ordered values $Z_1, \ldots, Z_n$ and

$$a_1 = a_1(n) = \text{largest integer} \leq 0.5(n - an^{0.5}),$$

$$a_2 = a_2(n) = \text{smallest integer} \geq 0.5(n + an^{0.5}).$$

Proof. As used in various proof schemes shown in this book, the idea of this proof is to rewrite the stated problem to a formulation in terms of sums of iid random variables and then to employ an appropriate theorem related to sums of iid random variables. In this case, we aim to use *the central limit theorem* (Section 2.4.5) via the following algorithm: Define the empirical distribution function $F_n(u) = \sum_{i=1}^{n} I(Z_i \leq u)/n$. The function $F_n(u)$ increases providing

$$\Pr\{Z_{a_1}^{(n)} \leq M\} = \Pr\{F_n(Z_{a_1}^{(n)}) \leq F_n(M)\} = \Pr\{a_1/n \leq F_n(M)\},$$

since $F_n(Z_{a_1}^{(n)}) = \sum_{i=1}^{n} I(Z_i \leq Z_{a_1}^{(n)})/n = \sum_{i=1}^{n} I(Z_i^{(n)} \leq Z_{a_1}^{(n)})/n = a_1/n$. Thus

$$\Pr\{Z_{a_1}^{(n)} \leq M\} = \Pr\{a_1/n \leq F_n(M)\} =$$

$$1 - \Pr\left\{\sum_{i=1}^{n} \{I(Z_i \leq M) - 0.5\}/(0.5n^{1/2}) < -a\right\},$$

where $I(Z_1 \leq M), \ldots, I(Z_n \leq M)$ are iid random variables with $E\{I(Z_1 \leq M)\} = \Pr(Z_1 \leq M) = 0.5$ and $\text{var}\{I(Z_1 \leq M)\} = E\{I(Z_1 \leq M) - 0.5\}^2 = 0.5^2$. Then

$\Pr\{Z_{a_1}^{(n)} \leq M\} \to 1 - \Phi(-a) = \Phi(a)$ as $n \to \infty$. Similarly, we have
$\Pr\{M \leq Z_{a_2}^{(n)}\} \to \Phi(a)$ as $n \to \infty$. Since

$$\Pr\{Z_{a_1}^{(n)} \leq M \leq Z_{a_2}^{(n)}\} = \Pr\{M \leq Z_{a_2}^{(n)}\} - \Pr\{M \leq Z_{a_1}^{(n)}\}$$

$$= \Pr\{M \leq Z_{a_2}^{(n)}\} - 1 + \Pr\{M > Z_{a_1}^{(n)}\}$$

$$\cong \Phi(a) - 1 + \Phi(a),$$

the proof is complete.

In order to construct a confidence sequence for M, we define

$$X_i = 1 \text{ if } X_i \leq M$$

$$= -1 \text{ if } X_i > M, \quad S_n = X_1 + \ldots + X_n$$

and

$$b_1 = b_1(n) = \text{largest integer } \leq 0.5(n - c_n)$$

$$b_2 = b_2(n) = \text{smallest integer } \geq 0.5(n + c_n),$$

where c_n is some sequence of positive constants.

Now we will obtain that

$$\Pr(Z_{b_1}^{(n)} \leq M \leq Z_{b_2}^{(n)} \text{ for every } n \geq m > 0) \geq 1 - \Pr\left(|S_n| \geq c_n \text{ for some } n \geq m > 0\right).$$

Towards this end, we consider the event

$A = \left\{ Z_{b_1}^{(n)} > M \text{ or } Z_{b_2}^{(n)} < M \right\} = \overline{\left\{ Z_{b_1}^{(n)} \leq M \leq Z_{b_2}^{(n)} \right\}}$ (here $\bar{A}$ is the complement of A).

If $Z_{b_1}^{(n)} > M$ then $M < Z_{b_1}^{(n)} \leq Z_{b_1+1}^{(n)} \leq Z_{b_1+2}^{(n)} \leq \ldots \leq Z_n^{(n)}$ and we have $(n - b_1)$ times

the value of (-1) present in $X_1, \ldots, X_n$. The values of the X's, which do not correspond to $Z_{b_1}^{(n)}, \ldots, Z_n^{(n)}$, can be equal to 1 or (-1) but must be ≤ 1. This implies

$$S_n = X_1 + \ldots + X_n \leq (-1)(n - b_1) + (1)b_1 = 2b_1 - n = -c_n.$$

If $Z_{b_2}^{(n)} < M$ then $Z_1^{(n)} < \ldots < Z_{b_2}^{(n)} < M$ and we have b_2 times the value of 1 present in $X_1, \ldots, X_n$. In this case, the values of the X's, which do not correspond to $Z_1^{(n)}, \ldots, Z_{b_2}^{(n)}$, can be equal to 1 or (-1) but must be $\geq (-1)$. This implies

$$S_n = X_1 + \ldots + X_n \geq (1)b_2 + (-1)(n - b_2) = c_n.$$

Therefore $A \subseteq \left\{ |S_n| \geq c_n \right\}$ leading to $\Pr(\bar{A}) = 1 - \Pr(A) \geq \Pr\left\{ |S_n| \geq c_n \right\}$, for all n. Thus

$$\Pr(Z_{b_1}^{(n)} \leq M \leq Z_{b_2}^{(n)} \text{ for every } n \geq m > 0) \geq 1 - \Pr(|S_n| \geq c_n \text{ for some } n \geq m > 0).$$

It is clear that $E\{\exp(uX_1)\} < \infty$, for all $0 < u < \infty$. Then, following Example 5 in Section 8.3, we use the sequence $c_n = [n(a^2 + \log(n/m))]^{1/2}$, obtaining $\Pr(|S_n| \geq c_n \text{ for some } n \geq m) \leq 2(1 - \Phi(a) + a\phi(a))$, which provides

$$\Pr(Z_{b_1}^{(n)} \leq M \leq Z_{b_2}^{(n)} \text{ for every } n \geq m > 0) \geq 1 - 2(1 - \Phi(a) + a\phi(a))$$

$$= 2\Phi(a) - 1 - 2a\phi(a).$$

Note that, comparing the method based on $\Pr\{Z_{a_1}^{(n)} \leq M \leq Z_{a_2}^{(n)}\} \cong 2\Phi(a) - 1$ with the result above, one can compute, for large m, that

a	$2\Phi(a) - 1$	$2\Phi(a) - 1 - 2a\phi(a)$
2	0.9546	0.7386
2.5	0.9876	0.9001
2.8	0.9948	0.9506
3	0.9947	0.971
3.5	0.9996	0.9933

We would like to emphasize again that, by virtue of the law of the iterated logarithm, we have

$$\Pr(Z_{a_1}^{(n)} \leq M \leq Z_{a_2}^{(n)} \text{ for every } n \geq m) = 0$$

and in many practical situations, we do not know if the sample size n is large enough to hold the asymptotic proposition $\Pr\{Z_{a_1}^{(n)} \leq M \leq Z_{a_2}^{(n)}\} \cong 2\Phi(a) - 1$.

8.4.3 Test with Power One

Assume that we can observe the independent and identically $N(\theta, 1)$-distributed data points $X_1, ..., X_n, X_{n+1}, ...$ in order to test for $H_0 : \theta \leq 0$ versus $H_1 : \theta > 0$. Define

$$N = \begin{cases} \text{first } n \geq 1 \text{ such that } S_n = X_1 + ... + X_n \geq c_n \\ \infty \text{ if no such } n \text{ occurs} \end{cases}$$

to apply the test procedure: when $N < \infty$, we stop sampling with X_N and reject H_0 in favor of H_1; if $N = \infty$, we continue sampling indefinitely and do not reject H_0. In this case, the Type I error rate has the form

$$\Pr_{\theta \leq 0}(\text{we reject } H_0) = \Pr_{\theta \leq 0}(N < \infty) = \Pr_{\theta \leq 0}\left\{ \max_{1 \leq k < \infty} \left(\sum_{i=1}^{k} X_i - c_k \right) \geq 0 \right\}$$

$$= \Pr_{\theta \leq 0}\left\{ \max_{1 \leq k < \infty} \left(\sum_{i=1}^{k} (X_i - \theta) + \theta k - c_k \right) \geq 0 \right\}.$$

That is to say

$$\Pr_{\theta \leq 0}(\text{we reject } H_0) \leq \Pr_{\theta \leq 0}\left\{ \max_{1 \leq k < \infty} \left(\sum_{i=1}^{k} (X_i - \theta) - c_k \right) \geq 0 \right\},$$

since $\theta k \leq 0$. Then

$$\Pr_{\theta \leq 0}(\text{we reject } H_0) \leq \Pr_{\theta=0}\left\{\max_{1 \leq k < \infty}\left(\sum_{i=1}^{k}(X_i) - c_k\right) \geq 0\right\} = \Pr_{\theta=0}(N < \infty).$$

As in Section 8.4.1, here we changed the measure $\Pr_\theta$ to be $\Pr_{\theta=0}$. If we are using $c_n = [(n+m)(a^2 + \log(n/m+1))]^{1/2}$, as presented in Example 5 of Section 8.3, then we have

$$\Pr_{\theta \leq 0}(\text{we reject } H_0) \leq \Pr_{\theta=0}\left\{\max_{1 \leq k < \infty}\left(\sum_{i=1}^{k}(X_i) - c_k\right) \geq 0\right\}$$

$$= \Pr_{\theta=0}(S_n \geq c_n \text{ for some } n \geq 1) \leq \frac{1}{2\Phi(a)}e^{-a^2/2},$$

which controls the Type I error probability of the test.

The Type II error probability of the test is

$$\Pr_{\theta>0}(\text{we do not reject } H_0) = \Pr_{\theta>0}(S_n < c_n \text{ for all } n \geq 1)$$

$$= \Pr_{\theta>0}(S_n/n < c_n/n \text{ for all } n \geq 1).$$

By virtue of the law of large numbers, under the alternative hypothesis, we have $S_n/n \to \theta > 0$, whereas $c_n/n \to 0$ as $n \to \infty$. Then one can find K such that for $n > K$, $\Pr_{\theta>0}(S_n/n < c_n/n) = 0$ (see Section 1.2 for details). Thus

$$1 - \text{Power} = \Pr_{\theta>0}(\text{we do not reject } H_0) = \Pr_{\theta>0}(S_n/n < c_n/n \text{ for all } n \geq 1) = 0$$

and the test has power one against the alternative $\theta > 0$.

Regarding the expected sample size $E_{\theta>0}(N)$, it can be shown that for any stopping rule N based on $X_1, \ldots$ the inequality $E_{\theta>0}(N) \geq -2\log(\Pr_0(N < \infty))/\theta^2$ must hold for every $\theta > 0$ (see Chapter 6). Thus if we are willing to tolerate an N for which $\Pr_0(N < \infty) = 0.05$, then necessarily $E_{\theta>0}(N) \geq 6/\theta^2$ for every $\theta > 0$; however, no such N will minimize $E_\theta(N)$ uniformly for all $\theta > 0$. For N applied in this section, where $c_n = [(n+m)(a^2 + \log(n/m+1))]^{1/2}$, a simple Monte Carlo study can evaluate $E_{\theta>0}(N)$ for different values of $\theta > 0$ and fixed $m > 0$.

9

Brief Comments on Confidence
Intervals and p-Values

9.1 Confidence Intervals

We assume the reader is familiar with the conventional principles of *confidence interval* estimation that is of a type given by an interval of a scalar parameter, which in turn can be generalized to the concept of a confidence region for a set of parameters (or a vector of parameters).

In this section, we will essentially focus on the Bayesian approach for confidence interval estimation because of its efficiency and natural interpretation, which provides wide applicability in statistical practice. However, the comments shown in this chapter can be easily adapted to the frequentist framework of confidence interval (or region) estimation. Two suggested detailed references pertaining to the core frequentist theory, as put forward by R.A. Fisher and J. Neman, are Schweder and Hjort (2002) and Singh et al. (2005).

The Bayesian display of the upper and lower bounds, which contains a large fraction of the posterior mass (typically 95%) related to a functional parameter, is an analog of the frequentist confidence interval and commonly termed in the literature as a *credible set* or simply "confidence interval" (e.g., Carlin and Louis, 2011). There is a rich statistical literature regarding the theoretical and applied aspects of the Bayesian confidence interval estimation (e.g., Broemeling, 2007; Gelman et al., 2013). To outline this technique, we assume that the dataset X consists of n independent and identically distributed observations $X = (X_1, ..., X_n)$ from density function $f(x \mid \theta)$ with an unknown parameter θ of interest. For simplicity, we suppose θ is scalar. In the Bayesian framework (Chapter 5) we define the prior distribution $\pi(\theta)$, which represents the prior information about θ mapped onto a probability space. The prior information is updated conditionally on the observed data using the likelihood function $\prod_{i=1}^{n} f(X_i \mid \theta)$ via Bayes theorem to obtain the posterior density function of θ,

$$h(\theta \mid X) = \prod_{i=1}^{n} f(X_i \mid \theta)\pi(\theta) \Big/ \int \prod_{i=1}^{n} f(X_i \mid \theta)\pi(\theta)d\theta.$$

We assume that $h(\theta \mid X)$ is unimodal. The $(1 - \alpha)100\%$ Bayesian confidence interval estimate for θ can be presented as an interval $[q_L, q_U]$ such that the posterior probability $\Pr(q_L < \theta < q_U \mid X) = 1 - \alpha$ (or simply $\Pr(q_L < \theta < q_U) = 1 - \alpha$ in this section) at a fixed significant level α, that is, $\int_{q_L}^{q_U} h(\theta \mid X)d\theta = 1 - \alpha$. In this case, the problem is that we have only one equation to find values of the two unknown quantities q_L, q_U. Consider, for example, Figure 9.1, where, for $\alpha = 0.05$, we display the scenarios related to the intervals $[q_L, q_U]$ that satisfy

$$\text{Panel (a)}: \frac{\alpha}{2} = \int_{-\infty}^{q_L} h(\theta \mid X)d\theta, \quad \frac{\alpha}{2} = \int_{q_U}^{\infty} h(\theta \mid X)d\theta;$$

$$\text{Panel (b)}: \frac{\alpha}{1.2} = \int_{-\infty}^{q_L} h(\theta \mid X)d\theta, \quad \alpha\left(1 - \frac{1}{1.2}\right) = \int_{q_U}^{\infty} h(\theta \mid X)d\theta$$

and

$$\text{Panel (c)}: \int_{q_L}^{q_U} h(\theta \mid X)d\theta = 1 - \alpha, \quad h(q_L \mid X) = h(q_U \mid X).$$

Warning: *Similar to the issue regarding the general Type I error rate definition mentioned in Section 4.4.4, it is reasonable to raise the question, "What kind of confidence interval definition do you use?" in terms of what is actually presented.*

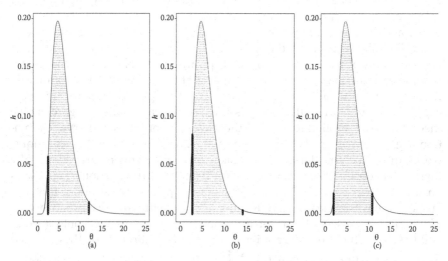

FIGURE 9.1
The confidence interval definitions related to the following scenarios: (a) the posterior probabilities $\Pr(\theta \le q_L) = \Pr(\theta \ge q_U) = \alpha/2$ and (b) the posterior probabilities $\Pr(\theta \le q_L) = \alpha/1.2$, $\Pr(\theta \ge q_U) = \alpha(1 - 1/1.2)$, where $\alpha = 0.05$. Panel (c) presents the interval $[q_L, q_U]$ calculated using the equations $\Pr(q_L < \theta < q_U) = 1 - \alpha$ and $h(q_L \mid X) = h(q_U \mid X)$.

In order to calculate the interval $\left[q_L, q_U\right]$ a common approach found in the statistical literature suggests employing the following two strategies:

Method (I): The bounds q_L and q_U are computed as roots of the equations

$$\frac{\alpha}{2} = \int_{-\infty}^{q_L} h(\theta \mid X) d\theta \text{ and } \frac{\alpha}{2} = \int_{q_U}^{\infty} h(\theta \mid X) d\theta.$$

This implies the Bayesian *equal-tailed confidence interval* estimation

Method (II): We can derive values for the bounds q_L and q_U as roots of the equations

$$h(q_L \mid X) = h(q_U \mid X) \text{ and } \int_{q_L}^{q_U} h(\theta \mid X) d\theta = 1 - \alpha.$$

This implies the Bayesian *highest posterior density confidence interval* estimation (see, e.g., panel (c) of Figure 9.1). Method (I) is computationally simple and oftentimes used in practice. The practical implementation of Method (II) usually requires using complicated computation schemes based on Markov Chain Monte Carlo techniques (e.g., Chen and Shao, 1999).

The length $q_U - q_L$ can characterize a quality of the confidence interval estimation. This means that the rule for constructing the confidence interval should make as much use of the information in the data set and prior as possible. In this case, one way of assessing optimality is by the length of the interval so that a rule for constructing a confidence interval is judged better than another if it leads to intervals whose lengths are typically shorter. For example, it seems that panel (c) of Figure 9.1 depicts the shorter confidence interval. Let us derive q_U and q_L that minimize $q_U - q_L$, satisfying $\int_{q_L}^{q_U} h(\theta \mid X) d\theta = 1 - \alpha$. To this end, we employ the Lagrange method that implies solving the equations

$$\frac{\partial}{\partial q_U}\left[q_U - q_L + \lambda\left(1 - \alpha - \int_{q_L}^{q_U} h(u \mid X) du\right)\right] = 0,$$

$$\frac{\partial}{\partial q_L}\left[q_U - q_L + \lambda\left(1 - \alpha - \int_{q_L}^{q_U} h(u \mid X) du\right)\right] = 0,$$

where λ is the Lagrange multiplier, with respect to q_U and q_L. Then we have $1 - \lambda h(q_U \mid X) = 0$, $-1 + \lambda h(q_L \mid X) = 0$, obtaining $h(q_L \mid X) = h(q_U \mid X)$.

Thus, we conclude that (a) in general, the highest posterior density confidence interval does have the shortest length, and (b) in the case, where h is a symmetric function, the equal-tail setup is the optimal definition of the confidence interval in the context of its length.

Warning: *In order to apply the above methods in practice, the form of the density function $f(x|\theta)$ needs to be specified. Daniels and Hogan (2008) showed significant issues relative to verifying the parametric assumptions for various cases as to when the Bayesian confidence interval estimation can be applied efficiently. Zhou and Reiter (2010) demonstrated that when parametric assumptions are not met exactly, the posterior estimators are generally biased. The statistical literature has displayed many examples when parametric forms of data distributions are not available and there are vital concerns relative to using the Bayesian parametric confidence interval approach. In this context, Vexler et al. (2016b) developed a robust nonparametric method for confidence interval estimation in the Bayesian manner. Toward this end, **empirical likelihood** functions (Chapter 10) were employed to replace the corresponding unknown parametric likelihood functions in the posterior probability construction.*

In the frequentist framework, the use of confidence intervals or regions for decision making has a one-to-one mapping to hypothesis testing about a parameter, set of parameters or functions. For a single parameter, e.g., the population mean, one can construct a confidence interval based on manipulating the probability statement that a parameter lies between a lower and upper bound, which are functions of the data (e.g., Section 3.3). In many instances the concept of a pivot can be used to manipulate the terms of the probability statement in order to obtain a confidence interval. Confidence intervals can be based on both parametric and nonparametric approaches, as well as large sample approximations.

In terms of confidence intervals and their relationship to hypothesis tests, we would reject H_0 for a two-sided test if the parameter under H_0 fell outside the confidence interval bounds. Consider, for example, a simple scenario when a test statistic $TS(\theta_0)$, as a function of θ_0 based on data, is proposed for testing the hypothesis $H_0 : \theta = \theta_0$, where θ is the parameter of interest. Assume we reject the null hypothesis for large values of $TS(\theta_0)$. In order to control the Type I error rate, we should derive an exact or asymptotic distribution of $TS(\theta_0)$ under H_0, say $\Pr_{H_0}\{TS(\theta_0) \le C\} \underset{\text{(or converges to)}}{=} G(C)$, for a fixed argument C. Then we reject the hypothesis H_0 when $TS(\theta_0) \ge g_{1-\alpha}$, where $g_{1-\alpha}$ is the $100(1-\alpha)\%$ percentile of the distribution G, and α is the significance level. By virtue of the relation between the testing and confidence interval estimation, we can obtain the confidence interval estimator of θ in the form of $CI_{1-\alpha} = \{\theta : TS(\theta) \le g_{1-\alpha}\}$, assuming that the nominal coverage probability is specified as $1-\alpha$. In this context, shorter confidence intervals can correspond to greater statistical power in the parallel statistical hypothesis test.

In various situations, *Monte Carlo* experiments (Section 2.4.5.1) can be used to evaluate and compare the qualities of proposed confidence interval estimators. In such cases, commonly, the Monte Carlo coverage probabilities (e.g., the average value of indicators $I\{\theta_0 \in CI_{1-\alpha}\}$ based on Monte Carlo generated data under H_0, in the terms of the example mentioned above) and the Monte Carlo average lengths of the considered confidence intervals (e.g., the average value of $\max\{\theta : TS(\theta) \leq g_{1-\alpha}\} - \min\{\theta : TS(\theta) \leq g_{1-\alpha}\}$ based on Monte Carlo generated data under H_0) are basic factors to be computed. The Monte Carlo cover probabilities can be compared to the expected coverage probability $1 - \alpha$.

9.2 *p*-Values

The *p*-value has long played a role in scientific research as a key decision-making tool with respect to hypothesis testing and dates back to Laplace in the 1770s (Stigler, 1986). The concept of the *p*-value was popularized by Fisher as an inferential tool and is where the first occurrence of the term "statistical significance" is found (Fisher, 1925). In the frequentist hypothesis testing framework a test is deemed statistically significant if the *p*-value, which is a statistic having support over the real line in (0,1) space, is below some threshold known as the critical value. In a vast majority of studies the critical value is set at 0.05.

A majority of traditional testing procedures are designed to draw a conclusion (or make an action) with respect to the binary decision of rejecting or not rejecting the null hypothesis H_0, depending on locations of the corresponding values of the observed test statistics, that is, detecting whether test statistic values belong to a fixed sphere or interval. In simple cases, test procedures require us to compare corresponding test statistics values based on observed data with test thresholds. P-values can serve as an alternative data-driven approach for testing statistical hypotheses based on using the observed values of test statistics as the thresholds in the theoretical probability of the Type I error. P-values can themselves also serve as a summary type result based on data in that they provide meaningful experimental data-based evidence about the null hypothesis.

For example, suppose that the test statistic L has a distribution function F under H_0. Under a one-sided upper-tailed alternative H_1 the *p*-value is the random variable $1 - F(L)$, which is uniformly distributed under H_0 (e.g., Vexler et al., 2016a).

The obvious correct use of the *p*-value is to simply draw a conclusion of reject or do not reject the null hypothesis. This principle simplifies and *standardizes* statistical decision-making policies. In this manner, for example, different algorithms for combining decision-making rules using their *p*-values as test statistics can be naturally derived (e.g., Vexler et al., 2017).

Warning: *The p-value is oftentimes misused and misinterpreted in the applied scientific literature where statistical decision-making procedures are involved. Many scientists misinterpret smaller p-values as providing stronger theoretical evidence against a null hypothesis relative to larger p-values. For example, some researchers draw conclusions regarding comparisons of associations between a disease and different factors using values of the corresponding p-values. In a hypothetical study, consider evaluating associations between a disease, say D, and two biomarkers, say A and B. It is not uncommon for scientists to conclude that the association between D and A is stronger than that between D and B if the p-value regarding the association between A and D is smaller than that of the association between B and D. This example demonstrates the noncareful use of the p-value's concept, since perhaps data obtained in a different but relevant experiment might provide the contradicting conclusion simply due to the stochastic nature of the p-value. These types of issues have led several scientific journals to discourage the use of p-values, with some scientists and statisticians encouraging their abandonment (Wasserstein and Lazar, 2016). For example, the editors of the journal entitled Basic and Applied Social Psychology announced that the journal would no longer publish papers containing p-value-based studies since the statistics were too often used to support lower-quality research (Trafimow and Marks, 2015). Misinterpreting the magnitude of the p-value as strength for or against the null hypothesis or as a probability statement about the null hypothesis can lead to a misinterpretation of the results of a statistical test. Several common weaknesses or misinterpretations of the p-value are as follows: (1) employing the p-value as the probability that the null hypothesis is true can be wrong or even far from reasonable, as the p-value strongly depends on current data in use; (2) the p-value is not very useful for large sample sizes, because almost no null hypothesis is exactly true when examined using real data, and when the sample size is relatively large, almost any null hypothesis will have a tiny p-value, leading to the rejection of the null at conventional significance levels; and (3) model selection is difficult, e.g., simply choosing the wrong model among a class of models or using a model that is not robust to statistical assumptions will lead to an incorrect p-value and/or inflated Type I error rates.*

The p-value is a function of the data and hence it is a random variable, which too has a probability distribution. The subtlety in terms of those that try to interpret the magnitude of the relative p-value is that the distribution of the p-value is conditional on either the null hypothesis being true or not. Under the null hypothesis, typically, p-values are exactly (or asymptotically) Uniform[0,1] distributed. However, if the null hypothesis is false p-values have a non-Uniform[0,1] distribution for which the shape of the distribution varies across several factors including sample size and the distance of the parameter of interest from the hypothesized value (null). Hence, for the same exact null and alternative values the distribution of the p-value may be small or large simply as a function of the sample size (statistical power). In the era of "big data" it would not be unusual to constantly find extremely small p-values simply as a function of a massively large sample size, with nothing really to do with the scientific question. Likewise a large observed p-value may simply be due to a very small sample size.

Statisticians have long recognized the deficiencies in terms of interpreting p-values relative to their stochastic nature and have tried to develop remedies to aid scientists in the interpretation of their data. For example, Lazzeroni et al. (2014) developed prediction intervals for p-values in replication studies. This approach has certain critical points regarding the following problems: (1) in the frequentist context it is uncommon to create confidence intervals of random variables; (2) under the null hypothesis p-values are distributed according to a Uniform[0,1] distribution, whereas in many scenarios, if we are sure the alternative hypothesis is in effect, the prediction interval for the p-value is not needed; and (3) prediction intervals for p-values can be directly associated with those for corresponding test statistic values, linking to just rejection sets of the test procedures.

The stochastic aspect of the p-value has been well studied by Dempster and Schatzoff (1965), who introduced the concept of the *expected significance level*. Sackrowitz and Samuel-Cahn (1999) developed the approach further and renamed it as the *expected p-value* (EPV). The authors presented the great potential of using EPVs in various aspects of hypothesis testing.

Comparisons of different test procedures, e.g., a Wilcoxon rank-sum test versus Student's t-test, based on their statistical power is oftentimes problematic in terms of deeming one method being the preferred test over a range of scenarios. One reason for this issue to occur is that the comparison between two or more testing procedures is dependent upon the choice of a prespecified significance level α. One test procedure may be more or less powerful than the other one depending on the choice of α. Alternatively, one can consider the EPV concept in order to compare test procedures. In this chapter, we show that the EPV corresponds to the integrated power of a test via all possible values of $\alpha \in (0,1)$. Thus, the performance of the test procedure can be evaluated globally using the EPV concept. Smaller values of EPV show better test qualities in a more universal fashion. This method is an alternative approach to the Neyman–Pearson concept of testing statistical hypotheses. The famous Neyman–Pearson lemma (Section 3.4) introduced us to the concept that a reasonable statistical testing procedure controls the Type I error rate at a prespecified significance level, α, in conjunction with maximizing the power in a uniform fashion. Thus, for different values of α we may obtain different superior test procedures. On the other hand, the EPV-based approach allows us to compare between decision-making rules in a more objective manner. The global test performance of testing procedures can be measured by one number, the EPV, and hence tests can be more easily rank-ordered.

We further advance the concept of the EPV. We prove that there is a strong association between the EPV concept and the well-known receiver operating characteristic (ROC) curve methodology (Chapter 7). It turns out that we can use well-established ROC curve and AUC methods to evaluate and visualize the properties of various decision-making procedures in the *p*-value-based context. Further, in parallel with partial AUCs (Section 7.6), we develop a *partial expected* **p-value** (pEPV) and introduce a novel method for visualizing the properties of statistical tests in an ROC curve framework. We prove that the conventional power characterization of tests is a partial aspect of the presented EPV/ROC technique.

In order to exemplify additional applications of the EPV/ROC methodology, we refer the reader to Vexler et al. (2017).

9.2.1   The EPV in the Context of an ROC Curve Analysis

In this section we present the following material: the formal definition of the EPV and the association between the EPV and the AUC. We also provide a new quantity called the partial EPV (pEPV), which characterizes a property of decision-making procedures using the concept of partial AUCs (see Section 7.6).

Let the random variable $T(D)$ represent a test statistic depending on data D. Assume F_i defines the distribution function of $T(D)$ under the hypothesis H_i, $i = 0,1$, where the subscript i indicates the null ($i = 0$) and alternative ($i = 1$) hypotheses, respectively. Given F_i is continuous we can denote F_i^{-1} to represent the inverse or quantile function of F_i, such that $F_i(F_i^{-1}(\gamma)) = \gamma$, where $0 < \gamma < 1$ and $i = 0,1$. In this setting, in order to concentrate upon the main issues, we will only focus on tests of the form: the event $T(D) > C$ rejects H_0, where C is a prefixed test threshold. Thus the *p*-value has the form $1 - F_0(T(D))$. Sackrowitz and Samuel-Cahn (1999) proved that the expected *p*-value $E(1 - F_0(T(D)) \mid H_1)$ is

$$\text{EPV} = \Pr(T^0 \geq T^A), \tag{9.1}$$

where independent random variables T^0 and T^A are distributed according to F_0 and F_1, respectively.

Proof. We have $E(1 - F_0(T(D)) \mid H_1) = \int \{1 - F_0(u)\} dF_1(u) = \int \Pr(T^0 \geq u) dF_1(u) = \Pr(T^0 \geq T^A)$, which completes the proof.

The simple example of the EPV is when $T^0 \sim N(\mu_1, \sigma_1^2)$ and $T^A \sim N(\mu_2, \sigma_2^2)$. Then the EPV can be expressed as

$$\text{EPV} = \Phi\left((\mu_1 - \mu_2)(\sigma_1^2 + \sigma_2^2)^{-1/2}\right),$$

where Φ is the cumulative standard normal distribution.

Note that the formal notation (9.1) is similar to that for the area under the corresponding ROC curve (Section 7.3). In this case, the ROC curve can assist in measuring a distance between the distribution functions F_0 and F_1. In this context, one can reconsider the EPV in terms of the area under the ROC curve (AUC), obtaining that the EPV is $1 - $ AUC. This connection between the EPV and the AUC induces new techniques for evaluating statistical test qualities via the well-established ROC curve methodology.

9.2.2 Student's *t*-Test versus Welch's *t*-Test

Consider, for illustrative purposes, the following example related to applications of Student's and Welch's *t*-tests. The recent biostatistical literature has extensively discussed which test, Student's *t*- or Welch's *t*-test, to use in practical applications. The questions in this setting are: What is the risk of using Student's *t*-test when variances of the two populations are different? Also, what is the loss in power when using Welch's *t*-test when the variances of the two populations are equal (Julious, 2005; Zimmerman and Zumbo, 2009)? In order to apply the ROC curve analysis based on the EPV concept, we denote Student's *t*-test statistic as

$$T_S = \left(\bar{X} - \bar{Y} \right) \left[S_p \left(n^{-1} + m^{-1} \right)^{1/2} \right]^{-1},$$

and Welch's *t*-test statistic as

$$T_W = \left(\bar{X} - \bar{Y} \right) \left(S_1^2 n^{-1} + S_2^2 m^{-1} \right)^{-1/2},$$

where $\bar{X}$ is the sample mean based on the independent normally distributed data points $X_1,...,X_n$, $\bar{Y}$ is the sample mean based on the independent normally distributed observations $Y_1,...,Y_m$, $S_1^2 = \sum_{i=1}^{n} (X_i - \bar{X})^2 /(n-1)$ and $S_2^2 = \sum_{j=1}^{m} (Y_i - \bar{Y})^2 /(m-1)$ are the unbiased estimators of the variances $\sigma_1^2 = Var(X_1)$ and $\sigma_2^2 = Var(Y_1)$, respectively, and $S_p^2 = \{(n-1)S_1^2 + (m-1)S_2^2\} / (n+m-2)$ is the pooled sample variance. Figure 9.2 depicts the ROC curves, $ROC(t) = 1 - F_1\{F_0^{-1}(1-t)\}, t \in (0,1)$, for each test when the distribution functions F_0, F_1 of the *t*-test statistic (Student's *t*-test statistic or Welch's *t*-test statistic) are correctly specified corresponding to underlying distributions of observations with $\delta = EX_1 - EY_1 = 0.7$ and 1 under H_1. These graphs show that there are no significant differences between the relative curves. In the scenario $n = 10$, $m = 50$, $\sigma_1^2 = 4$, $\sigma_2^2 = 1$, $\delta = 1$ Student's *t*-test slightly demonstrates better performance than that of Welch's *t*-test. By using different values of n, m, σ_1^2, σ_2^2, δ, we attempt to detect cases when significant differences between the relevant curves are in effect. Applying different combinations of $n = 10,20,...,150$; $m = 10,20,...,150$; $\sigma_1^2 = 1,2^2,...,10^2$; and $\sigma_2^2 = 1$, we could not derive a scenario when one of the considered tests

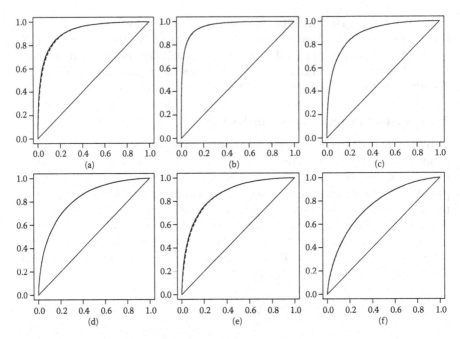

FIGURE 9.2

The ROC curves related to Student's t-test ("_____") and Welch's t-test ("- - - -"), where graph (a) represents the case of $n = 10$, $m = 50$, $\sigma_1^2 = 1$, $\sigma_2^2 = 1$, $\delta = 0.7$; graph (b) represents the case of $n = 20$, $m = 40$, $\sigma_1^2 = 1$, $\sigma_2^2 = 1$, $\delta = 0.7$; graph (c) represents the case of $n = 40$, $m = 20$, $\sigma_1^2 = 4$, $\sigma_2^2 = 1$, $\delta = 0.7$; graph (d) represents the case of $n = 40$, $m = 20$, $\sigma_1^2 = 9$, $\sigma_2^2 = 1$, $\delta = 0.7$; graph (e) represents the case of $n = 10$, $m = 50$, $\sigma_1^2 = 4$, $\sigma_2^2 = 1$, $\delta = 1$; and graph (f) represents the case of $n = 20$, $m = 40$, $\sigma_1^2 = 9$, $\sigma_2^2 = 1$, $\delta = 0.7$.

TABLE 9.1

The Areas Under the ROC Curves of the Student's t-Test (AUC_S) and Welch's
t-Test (AUC_W)

n	m	σ_1^2	σ_2^2	δ	AUC_S	AUC_W
10	50	1	1	0.7	0.9217	0.9172
20	40	1	1	0.7	0.9619	0.9611
40	20	4	1	0.7	0.8959	0.8962
40	20	9	1	0.7	0.8269	0.8271
10	50	4	1	1.0	0.8614	0.8569
20	40	9	1	0.7	0.7631	0.7626

clearly outperforms the other one with respect to the EPV. The corresponding AUC = (1 – EPV) values are given in Table 9.1. Thus, if the Type I error rates of the tests are correctly controlled, there are no critical differences between Student's t-test and Welch's t-test.

The results shown above can be obtained analytically, since the distribution functions of the statistics T_S and T_W under H_0 and H_1 have specified forms. Alternatively, we provide the following R code that can be easily modified in order to evaluate various decision-making procedures using the accurate Monte Carlo approximations to the EPV/ROC instruments.

```
library(pROC)
N<-75000 # Number of Monte Carlo generations
n<-20
m<-20
T0E<-array() #Values of T_S under H_0
T0NE<-array() #Values of T_W under H_0
T1E<-array() #Values of T_S under H_1
T1NE<-array() #Values of T_W under H_1

for(i in 1:N){
x0<-rnorm(n,0,1)# X's under H_0
y0<-rnorm(m,0,1)# Y's under H_0

x1<-rnorm(n,1,1) #X's under H_1
y1<-rnorm(m,0,4) #Y's under H_1

T0E[i]<-t.test(x0,y0,alternative = c("greater"),var.equal = TRUE)$stat[[1]]
T1E[i]<-t.test(x1,y1,alternative = c("greater"),var.equal = TRUE)$stat[[1]]

T0NE[i]<-t.test(x0,y0,alternative = c("greater"),var.equal = FALSE)$stat[[1]]
T1NE[i]<-t.test(x1,y1,alternative = c("greater"),var.equal = FALSE)$stat[[1]]
}
par(mfrow=c(1,3))
Ind<-c(array(1,N),array(0,N))
TE<-c(T0E,T1E)
TNE<-c(T0NE,T1NE)
plot.roc(Ind, TE, legacy.axes=TRUE) #ROC curve (1-EPV) for T_S
lines.roc(Ind,TNE,col='red') #ROC curve (1-EPV) for T_W

TEroc<-roc(Ind, TE) #ROC curve (1-EPV) for T_S
TNEroc<-roc(Ind, TNE) #ROC curve (1-EPV) for T_S

##############Partial EPVs
#Values of (1-the partial EPVs) for T_S depending on alpha:
TEauc<-function(alpha) 1-auc(TEroc, partial.auc=c(0, alpha))
#Values of (1-the partial EPVs) for T_W depending on alpha:
TNEauc<-function(alpha) 1-auc(TNEroc, partial.auc=c(0, alpha))
TEaucV<-Vectorize(TEauc)
TNEaucV<-Vectorize(TNEauc)
plot(TEaucV,0,1)
plot(TNEaucV,0,1,col='red')
```

9.2.3 The Connection between EPV and Power

The value of $1 - \mathrm{EPV}$ can be expressed in the form of the statistical power of a test through integration uniformly over the significance level α from 0 to 1; that is,

$$EPV = \Pr(T^0 \geq T^A) = \int_{-\infty}^{\infty} \Pr(T^A \leq t) dF_0(t) = \int_{-\infty}^{\infty} \Pr\{F_0(T^A) \leq F_0(t)\} dF_0(t)$$

$$= \int_1^0 \Pr\{1 - F_0(T^A) \geq \alpha\} d(1-\alpha) = \int_0^1 \left[1 - \Pr\{1 - F_0(T^A) \leq \alpha\} \right] d\alpha = 1 - \int_0^1 \Pr(p\text{-}value \leq \alpha \mid H_1) d\alpha.$$

The above expression of the EPV considers the weight of the significance level α from 0 to 1. It may appear to suffer from the defect of assigning most of its weight to relatively uninteresting values of α not typically used in practice, e.g., $\alpha \geq 0.1$. Alternatively, we can focus on significance levels of α in a specific interesting range by considering the pEPV; that is

$$pEPV = 1 - \int_0^{\alpha_U} \Pr\{p\text{-}value \leq \alpha \mid H_1\} d\alpha = 1 - \int_0^{\alpha_U} \Pr\{1 - F_0(T^A) \leq \alpha\} d\alpha$$

$$= 1 + \int_0^{\alpha_U} \Pr\{F_0(T^A) \geq 1 - \alpha\} d(1-\alpha) = 1 + \int_1^{1-\alpha_U} \Pr\{F_0(T^A) \geq z\} dz$$

$$= 1 - \int_{1-\alpha_U}^1 \Pr\{F_0(T^A) \geq z\} dz = 1 - \int_{F_0^{-1}(1-\alpha_U)}^{\infty} \Pr\{F_0(T^A) \geq F_0(t)\} dF_0(t)$$

$$= 1 - \int_{F_0^{-1}(1-\alpha_U)}^{\infty} \Pr\{T^A \geq t\} dF_0(t) = 1 - \Pr\{T^A \geq T^0, T^0 \geq F_0^{-1}(1-\alpha_U)\}$$

at a fixed upper level $\alpha_U \leq 1$. In the R code presented in Section 9.2.2, we provided an example of pEPV computations.

In general, one can define the function $pEPV(\alpha_L, \alpha_U) = 1 - \int_{\alpha_L}^{\alpha_U} \Pr\{p\text{-}value \leq u \mid H_1\} du$ and focus on $\frac{d}{d\alpha}\{-pEPV(0,\alpha)\}$. Then, in this case, the $\frac{d}{d\alpha}\{-pEPV(0,\alpha)\}$ implies the power at a significance level of α. An essential property of efficient statistical tests is unbiasedness (Lehmann and Romano, 2006). In this context, we can denote an ***unbiased statistical test*** when the probability of committing a Type I error is less than the significance level and we have a proper power function, that is, $\Pr(\text{reject } H_0 \mid H_0) \leq \alpha$ and $\Pr(\text{reject } H_0 \mid H_0 \text{ is not true}) \geq \alpha$. In parallel with this definition, it is natural to consider the inequality

$$pEPV(0,\alpha) \leq 1 - \int_0^{\alpha} \Pr\{p\text{-}value \leq u \mid H_0\} du = 1 - \alpha^2/2,$$

since $p\text{-}value \sim Uniform[0,1]$ (i.e., $\Pr\{p\text{-}value \leq u \mid H_0\} = u, u \in [0,1]$) under H_0 and we assume $H_1 \neq H_0$. In this case,

$$\frac{d}{d\alpha}\{pEPV(0,\alpha)\} = -\Pr(\text{reject } H_0 \mid H_0 \text{ is not true}) \text{ and } \frac{d}{d\alpha}\left\{1 - \alpha^2/2\right\} = -\alpha.$$

However, it is clear that the requirement $pEPV(0,\alpha) \le 1 - \alpha^2/2$ is weaker than that of $\Pr(\text{p-value} < \alpha \mid H_0 \text{ is not true}) \ge \alpha$.

Thus, the EPV based concept extends the conventional power characterization of tests.

Remark. The Neyman–Pearson lemma framework for comparing, for example, two test statistics, say M_1 and M_2, provides the following scheme: the Type I error rates of the tests should be fixed at a prespecified significance level α, $\Pr(M_1 \text{ rejects } H_0 \mid H_0) \le \alpha$ and $\Pr(M_2 \text{ rejects } H_0 \mid H_0) \le \alpha$; then M_1 is superior with respect to M_2, if $\Pr(M_1 \text{ rejects } H_0 \mid H_1) > \Pr(M_2 \text{ rejects } H_0 \mid H_1)$. In general the power functions, $\Pr(M_1 \text{ rejects } H_0 \mid H_1)$ and $\Pr(M_2 \text{ rejects } H_0 \mid H_1)$, depend on α. Thus, for different values of α we may theoretically obtain diverse conclusions regarding the preferable test procedure. The EPV and pEPV methods make the comparison more objective in a global sense. The test performance can be measured employing just the EPV or pEPV value by itself. Smaller values of the EPV or pEPV indicate a more preferable test procedure when comparing two or more tests. The definitions of EPV and pEPV show that for a most powerful test (e.g., the likelihood ratio test), the EPV and pEPV will be the minimum as compared to any other tests with the same H_0 versus H_1.

9.2.4 *t*-Tests versus the Wilcoxon Rank-Sum Test

In this section we compare and contrast the properties of two well-known two-sample test statistics, namely Welch's *t*-test and the Wilcoxon rank-sum test. In order to be concrete, we exemplify our points using a case-control study's statement of problem. The central idea of the case-control study is the comparison of a group having the outcome of interest to a control group with regard to one or more characteristics. In health-related experiments, the case group usually consists of individuals with a given disease, whereas the control group is disease-free. In such instances, the use of biomarkers to assist medical decision making and/or the diagnosis and prognosis of individuals with a given disease, is increasingly common in both clinical settings and epidemiological research. This has spurred an increase in exploration for and development of new biomarkers. For example, myocardial infarction (MI) is commonly caused by blood clots blocking the blood flow of the heart leading to heart muscle injury. Heart disease is a leading cause of death, affecting about 20% of population, regardless of ethnicity, according to the Centers for Disease Control and Prevention (e.g., Schisterman et al., 2001a, 2002). The biomarker "high density lipoprotein (HDL) cholesterol" is often used as a discriminant factor between individuals with and without MI disease. The HDL cholesterol levels can be examined from a 12-hour fasting blood specimen for biochemical analysis at baseline, providing values of measurements regarding HDL biomarkers to be collected on cases who survived an MI and on controls who had no previous MI. Note that oftentimes measurements related to biological processes follow a log-normal distribution (see for details Limpert et al., 2001; Vexler et al., 2016a, pp. 13–14). Thus, one may be interested in how often a log-transformed HDL cholesterol level of the case group, say X, "outperforms" a log-transformed HDL cholesterol level of the case group, Y. Typically, this research statement is associated with the measure $\Pr(X > Y)$ that is assumed to be examined using n independent and normally distributed data points $X_1, ..., X_n$ as well as m independent and normally distributed observations $Y_1, ..., Y_m$ (e.g., Vexler et al., 2008a&b). In this scenario, in order to test the hypothesis $H_0 : \Pr(X > Y) = 0.5$ versus $H_1 : \Pr(X > Y) > 0.5$ the traditional statistical literature strongly suggests using t-test type procedures (e.g., Browne, 2010). It is common that scholars are encouraged to apply t-test-type decision-making mechanisms when the underlying data follow a normal distribution.

We compare the one-sided two-sample Student's t- and Welch's t-tests with the corresponding Wilcoxon rank-sum test (e.g., Ahmad, 1996) in terms of their relative strengths and weaknesses. The Wilcoxon rank-sum test, which is a permutation test, is generally recommended when the data are assumed to be from a nonnormal distribution. In order to compare the tests we provide the following R code (R Development Core Team, 2014) that can be easily modified and applied to evaluate various decision-making procedures using accurate Monte Carlo approximations to the EPV/ROC instruments.

```
library(pROC)
N<-100000 #Number of Monte Carlo data generations
W0<-array()
T0<-array()
W1<-array()
T1<-array()
n<-25 #The sample size n
m<-25 #The sample size m

for(i in 1:N){
x0<-rnorm(n,0,1) #Values of X from N(0,1) generated under the hypothesis H0
y0<-rnorm(m,0,1) #Values of Y from N(0,1) generated under the hypothesis H0
x1<-rnorm(n,0,1) #Values of X from N(0,1) generated under the hypothesis H1
```

```
y1<-rnorm(m,-0.5,10) #Values of Y from N(-0.5,10) generated under the hypothesis H1

W0[i]<-wilcox.test(x0,y0,alternative = c("greater"))$stat[[1]]/(n*m)
#Values of the Wilcoxon test statistic under H0
W1[i]<-wilcox.test(x1,y1,alternative = c("greater"))$stat[[1]]/(n*m)
#Values of the Wilcoxon test statistic under H1

EV<-FALSE #This parameter indicates the use of Welch's t-test statistic
#EV<-TRUE #This parameter indicates the use of Student's t-test statistic

T0[i]<-t.test(x0,y0,alternative = c("greater"),var.equal = EV)$stat[[1]]
#Values of the t-test statistic under H0
T1[i]<-t.test(x1,y1,alternative = c("greater"),var.equal = EV)$stat[[1]]
#Values of the t-test statistic under H1
}

#Plotting the ROC cureves
Ind<-c(array(1,N),array(0,N))
W<-c(W0,W1)
T<-c(T0,T1)
plot.roc(Ind, W,type="l", legacy.axes=TRUE,xlab="t",ylab="ROC(t)")
lines.roc(Ind,T,col="red",lty=2)
```

To exemplify the proposed approach for comparing the test statistics, this R code provides simulation-based evaluations of the ROC curves based on values of the test statistics related to the null and alternative hypotheses, using the R built-in procedure *pROC*. In this scenario, we assume, for example, that $X_1,...,X_n \sim N(0,1)$ and $Y_1,...,Y_m \sim N(0,1)$ under H_0, whereas $X_1,...,X_n \sim N(0,1)$ and $Y_1,...,Y_m \sim N(-0.5,10)$. Figure 9.3 shows the ROC curves $(ROC_T(t),t)$ and $(ROC_W(t),t)$, where

$$ROC_T(t) = 1 - F_{T_1}\{F_{T_0}^{-1}(1-t)\} \quad \text{and} \quad ROC_W(t) = 1 - F_{W_1}\{F_{W_0}^{-1}(1-t)\}, t \in (0,1)$$

with the distribution functions F_{T_k} and F_{W_k} that correspond to the *t*-test statistic and the Wilcoxon rank-sum test statistic distributions under $H_k, k = 0,1$, respectively.

According to the executed R Code (the parameter EV<-FALSE), we focus on Welch's *t*-test statistic, which is reasonable in the considered setting of data distributions' parameters. It is interesting to remark that when examining Student's t-test statistic, setting the parameter EV<-TRUE the graphs show that there are no significant differences between the relative curves. Similar observations are in effect regarding the considerations shown below.

Analyzing EPVs for the one-sided, two-sample *t*- and Wilcoxon tests based on normally distributed data points ($n = m = 10, 20, 50$), Sackrowitz and Samuel-Cahn (1999) concluded that *"The t test is best both for the Normal*

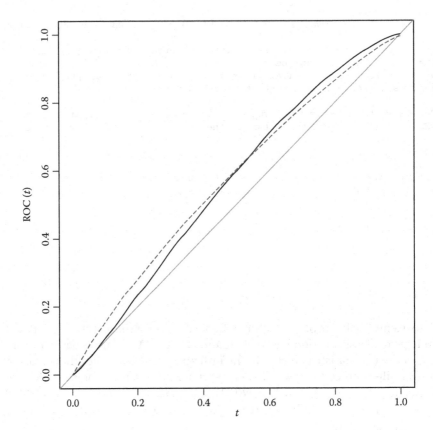

FIGURE 9.3
Values of the functions $ROC_T(t)$ (curve "- - - -") and $ROC_W(t)$ (curve "------") plotted against $t \in (0,1)$.

distribution (not surprising!) and the Uniform distribution." In order to compute the EPVs corresponding to the considered example, we can execute the code

```
Troc<-roc(Ind, T)
Wroc<-roc(Ind, W)
EPV_t<-1-auc(Troc) # EPV of the t-test
EPV_W<-1-auc(Wroc) # EPV of the Wilcoxon test
```

Indeed, the computed EPV of the *t*-test is 0.431, which is smaller than the 0.439 of that related to the Wilcoxon rank-sum test. However, Figure 9.3 demonstrates that for $t \in (0,0.5)$ the Wilcoxon test is somewhat better that the *t*-test. This motivates us to employ the pEPV for this analysis. Toward this end, we denote the function

$$G(\alpha) = \{pEPV_W(0,\alpha) - pEPV_t(0,\alpha)\}/pEPV_t(0,\alpha),$$

where $pEPV_T(0,\alpha)$ and $pEPV_W(0,\alpha)$ are the function $pEPV(0,\alpha)$ defined in Section 9.2.3 and computed with respect to the t-test and the Wilcoxon test, respectively. In order to depict the result we use the following code:

```
pEPV_t<-function(u) 1-auc(Troc, partial.auc=c(0,u))[[1]]
pEPV_W<-function(u) 1-auc(Wroc, partial.auc=c(0,u))[[1]]
G<-function(u) (pEPV_W(u)-pEPV_t(u))/(pEPV_t(u))
GV<-Vectorize(G)
plot(GV,0,1,xlab='alpha',ylab='G(alpha)')
```

Figure 9.4 presents the curve of $G(\alpha)$.
In this case, it is clear that the Wilcoxon test outperforms the t-test, when the significance level $\alpha < 0.8$.

Let us fix $\alpha = 0.05$ and calculate the corresponding powers of the tests using the following code:

```
Wc<-quantile(W0,0.95) # the 95% critical value of the Wilcoxon test
Tc<-quantile(T0,0.95) # the 95% critical value of the t-test
PowW<-mean(1*(W1>=Wc)) #the power of the Wilcoxon test
PowT<-mean(1*(T1>=Tc)) #the power of the t-test
print(c(PowT,PowW))
```

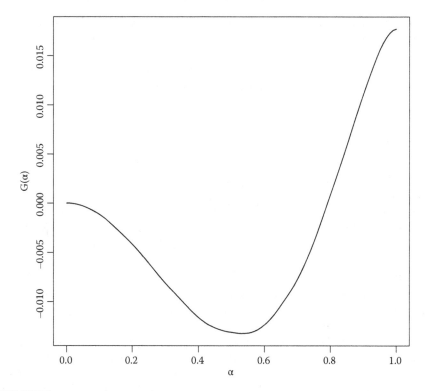

FIGURE 9.4
The relative comparison between the t-test and the Wilcoxon test using their pEPVs via the function $G(\alpha)$ plotted against $\alpha \in (0,1)$.

We obtain that the power of the Wilcoxon test is 0.12, whereas the power of the t-test is 0.08.

Remark 1. Assume we are interested in the measure $\Pr(X > Y)$. A fast way to evaluate $\Pr(X > Y)$ can be based on the R command *wilcox.test(X,Y,alternative = c("greater"))$stat[[1]]*. For example, in the setting of the example mentioned in this section, one can use

```
nn<-5000000
x1<-rnorm(nn,0,1)
y1<-rnorm(nn,-0.5,10)
wilcox.test(x1,y1,alternative = c("greater"))$stat[[1]]/(nn*nn)
```

to obtain the approximated value of $\Pr(X > Y)$ under H_1 as 0.5192665, which corresponds to $\Pr(X > Y) = (2\pi)^{-1/2} \int_{-\infty}^{0.5} e^{-z^2/2} dz \approx 0.5181275$.

Remark 2. In various scenarios with $Var(X_1) = Var(Y_1)$ under H_1, it was observed using the function $G(\alpha), \alpha < 0.1$, that the t-test procedures and the Wilcoxon rank-sum test provide approximately the same properties.

Remark 3. The R code presented in this section can be easily modified to provide the EPV/ROC analysis based on a real data. To this end the variables x0, y0 can be simulated corresponding to H_0 (e.g., as $X_1,...,X_n \sim N(0,1)$ and $Y_1,...,Y_m \sim N(0,1)$) and the variables x1, y1 can be sampled from observed $X_1,...,X_n$ and $Y_1,...,Y_m$ in a bootstrap manner at each loop iteration in *"for(i in 1:N){..."* (see for details Vexler et al., 2017 as well as Chapter 11).

9.2.5 Discussion

We have seen that the EPV is a very useful and succinct measurement tool of the performance of decision-making mechanisms. We have demonstrated a novel methodology to analyze and visualize characteristics of test procedures. Toward this end the "EPV/ROC" concept has been introduced. This approach provides us new and efficient perspectives toward developing and examining statistical decision-making policies, including those related to the partial EPVs, associations between the EPV and the power of tests, visualization of properties of testing mechanisms, development of optimal tests based on minimizing the EPVs, and creation of new methods for optimally combining multiple test statistics. Many possible avenues of research can be done based on the concept we introduced in this chapter. For example, a large sample theory can be developed to evaluate the EPVs in several parametric and nonparametric scenarios. In addition, Bayesian-type methods can be developed in order to evaluate test properties in the "EPV/ROC" frame. The proposed technique can be easily applied to obtain confidence region estimation of vector parameters based on confidence interval estimates for the individual elements. These topics warrant further strong empirical and methodological investigations.

Remark. We shall note that there are different approaches to define p-value type mechanisms, see, for example, Bayarri and Berger (2000), Berger and Boos (1994), Berger (2003), Hwang and Yang (2001).

10

Empirical Likelihood

10.1 Introduction

Over the long course of statistical methodological developments there been a shift from classic parametric likelihood methods to a focus towards robust and efficient nonparametric and semiparametric developments of various "artificial" or "approximate" likelihood techniques. These methods have a wide variety of applications related to biostatistical experiments. Many nonparametric and semiparametric approximations to powerful parametric likelihood procedures have been used routinely in both statistical theory and practice. Well-known examples include the quasi-likelihood method, which are approximations of parametric likelihoods via orthogonal functions, techniques based on quadratic artificial likelihood functions, and the local maximum likelihood methodology (e.g., Wedderburn, 1974; Claeskens and Hjort, 2004; Fan et al., 1998). Various studies have shown that artificial or approximate likelihood-based techniques efficiently incorporate information expressed through the data, and have many of the same asymptotic properties as those derived from the corresponding parametric likelihoods. The *empirical likelihood* (EL) method is one of a growing array of artificial or approximate likelihood-based methods currently in use in statistical practice (e.g., Owen, 2001; Vexler et al., 2009a, 2014). Interest and the resulting impact in EL methods continue to grow rapidly. Perhaps more importantly, EL methods now have various vital applications in an expanding number of health related studies.

In Sections 10.2 and 10.3, we outline basic components related to EL techniques and their theoretical evaluations. Sections 10.4 and 10.5 demonstrate valuable examples of EL applications. In Section 10.6, we provide arguments that can be accepted in favor of EL methods in order to be applied in statistical practice.

10.2 Empirical Likelihood Methods

As background for the development of EL-type techniques, we first outline the conventional EL approach. The classical EL takes the form

$\prod_{i=1}^{n} (F(X_i) - F(X_i-))$, which is a functional of the cumulative distribution function F and iid observations X_i, $i = 1, \ldots, n$. In the distribution-free setting, an empirical estimator of the likelihood takes the form of $L_p = \prod_{i=1}^{n} p_i$, where the components p_i, $i = 1, \ldots, n$, estimators of the probability weights, should maximize the likelihood L_p, provided that $\sum_{i=1}^{n} p_i = 1$ and empirical constraints based on $X_1, \ldots, X_n$ hold. For example, suppose we would like to test the hypothesis

$$H_0 : E\{g(X_1, \theta)\} = 0 \quad \text{versus} \quad H_1 : E\{g(X_1, \theta)\} \neq 0,$$

where $g(.,.)$ is a given function and θ is a parameter. Then, in a nonparametric fashion, we define the EL function of the form $EL(\theta) = L(X_1, \ldots, X_n \mid \theta) = \prod_{i=1}^{n} p_i$, where $\sum_{i=1}^{n} p_i = 1$.

Under the null hypothesis, the maximum likelihood approach requires one to find the values of $0 < p_1, \ldots, p_n < 1$ that maximize the EL given the empirical constraints $\sum_{i=1}^{n} p_i = 1$ and $\sum_{i=1}^{n} p_i g(X_i, \theta) = 0$ that present an empirical version of the condition under H_0 that $E\{g(X_1, \theta)\} = 0$. In situations, when there are no $0 < p_1, \ldots, p_n < 1$ to satisfy the empirical constraints, it is assumed that the null hypothesis is rejected in this stage. Further, following the Lagrange method, we define the function

$$W(p_1, \ldots, p_n) = \sum_{i=1}^{n} \log(p_i) + \lambda_1 \left(1 - \sum_{i=1}^{n} p_i\right) + \lambda \left(-\sum_{i=1}^{n} p_i g(X_i, \theta)\right),$$

where λ_1 and λ are Lagrange multipliers. Then we have $\partial W(p_1, \ldots, p_n) / \partial p_k = p_k^{-1} - \lambda_1 - \lambda g(X_k, \theta)$. Hence, to maximize $W(p_1, \ldots, p_n)$, $0 < p_1, \ldots, p_n < 1$ should satisfy $\partial W(p_1, \ldots, p_n) / \partial p_k = 0$ or equivalently $p_k \partial W(p_1, \ldots, p_n) / \partial p_k = 0$, $k = 1, \ldots, n$. This implies $\sum_{k=1}^{n} p_k \{\partial W(p_1, \ldots, p_n) / \partial p_k\} = 0$. Thus, since $\sum_{k=1}^{n} p_k = 1$, we obtain $n - \lambda_1 - \lambda \sum_{k=1}^{n} p_k g(X_k, \theta) = 0$, where, under H_0, it is assumed that $\sum_{k=1}^{n} p_k g(X_k, \theta) = 0$. This leads to $n - \lambda_1 = 0$. Therefore, using the equation $\partial W(p_1, \ldots, p_n) / \partial p_k = 0$, we obtain $p_k = (n + \lambda g(X_k, \theta))^{-1}$, $k = 1, \ldots, n$. That is to say, the Lagrange method provides

$$EL(\theta) = \sup_{0 < p_1, p_2, \ldots, p_n < 1, \sum p_i = 1, \sum p_i g(X_i, \theta) = 0} \prod_{i=1}^{n} p_i = \prod_{i=1}^{n} (n + \lambda g(X_i, \theta))^{-1},$$

where λ is a root of $\sum g(X_i, \theta)(n + \lambda g(X_i, \theta))^{-1} = 0$. Note that the derivate

$$\frac{\partial}{\partial\lambda}\sum g(X_i,\theta)\big(n+\lambda g(X_i,\theta)\big)^{-1} = -\sum g(X_i,\theta)^2\big(n+\lambda g(X_i,\theta)\big)^{-2} \leq 0.$$

Then, with respect to λ, the function $\sum g(X_i,\theta)\big(n+\lambda g(X_i,\theta)\big)^{-1}$ monotonically decreases. Taking into account this fact, one can show that if $\min_{i=1,...,n}\big(g(X_i,\theta)\big) < 0 < \max_{i=1,...,n}\big(g(X_i,\theta)\big)$ then one unique solution for λ can be found (see Owen, 2001, for details). Commonly, a numerical method is required to solve the equation $\sum g(X_i,\theta)\big(n+\lambda g(X_i,\theta)\big)^{-1} = 0$ with respect to λ.

Since under H_1, the only constraint under consideration is $\sum p_i = 1$, in a similar manner to that shown above, we have

$$EL = \sup_{0<p_1,p_2,...,p_n<1,\sum p_i=1} \prod_{i=1}^{n} p_i = \prod_{i=1}^{n} n^{-1} = (n)^{-n}.$$

Finally, we obtain the **EL ratio** (ELR) test statistic

$$ELR(\theta) = EL / EL(\theta)$$

for the hypothesis test of H_0 versus H_1. For example, when the function $g(u,\theta) = u - \theta$, the null hypothesis corresponds to the expectation $E(X_1) = \theta$, for fixed θ. The EL ratio test strategy is that we reject H_0 for large values of $ELR(\theta)$.

Owen (1988, 1990, 1991) showed that the nonparametric test statistic $2\log\big(ELR(\theta)\big)$ has an asymptotic chi-square distribution under the null hypothesis when $E\big|g(X_1,\theta)\big|^3 < \infty$. This result illustrates that *Wilks' theorem*–type results continue to hold in the context of this infinite-dimensional problem (n, the number of $p_1,...,p_n$, is assumed to be large, $n \to \infty$). The proof of this proposition is outlined in Section 10.3. Thus, we reject H_0 when

$$2\log\{ELR(\theta)\} \geq \chi_1^2(1-\alpha),$$

where $\chi_1^2(1-\alpha)$ is the $100(1-\alpha)\%$ percentile of the chi-square distribution with degree of freedom one, and α is the significance level.

Consequently, there are techniques for correcting forms of ELRs to improve the convergence rate of the respective null distributions of the test statistics to chi-square distributions. These techniques are similar to those applied in the field of parametric maximum likelihood ratio procedures (Vexler et al., 2009a). The statement of the hypothesis testing above can easily be inverted with respect to providing nonparametric confidence interval estimators (Chapter 9).

In terms of the accessibility of this method, it should be noted that the number of EL software packages continues to expand, particularly the R-based software packages. For example, *library(emplik)* and *library(EL)* are R packages that include the R functions *el.test()* and *EL.test()*. These simple R functions can be very useful for the EL analysis of data from statistical studies.

10.3 Techniques for Analyzing Empirical Likelihoods

The analysis presented in this section is relatively clear, and has the basic ingredients for more general cases. We posit that the following results can be associated with deriving different properties of EL-type procedures including the power and Type I error rate analysis of the ELR test.

Properties of many statistical quantities based on parametric likelihoods can be studied by using the fact that parametric likelihood functions are often highly peaked about their maximum values (e.g., Chapters 3 and 5). The modern statistical literature considers a variety of semi- and nonparametric procedures created by proposing to employ EL functions in efficient parametric schemes instead of parametric likelihoods. For example, in this context, the results of Qin and Lawless (1994) have a remarkable use with respect to operations with ELs in a similar manner to those related to parametric maximum likelihoods.

The following lemma illustrates a strong similarity between behaviors of empirical and parametric likelihood functions. Suppose the function $g(x, \theta)$ appeared in the EL definition is once differentiable with respect to the second argument θ. We then have the following.

Lemma 10.3.1.

Let θ_M be a root of the equation $n^{-1} \sum_{i=1}^{n} g(X_i, \theta_M) = 0$, where $\partial g(X_i, \theta)/\partial \theta < 0$ (or $\partial g(X_i, \theta)/\partial \theta > 0$), for all $i=1, 2,..., n$. Then the argument θ_M is a global maximum of the function

$$EL(\theta) = \max \left\{ \prod_{i=1}^{n} p_i : \ 0 < p_i < 1, \sum_{i=1}^{n} p_i = 1, \sum_{i=1}^{n} p_i g(X_i, \theta) = 0 \right\},$$

which increases and decreases monotonically for $\theta < \theta_M$ and $\theta > \theta_M$, respectively.

Proof. It is clear that the argument θ_M, a root of $n^{-1} \sum_{i=1}^{n} g(X_i, \theta_M) = 0$, maximizes the function $EL(\theta)$, since in this case $EL(\theta_M) = n^{-n}$ with $p_i = n^{-1}, i = 1,...,n$, which maximizes $\prod_{i=1}^{n} p_i$ given the sole constraint $\sum_{i=1}^{n} p_i = 1, 0 \le p_i \le 1, i = 1,...,n$.

Using the Lagrange method, one can represent $EL(\theta)$ as

$$EL(\theta) = \prod_{i=1}^{n} p_i, \quad 0 < p_i = \frac{1}{n + \lambda g(X_i, \theta)} < 1, i = 1,...,n,$$

where the Lagrange multiplier λ is a root of the equation
$\sum g(X_i,\theta)(n+\lambda g(X_i,\theta))^{-1}=0$ (e.g., Owen, 2001). This then yields the following expression:

$$\frac{d\log(EL(\theta))}{d\theta}=-\lambda\sum_{i=1}^{n}\frac{\partial g(X_i,\theta)/\partial\theta}{n+\lambda g(X_i,\theta)}-\sum_{i=1}^{n}\frac{g(X_i,\theta)}{n+\lambda g(X_i,\theta)}\frac{\partial\lambda}{\partial\theta}=-\lambda\sum_{i=1}^{n}\frac{\partial g(X_i,\theta)/\partial\theta}{n+\lambda g(X_i,\theta)},$$

where without loss of generality we assume $\partial g(X_i,\theta)/\partial\theta>0, i=1,\ldots,n$.
Now define the function

$$L(\lambda)=\sum_{i=1}^{n}g(X_i,\theta)(n+\lambda g(X_i,\theta))^{-1}.$$

Since $dL(\lambda)/d\lambda<0$, the function $L(\lambda)$ decreases with respect to λ and has just one root relative to solving $L(\lambda)=0$. Consider the scenario with $\theta>\theta_M$. In this case when $\lambda_0=0$ we can conclude that

$$L(\lambda_0)=\sum_{i=1}^{n}g(X_i,\theta)(n)^{-1}\geq\sum_{i=1}^{n}g(X_i,\theta_M)(n)^{-1}=0,$$

since $g(X_i,\theta)$ increases with respect to θ ($\partial g(X_i,\theta)/\partial\theta>0$).

The function $L(\lambda)$ decreases. This implies that the root of $L(\lambda)=0$ should be located on the right side from $\lambda_0=0$ and then this root is positive. For a graphical representation of this case see Figure 10.1a below.

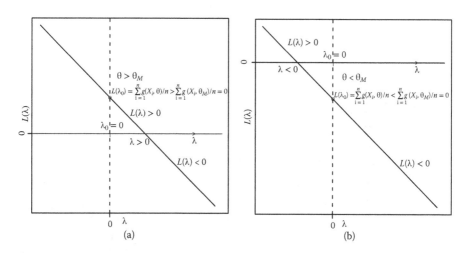

FIGURE 10.1
The schematic behaviors of $L(\lambda)$ plotted against λ (the axis of abscissa), when (a) $\theta>\theta_M$ and (b) $\theta<\theta_M$, respectively.

Thus, by virtue of

$$\frac{d\log(EL(\theta))}{d\theta} = -\lambda \sum_{i=1}^{n} \frac{\partial g(X_i,\theta)/\partial\theta}{n+\lambda g(X_i,\theta)},$$

we prove that the function $EL(\theta)$ decreases, when $\theta > \theta_M$.

Taking the same approach, one can show that the root of $L(\lambda) = 0$ should be to the left of $\lambda_0 = 0$, when $\theta < \theta_M$. For a graphical representation of this case see Figure 10.1b. This result combined with $\dfrac{d\log(EL(\theta))}{d\theta} = -\lambda \sum_{i=1}^{n} \dfrac{\partial g(X_i,\theta)/\partial\theta}{n+\lambda g(X_i,\theta)}$

completes the proof of Lemma 10.3.1.

Note that θ_M plays a role that is similar to that of parametric maximum likelihood estimators. For example, when $g(u,\theta) = u-\theta$, we obtain $\theta_M = \bar{X} = n^{-1}\sum_{i=1}^{n} X_i$; if, for a given function $z(u)$, $g(u,\theta) = z(u) - \theta^2, \theta > 0$ then

$$\theta_M{}^2 = n^{-1}\sum_{i=1}^{n} z(X_i).$$

Turning to the task of developing asymptotic methods based on ELs, we provide the proposition below. Without loss of generality and for simplicity of notation, we set $g(u,\theta) = u-\theta$ in the definition of the empirical likelihood ratio function $ELR(\theta)$. Thus, $EL(\theta) = \prod_{i=1}^{n} p_i$, $\log(ELR(\theta)) = \sum_{i=1}^{n} \log\{1+\lambda(X_i-\theta)/n\}$ with $p_i = \{n+\lambda(X_i-\theta)\}^{-1}$, where λ is a root of

$$\sum_{i=1}^{n} (X_i-\theta)(n+\lambda(X_i-\theta))^{-1} = 0.$$

Note that $\lambda = \lambda(\theta)$ is a function of θ. Then, defining $\lambda' = d\lambda(\theta)/d\theta$, $\lambda'' = d^2\lambda(\theta)/d\theta^2$, and $\lambda^{(k)} = d^k\lambda(\theta)/d\theta^k, k = 3,4$ and using $\sum_{i=1}^{n} (X_i-\theta)(n+\lambda(X_i-\theta))^{-1} = 0$, one can show:

Proposition 10.3.1. We have the following equations:

$$d\{\log ELR(\theta)\}/d\theta = -\lambda(\theta),\ \lambda' = -n\sum_{i=1}^{n} p_i^2 / \sum_{i=1}^{n} (X_i-\theta)^2 p_i^2,$$

$$\lambda'' = -\left\{2(\lambda')^2 \sum_{i=1}^{n} (X_i-\theta)^3 p_i^3 + 4n(\lambda')\sum_{i=1}^{n} (X_i-\theta)p_i^3 \right.$$

$$\left. -2n\lambda\sum_{i=1}^{n} p_i^3\right\}/\sum_{i=1}^{n} (X_i-\theta)^2 p_i^2,$$

$$\lambda^{(3)} = \left\{6\lambda'\lambda''\sum_{i=1}^{n} (X_i-\theta)^3 p_i^3 + 6n\lambda''\sum_{i=1}^{n} (X_i-\theta)p_i^3 - 6\lambda'^3\sum_{i=1}^{n} (X_i-\theta)^4 p_i^4 \right.$$

$$-18n(\lambda')^2 \sum_{i=1}^{n} (X_i-\theta)^2 p_i^4 + 12n(\lambda')\sum_{i=1}^{n} p_i^3$$

$$\left. -(18n^2(\lambda')+6n\lambda^2)\sum_{i=1}^{n} p_i^4\right\}/\sum_{i=1}^{n} (X_i-\theta)^2 p_i^2,$$

$$\lambda^{(4)} = \left\{ (8(\lambda')\lambda^{(3)} + 6(\lambda'')^2) \sum_{i=1}^{n} (X_i - \theta)^3 p_i^3 + 8n\lambda^{(3)} \sum_{i=1}^{n} (X_i - \theta)p_i^3 \right.$$

$$- 36(\lambda')^2 \lambda'' \sum_{i=1}^{n} (X_i - \theta)^4 p_i^4$$

$$- 72n\lambda'\lambda'' \sum_{i=1}^{n} (X_i - \theta)^2 p_i^4 - (36n^2\lambda'' - 18n\lambda\lambda') \sum_{i=1}^{n} p_i^4 + 24n\lambda'' \sum_{i=1}^{n} p_i^3$$

$$+ 24(\lambda')^4 \sum_{i=1}^{n} (X_i - \theta)^5 p_i^5 + 96n(\lambda')^3 \sum_{i=1}^{n} (X_i - \theta)^3 p_i^5 - 72n(\lambda') \sum_{i=1}^{n} (X_i - \theta)p_i^4$$

$$+ (144n^2(\lambda')^2 + 24n\lambda^2\lambda') \sum_{i=1}^{n} (X_i - \theta)p_i^5$$

$$\left. - (72n^2\lambda(\lambda') + 24n\lambda^3) \sum_{i=1}^{n} p_i^5 \right\} / \sum_{i=1}^{n} (X_i - \theta)^2 p_i^2.$$

The proof of Proposition 10.3.1 is based on technical computations.

This proposition can support a variety of evaluations of $ELR(\theta)$-type procedures. To show the relevant examples, we should note that $\log\{ELR(\theta_M)\} = 0$, since, in this case, $p_i = 1/n$, for all i, and $EL(\theta_M) = EL$. It is also clear that, when $\theta = \theta_M$, $\lambda(\theta) = 0$, since $p_i = 1/n$, $i = 1,...,n$ maximize $EL \geq EL(\theta)$, for all θ, and satisfy automatically the constraint $\sum p_i g(X_i, \theta) = 0$, when $\theta = \theta_M$, by virtue of the definition of θ_M. Thus, for example in the case of $g(u,\theta) = u - \theta$, one can use Proposition 10.3.1 to obtain the Taylor expansion for the function $\log\{ELR(\theta)\}$ at argument $\theta_M = \bar{X}$, in the form

$$\log ELR(\theta) \approx \log ELR(\bar{X}) + (\theta - \bar{X}) \frac{d \log ELR(\bar{X})}{d\theta} \bigg|_{\theta = \bar{X}}$$

$$+ \frac{(\theta - \bar{X})^2}{2!} \frac{d^2 \log ELR(\bar{X})}{d\theta^2} \bigg|_{\theta = \bar{X}} + \frac{(\theta - \bar{X})^3}{3!} \frac{d^3 \log ELR(\bar{X})}{d\theta^3} \bigg|_{\theta = \bar{X}}$$

$$= \frac{1}{2} \left(n^{0.5}(\theta - \bar{X}) \right)^2 / \left[\frac{1}{n} \sum_{i=1}^{n} (X_i - \bar{X})^2 \right]$$

$$+ \frac{1}{3} n(\theta - \bar{X})^3 / \left[\frac{1}{n} \sum_{i=1}^{n} (X_i - \bar{X})^2 \right]^3,$$

as $n \to \infty$. This approximation depicts Wilks' theorem when $\theta = EX_1$. (In the case of $\theta = EX_1$ and $n \to \infty$, $n^{0.5}(\theta - \bar{X})$ has a normal distribution, $n(\theta - \bar{X})^3 \xrightarrow{P} 0$, and $\sum_{i=1}^{n} (X_i - \bar{X})^2 / n \to \text{var}(X_1)$.) Using Proposition 10.3.1 to figure more terms in the Taylor expansion can provide high order approximations to the null distribution of the ELR test, e.g., to obtain the **Bartlett correction** of the ELR structure (e.g., Vexler et al., 2009a). Under the alternative hypothesis $\theta \neq EX_1$, the approximation above shows the power of the ELR test. In this context, we note that Lazar and Mykland (1999) considered a general form of ELRs and the case where $|\theta - EX_1| \sim O(n^{-0.5})$. The authors compared the local power of ELR to that of an ordinary parametric likelihood ratio. Their notable research shows that there is no loss of efficiency in using an EL model up to a second-order approximation.

In a similar manner to Proposition 10.3.1, more complicated ELR structures can be analyzed. For example, one can consider the null hypothesis: $H_0 : E(X_1) = \theta_1$ and $E(X_1^2) = \theta_2$. In this case, under the null hypothesis, the EL function is given as

$$EL(\theta_1, \theta_2) = \max\left\{ \prod_{i=1}^{n} p_i : \sum_{i=1}^{n} p_i = 1, \sum_{i=1}^{n} p_i X_i = \theta_1, \sum_{i=1}^{n} p_i X_i^2 = \theta_2 \right\}.$$

Then using the Lagrangian

$$\Lambda = \sum_{i=1}^{n} \log p_i + \lambda(1 - \sum_{i=1}^{n} p_i) + \lambda_1(\theta_1 - \sum_{i=1}^{n} p_i X_i) + \lambda_2(\theta_2 - \sum_{i=1}^{n} p_i X_i^2),$$

we obtain $p_i = \{n + \lambda_1(X_i - \theta_1) + \lambda_2(X_i^2 - \theta_2)\}^{-1}$, where λ_1 and λ_2 are roots of $\sum(X_i - \theta_1)p_i = 0$ and $\sum(X_i^2 - \theta_2)p_i = 0$. The Appendix presents several results that are similar to those related to the evaluations of $ELR(\theta)$ mentioned above.

To exemplify how close the empirical likelihood is to its parametric counterparts, we consider the following example. Let $\{X_1, ..., X_n\}$ denote a random sample from the following distributions: (1) normal distribution $N(\theta, 1)$, and (2) Exponential(θ), where θ is the rate parameter. Define, in the normal case, the minus maximum log-likelihood ratio test statistic as

$$M(\theta) = -\log\{MLR(\theta)\} = -\sum_{i=1}^{n}(X_i - \theta)^2/2 + \sum_{i=1}^{n}(X_i - \bar{X})^2/2$$

and the minus log-empirical likelihood ratio test statistic for $E(X_1) = \theta$ as

$$E(\theta) = -\log\{ELR(\theta)\} = -\sum_{i=1}^{n} \log\{1 + \lambda(X_i - \theta)/n\},$$

where λ is a root of $\sum_{i=1}^{n}(X_i - \theta)(n + \lambda(X_i - \theta))^{-1} = 0$ and $\bar{X} = n^{-1}\sum_{i=1}^{n} X_i$. In the case of the exponential distribution, the minus maximum log-likelihood ratio test statistic is

$$M(\theta) = -\log\{MLR(\theta)\} = n\log\theta - n\theta\bar{X} + n\log\bar{X} + n$$

and the minus log-empirical likelihood ratio test statistic for $E(X_1) = 1/\theta$ is

$$E(\theta) = -\log\{ELR(\theta)\} = -\sum_{i=1}^{n} \log\{1 + \lambda(X_i - 1/\theta)/n\}.$$

Generating $X_1, ..., X_n \sim N(1,1)$ and $X_1, ..., X_n \sim \text{Exp}(1)$, we obtained Figure 10.2. This figure presents the plots of the parametric maximum log-likelihood ratios and the log-empirical likelihood ratios versus values of the parameter θ based on samples of sizes $n = 25, 50, 150$, where the solid line and the dashed line represent the functions $E(\theta)$ and $M(\theta)$ when the underlying distribution is normal, respectively, while the dotted line and dot-dash line represent the functions $E(\theta)$ and $M(\theta)$ when the underlying distribution is exponential, respectively. Figure 10.2 illustrates Lemma 10.3.1. This figure shows that the empirical

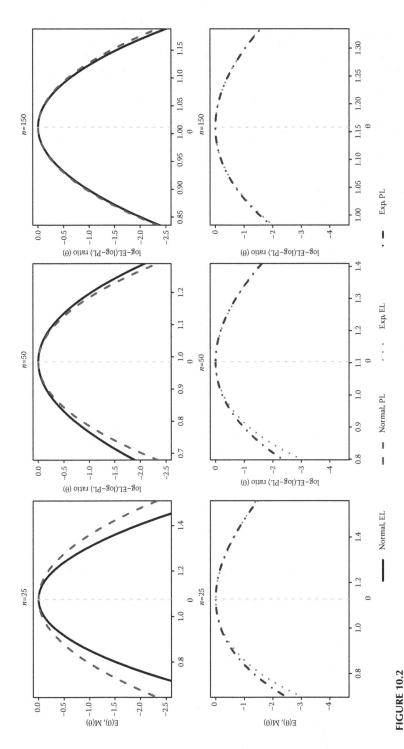

FIGURE 10.2

The log-empirical likelihood ratios and the maximum log-likelihood ratios based on samples of sample sizes $n = 25, 50, 150$, where the solid line and the dashed line correspond to the log-empirical likelihood ratios and the maximum log-likelihood ratios when the underlying distribution is normal, respectively, while the dotted line and the dot-dash line represent the log-empirical likelihood ratio and the maximum log-likelihood ratio when the underlying distribution is exponential, respectively.

likelihood ratio behaves in a similar manner to the parametric maximum likelihood ratio and approaches to the parametric maximum likelihood ratio asymptotically. Furthermore, as the sample size n increases, the log-empirical likelihood ratio approximates the maximum log-likelihood ratio well in the neighborhood of the maximum likelihood estimators. The log-empirical likelihood (ratio) increases monotonically up to the maximum likelihood estimator and then decreases monotonically.

The R code for implementation of the procedure is shown below.

```
library(emplik)
theta0<-1
n.seq<-c(25, 50, 150)

# normal
plot.norm<-function(X){
  get.elr<-function(theta) sapply(theta,function(pp) el.test(X,mu=pp)$'-2LLR'/(-2)) # log EL
  get.plr<-function(theta) sapply(theta,function(pp) sum(-(X-pp)^2/2)+sum((X-mean(X))^2/2)) #log(PL)
  rg<-6/sqrt(length(X))
  curve(get.elr,xlim=c(max(0,mean(X)-rg),mean(X)+rg),type="l",lty=1,lwd=2,add=TRUE,col=1)
  curve(get.plr,xlim=c(max(0,mean(X)-rg),mean(X)+rg),type="l",lty=2,lwd=2,add=TRUE,col=2)
}

#exponential
plot.exp<-function(X){
  get.elr.exp<-function(theta) sapply(theta,function(pp) el.test(X,mu=1/pp)$'-2LLR'/(-2)) #log EL
  get.l.exp<-function(theta) sum(log(dexp(X,rate=theta)))
  get.plr.exp<-function(theta) sapply(theta,function(pp) get.l.exp(pp)-get.l.exp(1/mean(X))) #log(PL)
  rg<-6/sqrt(length(X))
  curve(get.elr.exp,xlim=c(max(0.1,1/mean(X)-rg),1/mean(X)+rg)type="l",lty=3,lwd=2,add=TRUE,col=3)
  curve(get.plr.exp,xlim=c(max(0.1,1/mean(X)-rg),1/mean(X)+rg),type="l",lty=4,lwd=2,add=TRUE,col=4)
}

#add legend for the plot
add_legend <- function(...) {
  opar <- par(fig=c(0, 1, 0, 1), oma=c(0, 0, 0, 0),
          mar=c(0, 0, 0, 0), new=TRUE)
  on.exit(par(opar))
  plot(0, 0, type='n', bty='n', xaxt='n', yaxt='n')
  legend(...)
}
par(mar=c(5.5, 4, 3.5, 1.5),mfrow=c(2,3),mgp=c(2,1,0))

# normal
for (n in n.seq){
  rg<-2/sqrt(n)
  X<-rnorm(n,theta0,1)
  plot(theta0,1,xlim=c(max(0,mean(X)-rg),mean(X)+rg),xlab=expression(theta),            ylim=c(-
2.5,0.005),ylab=expression(paste("E(",theta,"),M(",theta,")")), main=paste0("n=",n),cex.axis=1.2)
  plot.norm(X)
  abline(v=mean(X),lty=2,col="grey")
}
# exponential
for (n in n.seq){
  rg<-2/sqrt(n)
  X<-rexp(n,rate=theta0)
  plot(theta0,1,xlim=c(max(0,1/mean(X)-rg),1/mean(X)+rg),xlab=expression(theta),            ylim=c(-
4.5,0.005),ylab=expression(paste("E(",theta,"),M(",theta,")")), main=paste0("n=",n),cex.axis=1.2)
  plot.exp(X)
  abline(v=1/mean(X),lty=2,col="grey")
}
add_legend("bottom", legend=c("Normal, EL","Normal, PL","Exp, EL","Exp, PL"), lwd=2,
      lty=1:4, col=1:4, horiz=TRUE, bty='n', cex=1.1)
```

10.3.1 Practical Theoretical Tools for Analyzing ELs

In this section we show several simple propositions that can assist in analyzing empirical likelihood type procedures. For example, the remainder term in the approximation

$$\log\left\{ELR(\theta)\right\} \approx \frac{1}{2}\left(n^{0.5}(\theta - \bar{X})\right)^2 / \left[\frac{1}{n}\sum_{i=1}^{n}(X_i - \bar{X})^2\right] + \frac{1}{3}n(\theta - \bar{X})^3 / \left[\frac{1}{n}\sum_{i=1}^{n}(X_i - \bar{X})^2\right]^3$$

mentioned below Proposition 10.3.1 can be evaluated using the propositions presented in this section. The analysis is relatively clear, and has the basic ingredients for more general cases.

Proposition 10.3.2. Assume $E\left(|X_1|^3\right) < \infty$. Then $\max_{i=1,...,n}|X_i| = o_p\left(n^{1/3+\epsilon}\right)$, for all $\epsilon > 0$.

Proof. Chebyshev's inequality (Chapter 1) provides that

$$\Pr\left(\max_{i=1,...,n}|X_i| \geq n^{1/3+\epsilon}\right) \leq \sum_{i=1}^{n}\Pr\left(|X_i| \geq n^{1/3+\epsilon}\right) \leq \sum_{i=1}^{n}\frac{E|X_i|^3}{n^{1+3\epsilon}} = \frac{E|X_1|^3}{n^{3\epsilon}} \xrightarrow[n\to\infty]{} 0.$$

This completes the proof.

In many cases, while analyzing EL-type procedures, we need to evaluate forms similar to $\lambda(\theta)X_i, \lambda'(\theta)X_i$, and so on for all θ. Proposition 10.3.2 shows $X_i = o_p\left(n^{1/3+\epsilon}\right), i = 1,...,n$. Proposition 10.3.1 connects $\lambda^{(k)}(\theta)$ with $\lambda(\theta), k = 1,..,4$. The following results examine $\lambda(\theta)$.

Consider as in Section 10.2 the empirical likelihood

$$EL(\theta) = \sup_{0<p_1,p_2,...,p_n<1,\sum p_i=1,\sum p_i g(X_i,\theta)=0} \prod_{i=1}^{n}p_i = \prod_{i=1}^{n}\left(n + \lambda g(X_i,\theta)\right)^{-1},$$

where λ is a root of $\sum g(X_i,\theta)\left(n + \lambda g(X_i,\theta)\right)^{-1} = 0$. Then we obtain the following propositions.

Proposition 10.3.3. We have that $\lambda \geq 0$ if and only if $\sum_{i=1}^{n} g(X_i,\theta) \geq 0$, and $\lambda < 0$ if and only if $\sum_{i=1}^{n} g(X_i,\theta) < 0$.

Proof. The forms of $p_i = \{n + \lambda g(X_i, \theta)\}^{-1}$, $i = 1,..,n$, and $n^{-n} \geq \prod_{i=1}^{n} p_i$ (here $p_i = n^{-1}, i = 1,..,n$, maximize $\prod_{i=1}^{n} p_i$ provided that only $0 < p_1,...,p_n < 1, \sum p_i = 1$) imply that

$$0 \leq \log\left(n^{-n}/\prod_{i=1}^{n} p_i\right) = \sum_{i=1}^{n} \log\{1 + \lambda g(X_i, \theta)/n\}.$$

Using the inequality $\log(1 + s) \leq s$ for $s > -1$, we obtain

$$0 \leq \sum_{i=1}^{n} \log\{1 + \lambda g(X_i, \theta)/n\} \leq \sum_{i=1}^{n} \lambda g(X_i, \theta)/n = \lambda \sum_{i=1}^{n} g(X_i, \theta)/n.$$

This completes the proof.

Proposition 10.3.4. The Lagrange multiplier λ satisfies

$$\lambda = \sum_{i=1}^{n} g(X_i, \theta)/\sum_{i=1}^{n} \{g(X_i, \theta)\}^2 p_i.$$

Proof. The constraint $\sum_{i=1}^{n} g(X_i, \theta) p_i = 0$ with $p_i = \{n + \lambda g(X_i, \theta)\}^{-1}$, $i = 1,..,n$, implies that

$$\begin{aligned}
\sum_{i=1}^{n} g(X_i, \theta) &= \sum_{i=1}^{n} \{g(X_i, \theta)(1 - p_i)\} + \sum_{i=1}^{n} \{g(X_i, \theta) p_i\} \\
&= \sum_{i=1}^{n} g(X_i, \theta)(1 - p_i) \\
&= \sum_{i=1}^{n} g(X_i, \theta)\left\{\frac{n + \lambda g(X_i, \theta) - 1}{n + \lambda g(X_i, \theta)}\right\} \\
&= n\sum_{i=1}^{n} g(X_i, \theta) p_i + \lambda \sum_{i=1}^{n} g(X_i, \theta)^2 p_i - \sum_{i=1}^{n} g(X_i, \theta) p_i \\
&= \lambda \sum_{i=1}^{n} \{g(X_i, \theta)\}^2 p_i.
\end{aligned}$$

This completes the proof.

Proposition 10.3.5. If $\lambda \geq 0$, we have $0 \leq \lambda \leq n \sum_{i=1}^{n} g(X_i, \theta) \left[\sum_{i=1}^{n} \{g(X_i, \theta)\}^2 I\{g(X_i, \theta) < 0\} \right]^{-1}$;

if $\lambda < 0$, we have $n \sum_{i=1}^{n} g(X_i, \theta) \left[\sum_{i=1}^{n} \{g(X_i, \theta)\}^2 I\{g(X_i, \theta) > 0\} \right]^{-1} \leq \lambda < 0$, where

$I\{\cdot\}$ is the indicator function.

Proof. With $\lambda \geq 0$, we obtain

$$\sum_{i=1}^{n} \{g(X_i, \theta)\}^2 p_i \geq \sum_{i=1}^{n} \left[g(X_i, \theta)^2 p_i I\{g(X_i, \theta) < 0\} \right] =$$

$$\sum_{i=1}^{n} \left[\{g(X_i, \theta)\}^2 \frac{I\{g(X_i, \theta) < 0\}}{n + \lambda g(X_i, \theta)} \right] \geq \sum_{i=1}^{n} \left[\{g(X_i, \theta)\}^2 \frac{1}{n} I\{g(X_i, \theta) < 0\} \right],$$

where $p_i = \{n + \lambda g(X_i, \theta)\}^{-1}$, $i = 1, \ldots, n$.

Applying this result and Proposition 10.3.3 to Proposition 10.3.4 yields

$$0 \leq \lambda < n \sum_{i=1}^{n} g(X_i, \theta) \left[\sum_{i=1}^{n} \{g(X_i, \theta)\}^2 I(g(X_i, \theta) < 0) \right]^{-1}.$$

It follows similarly that when $\lambda < 0$,

$$n \sum_{i=1}^{n} g(X_i, \theta) \left[\sum_{i=1}^{n} \{g(X_i, \theta)\}^2 I\{g(X_i, \theta) > 0\} \right]^{-1} < \lambda < 0.$$

This completes the proof.

Proposition 10.3.5 provides the exact non-asymptotic bounds for λ. Owen (1988) used complicated considerations to obtain the approximate bounds for λ as $n \to \infty$. Proposition 10.3.5 immediately demonstrates that, for all $\varepsilon > 0$, $\lambda = o_p\left(n^{1/2+\varepsilon}\right)$ under H_0, since the bounds presented in Proposition 10.3.5 are based on the sums of iid random variables. The propositions above can be useful in the context of numerical computations of ELs, providing, e.g., the exact bounds for λ, where λ is a numerical solution of

$$\sum g(X_i, \theta)(n + \lambda g(X_i, \theta))^{-1} = 0.$$

Proposition 10.3.6. Since the probability weights $p_i = (n + \lambda g(X_i, \theta))^{-1}, i = 1, \ldots, n,$
we have the properties $\sum g(X_i, \theta)^2 p_i^2 = -\frac{n}{\lambda^2} + \frac{n^2}{\lambda^2} \sum p_i^2$ and $\sum_{i=1}^{n} p_i^2 \geq n^{-1}.$

Proof. By virtue of $\sum p_i = 1$, it is clear that

$$
\begin{aligned}
0 \leq \sum g(X_i, \theta)^2 p_i^2 &= \frac{1}{\lambda^2} \sum \frac{\lambda^2 g(X_i, \theta)^2}{\{n + \lambda g(X_i, \theta)\}^2} \\
&= \frac{1}{\lambda^2} \sum \frac{\lambda^2 g(X_i, \theta)^2 + 2n\lambda g(X_i, \theta) + n^2}{\{n + \lambda g(X_i, \theta)\}^2} \\
&\quad - \frac{1}{\lambda^2} \sum \frac{2n\lambda g(X_i, \theta) + n^2}{\{n + \lambda g(X_i, \theta)\}^2} \\
&= \frac{n}{\lambda^2} - \frac{1}{\lambda^2} \sum \frac{2n\lambda g(X_i, \theta) + n^2}{\{n + \lambda g(X_i, \theta)\}^2},
\end{aligned}
$$

where

$$
\begin{aligned}
\frac{n}{\lambda^2} - \frac{1}{\lambda^2} &\sum \frac{2n\{\lambda g(X_i, \theta) + n\} - 2n^2 + n^2}{\{n + \lambda g(X_i, \theta)\}^2} \\
&= \frac{n}{\lambda^2} - \frac{2n}{\lambda^2} \sum p_i + \frac{n^2}{\lambda^2} \sum p_i^2 \quad \text{and} \quad \sum_{i=1}^{n} p_i = 1.
\end{aligned}
$$

Thus, we obtain $-\frac{n}{\lambda^2} + \frac{n^2}{\lambda^2} \sum p_i^2 \geq 0.$

This completes the proof.

For example, consider the equation $\sum g(X_i, \theta)(n + \lambda g(X_i, \theta))^{-1} = 0.$ We have

$$
\frac{d}{d\theta} \sum \frac{g(X_i, \theta)}{(n + \lambda g(X_i, \theta))} = 0,
$$

which implies that

$$
\sum \frac{g'(X_i, \theta)(n + \lambda g(X_i, \theta)) - \lambda' g(X_i, \theta)^2 - \lambda g'(X_i, \theta)g'(X_i, \theta)}{(n + \lambda g(X_i, \theta))^2} = 0.
$$

Then

$$
\sum \frac{g'(X_i, \theta)n - \lambda' g(X_i, \theta)^2}{(n + \lambda g(X_i, \theta))^2} = 0.
$$

This result leads to

$$\lambda' = \frac{n\sum_{i=1}^{n} g'(X_i,\theta)p_i^2}{\sum_{i=1}^{n} g(X_i,\theta)^2 p_i^2}.$$

In the case with $g(u,\theta) = u - \theta$, one can use Proposition 10.3.6 to obtain the inequality

$$\lambda' = -\frac{n\sum_{i=1}^{n} p_i^2}{\sum_{i=1}^{n}(X_i - \theta)^2 p_i^2} \leq -\frac{1}{\sum_{i=1}^{n}(X_i - \theta)^2 p_i^2}.$$

10.4 Combining Likelihoods to Construct Composite Tests and to Incorporate the Maximum Data-Driven Information

Strictly speaking, EL techniques and parametric likelihood methods are closely related concepts. This provides the impetus for an impressive expansion in the number of EL developments, based on combinations of likelihoods of different types (e.g., Qin, 2000).

Consider a simple example, where we assume to observe independent couples given as (X,Y). In this case, the likelihood function can be denoted as $L(X,Y)$. Suppose that the data points related to X's are observed completely, whereas a proportion of the observed data for the Y's is incomplete. Assume a model of Y given X, i.e., $Y \mid X$, is well defined, e.g., $Y_i = \beta X_i + \varepsilon_i$, where β denotes the model parameter and ε_i is a normally distributed error term, for $i = 1,\ldots,n$. Then, we refer to Bayes theorem to represent the joint likelihood $L(X,Y) = L(Y \mid X)L(X)$, where $L(X)$ can be substituted by the EL to avoid parametric assumptions regarding the distribution of X's.

In this context, Qin (2000) shows an inference on incomplete bivariate data, using a method that combines the parametric model and ELs. This method also incorporates auxiliary information from variables in the form of constraints, which can be obtained from reliable resources such as census reports. This approach makes it possible to use all available bivariate data, whether completely or incompletely observed. In the context of a group comparison, constraints can be formed based on null and alternative hypotheses, and these constraints are incorporated into the EL. This result was extended and applied to the following practical issues.

Malaria remains a major epidemiological problem in many developing countries. In endemic areas, an individual may have symptoms attributable either to malaria or to other causes. From a clinical viewpoint, it is important to attend to the next tasks: (1) to correctly diagnose an individual who has developed symptoms, so that the appropriate treatments can be given; and (2) to determine the proportion of malaria-affected cases in individuals who have symptoms, so that policies on intervention program can be developed. Once symptoms have developed in an individual, the diagnosis of malaria can be based on the analysis of the parasite levels in blood samples. However, even a blood test is not conclusive, as in endemic areas many healthy individuals can have parasites in their blood slides. Therefore, data from this type of study can be viewed as coming from a mixture distribution, with the components corresponding to malaria and nonmalaria cases. Qin and Leung (2005) constructed new EL procedures to estimate the proportion of clinical malaria using parasite-level data from a group of individuals with symptoms attributable to malaria.

Yu et al. (2010) proposed two-sample EL techniques based on incomplete data to analyze a Pneumonia Risk Study in an ICU setting. In the context of this study, the initial detection of ventilator-associated pneumonia (VAP) for inpatients at an intensive care unit requires composite symptom evaluation, using clinical criteria such as the clinical pulmonary infection score (CPIS). When CPIS is above a threshold value, bronchoalveolar lavage (BAL) is performed, to confirm the diagnosis by counting actual bacterial pathogens. Thus, CPIS and BAL results are closely related, and both are important indicators of pneumonia, whereas BAL data are incomplete. Yu et al. (2010) and Vexler et al. (2010c) derived EL methods to compare the pneumonia risks among treatment groups for such incomplete data.

In semi- and nonparametric contexts, including EL settings, Qin and Zhang (2005) showed that the full likelihood can be decomposed into the product of a conditional likelihood and a marginal likelihood, in a similar manner to the parametric likelihood considerations. These techniques augment the study's power by enabling researchers to use any observed data and relevant information.

10.5 Bayesians and Empirical Likelihood

The statistical literature has shown that Bayesian methods (e.g., Chapter 5) can be applied for various tasks for the analysis of health-related experiments. Commonly, the application of a Bayesian approach requires the assumption of functional forms corresponding to the distribution of the underlying data and parameters of interest. However, in cases with data subject to complex missing data problems, parametric estimation is complicated and formal tests for the relevant goodness-of-fit are often not available. The statistical literature has shown that tests derived from empirical likelihood methodology possess many of the same asymptotic properties as those based on parametric likelihoods. This leads naturally to the idea of using the empirical likelihood instead of the parametric likelihood as the basis for Bayesian inference.

Lazar (2003) demonstrated the potential for constructing nonparametric Bayesian inference based on ELs. The key idea is to substitute the parametric likelihood (PL) with the EL in the Bayesian likelihood construction relative to the component of the likelihood used to model the observed data. It is demonstrated that the EL function is a proper likelihood function and can serve as the basis for robust and accurate Bayesian inference. This Bayesian empirical likelihood method provides a robust nonparametric data-driven alternative to the more classical Bayesian procedures.

Vexler et al. (2014) developed the nonparametric Bayesian posterior expectation fashion by incorporating the EL methodology into the posterior likelihood construction. The asymptotic forms of the EL-based Bayesian posterior expectation are shown to be similar to those derived in the well-known parametric Bayesian and Frequentist statistical literature. In the case when the prior distribution function depends on unknown hyper-parameters, a nonparametric version of the empirical Bayesian method, which yields double empirical Bayesian estimators, can be obtained. This approach yields a nonparametric analog of the well-known *James–Stein estimation* that has been well addressed in the literature dealing with multivariate-normal observations (e.g., Stein, 1956).

Vexler et al. (2016b) provided an EL-based technique for incorporating prior information into the equal-tailed and highest posterior density confidence interval estimators (Chapter 9) in the Bayesian manner. It was demonstrated that the proposed EL Bayesian approach may correct confidence regions with respect to skewness of the data distribution.

The EL Bayesian procedures can serve as a powerful approach to incorporating external information into the inference process about given data, in a distribution-free manner.

10.6 Three Key Arguments That Support the Empirical Likelihood Methodology as a Practical Statistical Analysis Tool

One of the important advantages of EL techniques is their general applicability and an assessment of their performance under conditions that are commonly unrestricted by parametric assumptions. When one is in doubt about the best strategy for constructing statistical decision rules, the following arguments can be accepted in favor of EL methods:

Argument 1: The EL methodology employs the likelihood concept in a simple nonparametric fashion in order to approximate optimal parametric procedures. The benefit of using this approach is that the EL techniques are often robust as well as highly efficient. In this context, we also may apply EL functions to replace parametric likelihood functions in known and well-developed constructions.

Argument 2: Similarly to the parametric likelihood concept, the EL methodology gives relatively simple systematic directions for constructing efficient statistical tests that can be applied in various complex statistical experiments.

Argument 3: Perhaps the extreme generality of EL methods and their wide scope of usefulness partly follow from the ability to easily set up EL-type statistics as components of composite parametric, semiparametric, and nonparametric likelihood–based systems, efficiently attending to any observed data and relevant information. Parametric, semiparametric, and empirical likelihood methods play roles complementary to one another, providing powerful statistical procedures for complicated practical problems.

In conclusion, we note that EL-based methods are employed in much of modern statistical practice, and we cannot describe all relevant theory and examples. The reader interested in the EL methods will find more details and many pertinent articles across the statistical literature.

Appendix

$ELR(\theta_1, \theta_2)$: *Several results that are similar to those related to the evaluations of* $ELR(\theta)$.

One can show that the logarithm of the ELR test statistic for the null hypothesis: $H_0 : E(X_1) = \theta_1$ and $E(X_1^2) = \theta_2$ has the form

$$\log ELR(\theta_1, \theta_2) = \sum_{i=1}^{n} \log\{1 + \lambda_1(X_i - \theta_1)/n + \lambda_2(X_i^2 - \theta_2)/n\},$$

where λ_1 and λ_2 are Lagrange multipliers that satisfy the equations

$$\sum_{i=1}^{n} \frac{(X_i - \theta_1)}{n + \lambda_1(X_i - \theta_1) + \lambda_2(X_i^2 - \theta_2)} = 0 \text{ and } \sum_{i=1}^{n} \frac{(X_i^2 - \theta_2)}{n + \lambda_1(X_i - \theta_1) + \lambda_2(X_i^2 - \theta_2)} = 0.$$

In this case, $\partial \log(ELR) / \partial \theta_1 = -\lambda_1$ and $\partial \log ELR / \partial \theta_2 = -\lambda_2$. At point $\left(\theta_1 = \bar{X} = \sum_{i=1}^{n} X_i/n, \theta_2 = \bar{X}^2 = \sum_{i=1}^{n} X_i^2/n\right)$, we have $\log\{ELR(\theta_1, \theta_2)\} = \lambda_1 = \lambda_2 = 0$, $p_i = 1/n$ and the following derivative values:

$$\frac{\partial \lambda_1}{\partial \theta_1} = \frac{n^2 \sum_{i=1}^{n} (X_i^2 - \bar{X}^2)^2}{\Delta}, \quad \frac{\partial \lambda_2}{\partial \theta_2} = \frac{n^2 \sum_{i=1}^{n} (X_i - \bar{X})^2}{\Delta}, \quad \frac{\partial \lambda_1}{\partial \theta_2} = \frac{\partial \lambda_2}{\partial \theta_1} = \frac{n^2 \sum_{i=1}^{n} (X_i - \bar{X})(X_i^2 - \bar{X}^2)}{\Delta}.$$

$$\frac{\partial^2 \lambda_1}{\partial \theta_1^2} = \frac{1}{n\Delta} [2 \sum_{i=1}^{n} (X_i^2 - \bar{X}^2) \{ \frac{\partial \lambda_1}{\partial \theta_1} (X_i - \bar{X}) + \frac{\partial \lambda_2}{\partial \theta_1} (X_i^2 - \bar{X}^2) \}^2 \sum_{i=1}^{n} (X_i - \bar{X})(X_i^2 - \bar{X}^2)$$
$$- 2 \sum_{i=1}^{n} (X_i - \bar{X}) \{ \frac{\partial \lambda_1}{\partial \theta_1} (X_i - \bar{X}) + \frac{\partial \lambda_2}{\partial \theta_1} (X_i^2 - \bar{X}^2) \}^2 \sum_{i=1}^{n} (X_i^2 - \bar{X}^2)^2],$$

$$\frac{\partial^2 \lambda_2}{\partial \theta_1^2} = \frac{1}{n\Delta} [2 \sum_{i=1}^{n} (X_i - \bar{X}) \{ \frac{\partial \lambda_1}{\partial \theta_1} (X_i - \bar{X}) + \frac{\partial \lambda_2}{\partial \theta_1} (X_i^2 - \bar{X}^2) \}^2 \sum_{i=1}^{n} (X_i - \bar{X})(X_i^2 - \bar{X}^2)$$
$$- 2 \sum_{i=1}^{n} (X_i^2 - \bar{X}^2) \{ \frac{\partial \lambda_1}{\partial \theta_1} (X_i - \bar{X}) + \frac{\partial \lambda_2}{\partial \theta_1} (X_i^2 - \bar{X}^2) \}^2 \sum_{i=1}^{n} (X_i - \bar{X})^2],$$

$$\frac{\partial^2 \lambda_1}{\partial \theta_2^2} = \frac{\partial^2 \lambda_2}{\partial \theta_1 \partial \theta_2} = \frac{1}{n\Delta} [2 \sum_{i=1}^{n} (X_i^2 - \bar{X}^2) \{ \frac{\partial \lambda_1}{\partial \theta_2} (X_i - \bar{X}) + \frac{\partial \lambda_2}{\partial \theta_2} (X_i^2 - \bar{X}^2) \}^2 \sum_{i=1}^{n} (X_i - \bar{X})(X_i^2 - \bar{X}^2)$$
$$- 2 \sum_{i=1}^{n} (X_i - \bar{X}) \{ \frac{\partial \lambda_1}{\partial \theta_2} (X_i - \bar{X}) + \frac{\partial \lambda_2}{\partial \theta_2} (X_i^2 - \bar{X}^2) \}^2 \sum_{i=1}^{n} (X_i^2 - \bar{X}^2)^2],$$

$$\frac{\partial^2 \lambda_2}{\partial \theta_1^2} = \frac{\partial^2 \lambda_1}{\partial \theta_1 \partial \theta_2} = \frac{1}{n\Delta} [2 \sum_{i=1}^{n} (X_i - \bar{X}) \{ \frac{\partial \lambda_1}{\partial \theta_1} (X_i - \bar{X}) + \frac{\partial \lambda_2}{\partial \theta_1} (X_i^2 - \bar{X}^2) \}^2 \sum_{i=1}^{n} (X_i - \bar{X})(X_i^2 - \bar{X}^2)$$
$$- 2 \sum_{i=1}^{n} (X_i^2 - \bar{X}^2) \{ \frac{\partial \lambda_1}{\partial \theta_1} (X_i - \bar{X}) + \frac{\partial \lambda_2}{\partial \theta_1} (X_i^2 - \bar{X}^2) \}^2 \sum_{i=1}^{n} (X_i - \bar{X})^2],$$

where $\Delta = \{ \sum_{i=1}^{n} (X_i - \bar{X})(X_i^2 - \bar{X}^2) \}^2 - \sum_{i=1}^{n} (X_i - \bar{X})^2 \sum_{i=1}^{n} (X_i^2 - \bar{X}^2)^2$.

Then, in a similar manner to the analysis shown in Section 10.3, one can show that, under H_0, $2 \log ELR(\theta_1, \theta_2) \sim \chi_2^2$, as $n \to \infty$.

11

Jackknife and Bootstrap Methods

11.1 Introduction

Jackknife and *bootstrap* methods and other "computationally intensive" techniques of statistical inference have a long history dating back to the permutation test introduced in the 1930s by R.A. Fisher. Ever since that time there has been work towards developing efficient and practical nonparametric models that did not rely upon the classical normal-based model assumptions. In the 1940s Quenouille introduced the method of deleting "one observation at a time" for reducing a bias of estimation. This method was further developed by Tukey for standard error estimation and coined by him as the *"jackknife"* method (Tukey, 1958). This early work was followed by many variants up to the 1970s. The jackknife method was then extended to what is now referred to as the bootstrap method. Even though there were predecessors towards the development of the bootstrap method, e.g., see Hartigan (1969, 1971, 1975), it is generally agreed upon by statisticians that Efron's (1979) paper in which the term "bootstrap" was coined, in conjunction with the development of high-speed computers, was a cornerstone event towards popularizing this particular methodology. Following Efron's paper there was an explosion of research on the topic of bootstrap methods. At one time nonparametric bootstrapping was thought to be a statistical method that would solve almost all problems in an efficient easy-to-use nonparametric manner. So why do we not have a PROC BOOTSTRAP in SAS, and why are bootstrap methods not used more widely? One answer lies in the fact that there is not a general approach to bootstrapping along the lines of fitting a generalized linear model with normal error terms. Oftentimes the bootstrap approach to solving a problem requires writing new pieces of sometimes-difficult SAS code that only pertains to a specific problem. Another reason for the bootstrap method's failure to take off as a general approach is that it sometimes does not work well in certain situations, and that the method for correcting these deficient procedures are oftentimes difficult or tedious.

Our focus will be on problems where the simple bootstrap methods are known to work well. Even though the bootstrap method is primarily considered a nonparametric method, it can also be used in conjunction with parametric models as well. We will touch on how to employ the parametric bootstrap method as well.

Complicated problems in practice where the bootstrap method is a reasonable approach are situations such as repeated measures analyses, where one wishes to treat the correlation structure as a nuisance parameter, as opposed to assuming something unreasonable, or the case where there are unequal numbers of repeated measurements per subject.

The most common use of the bootstrap method is to approximate the sampling distribution of a statistic such as the mean, median, regression slope, correlation coefficient, and so on. Once the sampling distribution has been approximated via the bootstrap method, estimation and inference involving the given statistic follows in a straightforward manner. Note however that the bootstrap does not provide exact answers. It provides approximate variance estimates and approximate coverage probabilities for confidence intervals. As with most statistical methods these approximations improve for increasing sample sizes. The estimated probability distribution of a given statistic based upon the bootstrap method is obtained by conditioning on the observed dataset and replacing the population distribution function with its estimate in some statistical function such as the expected value. The method may be carried out using either a parametric or nonparametric estimate of the distribution function. For example, the parametric bootstrap distribution of the sample mean $\bar{x}$ under normality assumptions is given simply by $\hat{F}(x) = \Phi(\sqrt{n}(x - \bar{x}) / s)$, where Φ denotes the probit function, n is the sample size, and $\bar{x}$ and s are the sample mean and sample standard deviation, respectively. The 95% parametric bootstrap percentile confidence interval is given simply by the 2.5th and 97.5th percentiles of $\hat{F}(x)$ or simply $\bar{x} + s \times 1.96 / \sqrt{n}$. This should look familiar to anybody who has opened an introductory statistics book as the approximate normal theory confidence interval for the sample mean.

Oftentimes the calculations are not so straightforward or we wish to apply the bootstrap method in a nonparametric fashion, that is, we don't wish to constrain ourselves to a parametric functional form such as the normal distribution when specifying the distribution function $F(x)$. In the majority of cases we need to approximate the bootstrap method through the generation of *bootstrap replications* of the statistic of interest. Using a resampling procedure we will be able to approximate bootstrap estimates for quantities such as standard errors, p-values, and confidence intervals for a complicated statistic without relying on traditional approximations based upon asymptotic normality.

There are many well-known books on bootstrapping such as Efron and Tibshirani (1994), Davison and Hinkley (1997), and Shao and Tu (1995) that we can suggest to the reader who is interested in further details regarding jackknife and bootstrap methods.

This chapter will outline the following topics: jackknife bias estimation, jackknife variance estimation, confidence interval definition, approximate confidence intervals, variance stabilization, bootstrap methods, nonparametric simulation, resampling algorithms with SAS and R, bootstrap confidence intervals, use of the Edgeworth expansion to illustrate the accuracy of bootstrap intervals, bootstrap-t percentile intervals, further refinement of bootstrap confidence intervals, and bootstrap tilting (Sections 11.2 through 11.14, respectively).

11.2 Jackknife Bias Estimation

Quenouille (1949, 1956) developed a nonparametric estimate of the large sample bias of a given statistic that has first order bias of $1/n$. The methodology Quenouille developed was coined the *jackknife* method by Tukey (1958). In terms of demonstrating the method let $X_1, X_2,\ldots, X_n$ be a set of iid observations from a distribution function F with a density function $f(x;\theta)$ and let $\hat{\theta} = \hat{\theta}(X_1, X_2,\ldots, X_n)$ be an estimator of some population quantity $\theta = t(F)$, where $t(F)$ is what is referred to as a *statistical functional*, e.g., the expectation, quantile, etc. An estimate of $t(F)$ is given by $\hat{\theta} = t(\hat{F})$, where $\hat{F}(x) = \sum_{i=1}^{n} I(X_i \leq x)/n$ is the empirical distribution function and $I(.)$ denotes the indicator function. For example, if $t(F) = \int x dF$ is the expectation then $\hat{\theta} = t(\hat{F}) = \int x d\hat{F}(x) = \sum_{i=1}^{n} X_i / n$ is the sample mean (see also Section 1.6 in this context).

The bias of the statistic is given by

$$bias = E[t(\hat{F}) - t(F)].$$

Quenouille derived an estimate of the bias by deleting one observation X_i and then recalculating $\hat{\theta} = \theta(\hat{F})$, given as

$$\hat{\theta}_{(i)} = t(\hat{F}_i) = \hat{\theta}(X_1, X_2,\ldots, X_{i-1,}, X_{i+1,},\ldots, X_{n,})$$

along with the average $\hat{\theta}_{(.)} = \sum_{i=1}^{n} \hat{\theta}_{(i)} / n$. Then the estimate of the bias is given as $(n-1)(\hat{\theta}_{(.)} - \hat{\theta})$ such that the bias-corrected jackknife estimator for θ is given as

$$\tilde{\theta} = n \cdot \hat{\theta} - (n-1)\hat{\theta}_{(.)}.$$

Note however, there is a statistical price to pay for such a correction in terms of bias-variance trade-offs. This approach to bias correction is most useful for statistics that have expectations of the form

$$E\left(\hat{\theta}\right) = \theta + \frac{a_1(F)}{n} + \frac{a_2(F)}{n^2} + O(n^{-3}),$$

when the constants $a_1(F)$ and $a_2(F)$ do not depend on n. Oftentimes expectations of maximum likelihood estimators have values of the form above, e.g., see Firth (1993) for a general description of the problem.

The mechanism for which the jackknife method works follows by noting that

$$E\left(\hat{\theta}_{()}\right) = \theta + \frac{a_1(F)}{n-1} + \frac{a_2(F)}{(n-1)^2} + O(n^{-3}).$$

Hence,

$$E\left(\tilde{\theta}\right) = \theta - \frac{a_2(F)}{n(n-1)} + O(n^{-3})$$

such that $\tilde{\theta}$ has bias of order $O(n^{-2})$, whereas $\hat{\theta}$ has bias of order $O(n^{-1})$. As an example denote the population variance as

$$t(F) = \int \left(u - E(X)\right)^2 dF(u)$$

with the corresponding moment estimator given as

$$t(\hat{F}) = \int \left(u - \bar{X}\right)^2 d\hat{F}(u) = \sum_{i=1}^{n}(X_i - \bar{X})^2 / n,$$

where $\bar{X} = \sum_{i=1}^{n} X_i / n$. Then an estimate of the bias is given as $\sum_{i=1}^{n}\left(X_i - \bar{X}\right)^2 / (n(n-1))$ such that the jackknife bias-corrected estimator is given as $\tilde{\theta} = \sum_{i=1}^{n}\left(X_i - \bar{X}\right)^2 / (n-1)$. In this case $\tilde{\theta}$ is precisely unbiased.

A variant of the delete one observation at a time approach towards bias reduction is the **grouped jackknife** approach. Let $n = gh$, where g and h are integers such that we can remove g distinct blocks of size h from $X_1, X_2,..., X_n$ given as $X_1^*, X_2^*,... , X_h^*$ then

$$\tilde{\theta} = g\hat{\theta} - (g-1)\hat{\theta}_{()},$$

where $\hat{\theta}_{(.)} = \sum_i \hat{\theta}_i / \binom{n}{h}$ and $\sum_i$ denotes the summation over all possible subsets. The blocked jackknife biased corrected estimator has smaller variance than the leave one out at a time classic estimators (Shao and Wu, 1989).

11.3 Jackknife Variance Estimation

Tukey (1958) put forth the idea that the jackknife method is a useful tool for estimating the variance of $\hat{\theta} = \theta(\hat{F})$ in the iid setting. The variance estimate for $\hat{\theta}$ takes the form $\widehat{Var}(\hat{\theta}) = \sum_{i=1}^{n} (\hat{\theta}_{(i)} - \hat{\theta}_{(.)})^2 / n$. In general, the variance estimator works for a class of statistics that are so-called smooth statistics and not so well in other instances, that is, in many instances $\lim_{n \to \infty} \{n(Var(\hat{\theta}) - \widehat{Var}(\tilde{\theta}))\} \neq 0$, where $Var(X) = E(X - (EX)^2)^2$. In fact, $E\{\widehat{Var}(\hat{\theta})\} > Var(\hat{\theta})$. We outline the concept of smoothness in the bootstrap methods section below.

For a simple example, let $\hat{\theta} = t(\hat{F}) = \int x d\hat{F} = \sum_{i=1}^{n} X_i / n$ be the sample mean; then $\hat{\theta}_{(i)} = \dfrac{n\hat{\theta} - X_i}{n-1}$, $\hat{\theta}_{(.)} = \hat{\theta}$ and $\hat{\theta}_{(i)} - \hat{\theta}_{(.)} = \dfrac{\theta - X_i}{n-1}$. This yields $\widehat{Var}(\hat{\theta}) = \dfrac{1}{n(n-1)} \sum_{i=1}^{n} (X_i - \bar{X})^2 = \dfrac{S^2}{n}$. There may in general be a temptation to use $\hat{\theta} \pm t_{n-1,\alpha/2} \sqrt{\widehat{Var}(\hat{\theta})}$ for a confidence interval about θ. However, intervals of this type have notoriously poor coverage probabilities. We will illustrate that the bootstrap approach described below provides a more suitable approach for generating approximate confidence intervals.

11.4 Confidence Interval Definition

Let X denote a random variable and let a and b denote two positive real numbers. Then

$$\begin{aligned}
P(a < X < b) &= P(a < X \text{ and } X < b) \\
&= P\left(\frac{bX}{a} > b \text{ and } X < b\right) \\
&= P(X < b < \frac{bX}{a}).
\end{aligned}$$

The interval $G(X) = (X, \dfrac{bX}{a})$ is then a random interval and assumes the value $G(x)$ whenever X assumes the value x. The interval $G(X)$ contains the value b with a certain fixed probability. Now in this framework denote $\theta \in \Theta \subset R$. For $0 < \alpha < 1$ a function satisfying $P(\underline{\theta}(X) \le \theta) \ge 1 - \alpha$, $\forall \theta$ is called a lower *confidence band* at level α, where $\underline{\theta}(X)$ does not depend on θ and X is a random vector of observations. A similar definition holds for the upper confidence band $\overline{\theta}(X)$. A family of subsets $S(X)$ of Θ is said to constitute a family of confidence sets at confidence level $1 - \alpha$ if $P(S(X) \in \Theta) \ge 1 - \alpha$, $\forall \theta \in \Theta$. A special case $S(X) = (\underline{\theta}(X), \overline{\theta}(X))$ is called a *confidence interval* provided $P(\underline{\theta}(X) < \theta < \overline{\theta}(X)) \ge 1 - \alpha$, $\forall \theta$.

A key towards generating a standard confidence interval used in applications is to develop a so-called *pivot*. For example, let $X_1, X_2, \ldots, X_n$ be iid observations from a density function $f(x; \theta)$ and denote the statistic $T(X_1, X_2, \ldots, X_n; \theta) = T(X; \theta)$. The goal in confidence interval generation is to start by choosing λ_1 and λ_2 such that the probability statement

$$P(\lambda_1 < T(X; \theta) < \lambda_2) = 1 - \alpha$$

may be written in the form discussed above and given as

$$P(\underline{\theta}(X) < \theta < \overline{\theta}(X)) \ge 1 - \alpha.$$

This can be accomplished by finding a pivot within the form of the statistic $T(X; \theta)$ about the parameter θ. If the distribution function of $T(X; \theta)$ has a form that is independent of θ then $T(X; \theta)$ is called a pivot. For example, let $X_1, X_2, \ldots, X_n \sim N(\theta, \sigma)$; then the pivot $T(X; \theta) = \sqrt{n}(\overline{x} - \theta)\sigma^{-1} \sim N(0,1)$, where $\overline{x} = \displaystyle\sum_{i=1}^{n} X_i / n$, that is, $T(X; \theta)$ has a distribution that is θ free. Hence we can pivot about θ to arrive at the exact $1 - \alpha$ confidence interval for θ with the classic form $P_\theta(\overline{x} - z_{1-\alpha/2}\sigma / \sqrt{n} < \theta < \overline{x} + z_{1-\alpha/2}\sigma / \sqrt{n}) \ge 1 - \alpha$.

11.5 Approximate Confidence Intervals

When the distribution of the statistic $T(X; \theta)$ is unknown or analytically intractable oftentimes it can be approximated with large sample approximations given certain regularity conditions, e.g., the existence of moments. The reason as to why the distribution of $T(X; \theta)$ may be unknown is that we do not wish to assume a form for a density function $f(x;\theta)$ or we simply do not know what it may be based on experience.

A well-known approximation is the case when $T(X;\theta)$ takes the form of a sum of iid observations. Then we have in the general case the asymptotic approximation $T(X;\theta) \sim AN(\theta, \sigma^2_T/n)$, where $Var(T(X;\theta)) = \sigma^2_T/n$. The classic large sample confidence interval or *z-interval* then takes the form $T(X;\theta) \pm z_{1-\alpha/2}\sigma_T/\sqrt{n}$. The general problem with this approximate confidence interval is that in general the nuisance parameter σ^2_T is unknown.

Typically, some consistent estimator of σ^2_T is used in the confidence interval approximation. Now, however, unlike the classic case when $X_1, X_2, \ldots, X_n \sim N(\theta, \sigma^2)$ and we can apply the t-distribution given $\hat\sigma^2$ is the sample standard deviation to generate a precise confidence interval, the confidence interval $T(X;\theta) \pm z_{1-\alpha/2}\hat\sigma/\sqrt{n}$ is an approximation of an approximation. In general, if $T(X;\theta) \sim AN(\theta, \sigma^2_T/n)$ and $\hat\sigma^2 \overset{P}{\to} \sigma^2_T$ then $T(X;\theta) \pm z_{1-\alpha/2}\hat\sigma/\sqrt{n}$ has coverage probability that converges to $1-\alpha$ as the sample size $n \to \infty$. However, in many instances approximate confidence intervals of this type may have poor coverage in small finite samples and should be used with caution.

In certain instances these types of approximate intervals may be improved upon using some common techniques such as variance stabilization transformations, symmetry transformations (e.g., the log transform) or incorporating some functional knowledge about $f(x;\theta)$.

11.6 Variance Stabilization

When the large sample variance of the statistic $T(X;\theta) = \hat\theta$ depends on θ, that is, $\hat\theta \sim AN\left(\theta, \dfrac{h(\theta)\sigma^2_T}{n}\right)$, where $h(.)$ is a continuously differentiable function, then one may consider a function g such that $g(\hat\theta) \sim AN\left(\theta, \dfrac{c\sigma^2_T}{n}\right)$. For illustration purposes consider $X_1, X_2, \ldots, X_n$ to be iid data points from an exponential density function $f(x;\theta) = \exp(-x/\theta)/\theta$. Then we know $E(\bar{x}) = \theta$, $Var(\bar{x}) = \theta^2$, and $\bar{x} \sim AN(\theta, \theta^2/n)$. One variant of a $(1-\alpha)$ large sample confidence interval for θ would be $\bar{x} \pm z_{1-\alpha/2}\bar{x}/\sqrt{n}$ due to the variance being dependent on the parameter of interest. Alternatively, consider that $\log\bar{x} \sim AN(\log\theta, 1/n)$ with variance that does not depend on θ. Hence a $1-\alpha$ large sample confidence interval for $\log\theta$ would be $\log\bar{x} \pm z_{1-\alpha/2}1/\sqrt{n}$. This interval then can be back-transformed to the original scale by exponentiating the lower and upper bounds.

11.7 Bootstrap Methods

The term "bootstrap" was coined by Efron (1979). Hartigan (1969) first discussed what we now refer to as the bootstrap method. Bootstrap methods are a very valuable inference tool if properly used. The primary usage of this method is around bias estimation, variance estimation, and confidence interval generation and inference. In some sense, bootstrap methods generalize the jackknife described earlier. The bootstrap method is a resampling method based on sampling from the original dataset with replacement. For small samples we can enumerate all possible subsamples, which we will refer to as the exact bootstrap method. For larger samples Monte Carlo approaches are generally applied. The key idea is to extract "extra" information from the data via sampling with replacement. An alternative approach termed permutation methods will be described in a later section, which in its most basic form is a sampling without replacement approach.

For the purpose of introducing the method we will start with the univariate standard case where we assume $X_1, X_2, \ldots, X_n$ is a set of iid observations from $f(x; \theta)$. The empirical distribution function $\hat{F}(x) = \sum_{i=1}^{n} I(X_i \leq x)/n$ plays a key role in classic bootstrap methods. More formally, $\hat{F}(x) = \sum_{i=1}^{n} H(x - X_i)/n$, where $H(u)$ is the unit step function defined as

$$H(u) = \begin{cases} 0, & u < 0, \\ 1, & u \geq 0. \end{cases}$$

Note that $H(u)$ is in a sense also a discrete-valued distribution function. Hence, by convention the derivative of $H(u)$, $H'(u) = h(u)$, is a degenerate density function with point mass at $u = 0$. Note also that we will use the empirical quantile estimator as well to illustrate bootstrap methods and aid in resampling approaches. Let $X_{(1)} < X_{(2)} < \ldots < X_{(n)}$ denote the order statistic. Then the empirical quantile function estimator in the absolutely continuous case for $F^{-1}(u) = Q(u)$ is given as $\hat{Q}(u) = X_{([nu]+1)}$, where $[.]$ denotes the floor function. The alternative definition for the empirical distribution function about H provides a more formal method for calculating quantities, e.g., $\int g(x) d\hat{F}(x)$, which if done analytically provides so-called exact bootstrap solutions, where $g(x)$ denotes a generic function corresponding to the population quantity of interest, e.g., $g(x) = x$ corresponds to the calculation of $E(X)$.

The heart of bootstrap methods revolves around understanding statistical functionals. Notationally, a statistical functional has the form $\theta = t(F)$ such that the estimator has the form $\hat{\theta} = t(\hat{F})$. The function $\theta = t(F)$ is central to nonparametric estimation. The key assumption that we will operate under is that some characteristic of F is defined by θ. Note that F and θ may be multidimensional.

In general, bootstrap methods work well in terms of the performance character-istics when the statistical functional of interest has the form $\theta = t(F)$. In other scenarios caution must be taken when using bootstrap methods, e.g., estimat-ing properties of a threshold parameter. As a general rule-of-thumb if $\hat{\theta} = t(\hat{F})$ can be assumed to be asymptotically normal and consistent then the bootstrap methods that we will outline will work well.

As a straightforward example of the relationship between a statistical functional and its corresponding estimator, consider the statistical func-tional $\theta = t(F) = \int x dF$, which is the expectation. Then the estimator is given by "plugging-in" $\hat{F}$ for F and given as

$$
\begin{aligned}
\hat{\theta} = t(\hat{F}) &= \int x d\hat{F}(x) \\
&= \int x d(\sum_{i=1}^{n} H(x - X_i)/n) \\
&= \frac{1}{n}\sum_{i=1}^{n} \int x dH(x - X_i) \\
&= \frac{1}{n}\sum_{i=1}^{n} X_i = \bar{X},
\end{aligned}
$$

that is, the sample average. Oftentimes in terms of direct calculations the quantile form of the statistical functional is worth considering, e.g., for the average we have

$$
\theta = t(F) = \int x dF = \int_0^1 Q(u) du
$$

and hence $\hat{\theta} = \int_0^1 \hat{Q}(u) du = \frac{1}{n}\sum_{i=1}^{n} \int_{(i-1)/n}^{i/n} \hat{Q}(u) du = \frac{1}{n}\sum_{i=1}^{n} X_{(i)} = \bar{X}$, where $\hat{Q}(u) = X_{([nu]+1)}$

and [.] denotes the floor function.

11.8 Nonparametric Simulation

In many scenarios $\theta = t(F)$ can be estimated directly via the plug-in method by $\hat{\theta} = t(\hat{F})$ or via Monte Carlo simulation. The reason one may wish to use simulation is that direct calculations may be complex. Many quantities of interest around the statistical functional such as confidence intervals are difficult to calculate directly. For example, say we are interested in the statistical functional pertaining to the quantile of the sample average. In this case

$$\theta = t(F) = \min_{\theta} E[\,|\bar{X} - \theta| + (2\alpha - 1)(\bar{X} - \theta)],$$

where α denotes the quantile of $\bar{X}$, $0 < \alpha < 1$. This quantity can be calculated directly for small samples, but becomes computationally, analytically infeasible for even moderate sample size. Or as another complex example say we were interested in the statistical functional of $t(F) = Var(S/\bar{x})$ where S is the sample standard deviation. In this case, direct calculation is not possible. However a simulation approached based on sampling with replacement provides a powerful tool for calculating such quantities.

Let us take a simple example of estimating the variance for the coefficient of variation. In this case $\theta = t(F) = 100 \times \sqrt{Var(X)}/E(X)$ such that $\hat{\theta} = t(\hat{F}) = 100 \times S/\bar{X}$. Deriving the estimator $\widehat{Var}(100 \times S/\bar{X})$ of the coefficient of variation is nontrivial even when the parametric form of the density is assumed known. Suppose we observe a sample of size $n = 10$ with observed data X={0.25, 0.40, 0.46, 0.27, 2.51, 1.24, 4.11, 6.11, 0.46, 1.35}. The estimate in this case is $\hat{\theta} = t(\hat{F}) = 114.6$. For the nonparametric bootstrap approach we sample with replacement from $\hat{F}$ in order to form bootstrap replicates. One single randomly sampled bootstrap replicate in this example was x* ={0.25, 0.40, 0.46, 0.27, 1.29, 1.29, 4.11, 6.11, 0.25, 1.37} such that the bootstrap replicate statistics was $\hat{\theta}^* = t(\hat{F}^*) = 124.29$, where $\hat{F}^*$ is the empirical distribution function based on the resampled values. If we repeat this process say with $B = 10,000$ bootstrap replications we obtain the approximate distribution for $\hat{\theta} = t(\hat{F}) = 100 \times S/\bar{X}$ illustrated in Figure 11.1. Similar to the jackknife a nonparametric estimate of the variance of $\hat{\theta} = t(\hat{F})$ is $\widehat{Var}(t(\hat{F})) \approx \frac{1}{B-1}\sum_{i=1}^{B}(t_i(\hat{F}^*) - \bar{t}(\hat{F}^*))^2$, where $\bar{t}(\hat{F}^*) = \frac{1}{B}\sum_{i=1}^{B} t_i(\hat{F}^*)$. For our example, $\widehat{Var}(t(\hat{F})) = 514.6$. Note that there are two sources of variance in the approximation, Monte Carlo error and stochastic error. The Monte Carlo error goes to 0 as $B \rightarrow \infty$. We will demonstrate that this resampling approach can be extended to generating approximate bootstrap confidence intervals for $\theta = t(F)$.

The general steps one needs to follow in order to utilize the power of classic bootstrap methods are as follows:

(1) Have a clear definition of $\theta = t(F)$.
(2) Ensure that the estimator for $\theta = t(F)$ has the form $\hat{\theta} = t(\hat{F})$.

(3) Generate B bootstrap samples of size n from $\hat{F}$ with replacement denoted $X_1^*, X_2^*, \ldots, X_n^*$.

(4) Calculate bootstrap replicates of the statistic $t_1(\hat{F}^*), t_2(\hat{F}^*), \ldots, t_B(\hat{F}^*)$.

(5) Utilize $t_1(\hat{F}^*), t_2(\hat{F}^*), \ldots, t_B(\hat{F}^*)$ to approximate the distribution of $\hat{\theta} = t(\hat{F})$ to calculate the quantity of interest, e.g., an estimate of the variance for $\hat{\theta} = t(\hat{F})$.

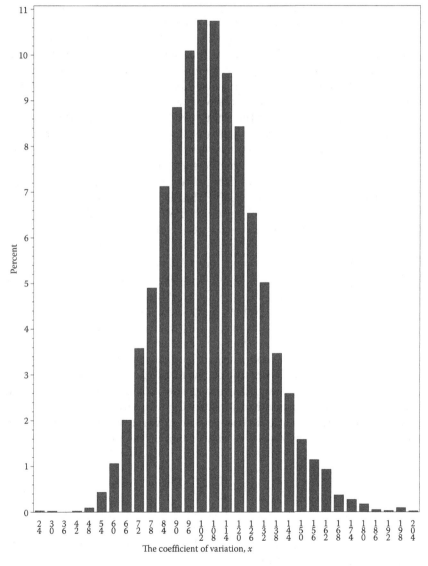

FIGURE 11.1
$B = 10{,}000$ bootstrap replications for the coefficient of variation example.

11.9 Resampling Algorithms with SAS and R

The majority of nonparametric bootstrap procedures discussed from this point forward rely upon the ability to sample from the data with replacement. In this chapter we will discuss the pieces of code needed to carry out the simple bootstrap in the univariate setting. When we get to more complicated repeated measures and cluster-related datasets later in the book we will use the code provided below as a jumping off point. The basic idea is that once you understand the syntax provided in this chapter you should be able to easily modify it for most bootstrap-related problems that would be encountered in practice.

It turns out that resampling from the data with replacement can be accomplished relatively easily through the generation of a vector or set of multinomial random variables. The algorithms outlined below will be the "front-end" for most of the bootstrap procedures we intend to discuss. The key to programming the nonparametric bootstrap procedure is to consider carefully how data is managed internally within SAS. The point of the procedures outlined below is to avoid having to create a multitude of arrays or specialized macros, and to try maximize efficiency, thus making it easier for the novice to carry out the bootstrap procedures. In other instances we will be able to take advantage of PROC SURVEYSELECT, which is an already built-in procedure that allows us to resample the data with replacement. Note however, for certain problems one may not be able to avoid using macros or arrays. We will deal with a few specialized cases later in the book.

Let us start with an example dataset $\mathbf{X} = \{0.5, 0.4, 0.6, 0.2\}$ of size $n = 4$. If we sample from this dataset once with replacement, we might obtain a bootstrap replication denoted $\mathbf{x}^* = \{0.5, 0.4, 0.6, 0.2\}$. Note that this is equivalent to keeping track of the set of multinomial counts $c = \{2,1,0,1\}$ corresponding to the original dataset $\mathbf{x}$ as listed and outputting each observation X_i the corresponding c_i number of times, where X_i denotes the ith observation and c_i denotes the corresponding count, e.g., $X_2 = 0.4$ and $c_2 = 1$. In other words sampling with replacement is *exactly* equivalent to generating a set of random multinomial counts with marginal probabilities $1/n$, and outputting the data value the corresponding number of times. One way to do this in SAS easily and efficiently is to generate random binomial variables conditioned on the margins as described in Davis (1993) and given by the following formula:

$$C_i \sim B\left(n - \sum_{j=0}^{i-1} C_j, \frac{1}{n-i+1}\right) \qquad (11.1)$$

for $i = 1, \ldots, n-1$, where $C_0 = p_0 = 0$, $C_n = n - \sum_{j=0}^{n-1} C_j$, and $B(n,p)$ denotes a standard binomial distribution. Random binomial variables may be generated using the RANBIN function in SAS. Even though this formula may look intimidating at first glance, it is relatively straightforward to program. Again, note that we are sticking with the convention that a capital "C" represents a random quantity, and a lowercase "c" represents an observed value. Therefore, in bootstrap parlance, the data X is considered fixed or observed for a given bootstrap resampling procedure, and the multinomial counts C vary randomly every bootstrap replication. The theoretical properties of bootstrap estimators can be examined fairly straightforward within this framework by noting that the multinomial counts C are independent of the data X. For our simple example of $n = 4$ observations we would have for a single bootstrap resample:

(1) C_1 is a random binomial variable $B(4, 1/4)$.
(2) C_2 is a random binomial variable $B(4 - C_1, 1/3)$.
(3) C_3 is a random binomial variable $B(4 - C_1 - C_2, 1/2)$.
(4) $C_4 = 4 - C_1 - C_2 - C_3$.

We would then want to output the value X_i C_i number of times for one bootstrap resample. Note that if $n - \sum_{j=0}^{i-1} C_i < 0$ then stop; all subsequent C_i's should be set to "0". The algorithm is easily accomplished in SAS a multiple number of times in a variety of ways. For the first example let us focus on the most straightforward approach. Let us generate counts for $X=\{0.5, 0.4, 0.6, 0.2\}$, $B = 3$ bootstrap replications without doing anything fancy. We need to generate random binomial variables using the function RANBIN(seed, n, p), where n and p are the parameters of the binomial distribution. The seed dictates the random number stream; a "0" produces a different random number stream each successive run of the program. Note that there are practical reasons for choosing a nonzero seed, such as the need to re-create a given analyses. In this case one may choose a positive integer such as 123453. Seeds less than "0" may also be employed. We refer the reader to the SAS technical documents for further details (see Section 1.11).

In order to understand the basic resampling code written below, one must be familiar with the SORT command, in conjunction with the FIRST and LAST command. In addition, knowledge of the RETAIN command is needed. The function RANBIN will be used to generate random binomial variables.

```
data original;
n=4;            /*set the sample size*/
input x_i @@;
do b=1 to 3;   /*output the data B times*/
 output;
end;
cards;
0.5 0.4 0.6 0.2;
proc sort;by b;
```

This first piece of code in `data original` just outputs the same data-set three times in a row. We then need to sort the values by b. Now all we do in the next set of code is carry out the generation of multinomial random variables sequentially via a marginal random binomial number generator.

```
/*SAS PROGRAM 11.1*/
data resample;
set original;by b;
retain sumc i;    /*need to add the previous
            count to the total */
if first.b then do;
 sumc=0;
 i=1;          /*set counters*/
end;
p=1/(n-i+1);   /*p is the probability of a "success"*/

if ^last.b then do;
if n>sumc then c_i=ranbin(0,n-sumc,p); /*generate the binomial variate*/
 else c_i=0;
 sumc=sumc+c_i;
end;
i=i+1;
if last.b then c_i=n-sumc;
proc print;
var b  c_i x_i;
```

The statement "else c_i=0" is just a shortcut needed for the cases where we hit the limit of the constraint that $n - \sum_{j=0}^{i-1} C_j$ must be positive. All the other statements are needed for counting purposes and updating the marginal binomial probabilities.

Basically what we have done is keep track of $n - \sum_{j=0}^{i-1} C_j$ and $\dfrac{1}{n-i+1}$ for $B = 1$, and then we repeated the resampling scheme for $B = 2$, and for $B = 3$. The output for a given run is below.

OBS	B	C_I	X_I
1	1	3	0.5
2	1	0	0.4
3	1	0	0.6
4	1	1	0.2
5	2	2	0.5
6	2	0	0.4
7	2	0	0.6
8	2	2	0.2
9	3	1	0.5
10	3	0	0.4
11	3	0	0.6
12	3	3	0.2

What this program above does is basically the nuts and bolts of most univariate bootstrapping procedures. It is easily modified for the multivariate procedures. Note that if there are missing values they should be eliminated within the first data step.

As an example consider how the program would work for a simple statistic such as the sample mean $\bar{X} = \sum_{i=1}^{n} X_i / n$. A bootstrap replication of the mean would simply be $\bar{x}^* = \sum_{i=1}^{n} C_i X_i / n$, or for our example $\bar{x}_1^* = (3 \times 0.5 + 1 \times 0.2) / 4 = 0.426$, or for those of you who prefer matrix notation $\bar{X}^* = \dfrac{XC'}{n}$. To carry out this process in SAS simply add the following code to the end of SAS PROGRAM 11.1:

```
proc means;by b;
var x_i;
weight c_i;
output out=bootstat mean=xbarstar;
```

For the sample mean we can take advantage of the WEIGHT statement built in to PROC MEANS. Since the sample size of $n = 4$ is small we would basically only need to increase the value of B up to say $B = 100$ in this example in order to get a very accurate approximation of the distribution of the sample mean for this dataset. Guidelines for the number of resamples will be discussed later. Through the use of the WEIGHT statement PROC MEANS is "automatically" calculating $\bar{x}^* = \sum_{i=1}^{n} C_i X_i / n$ for each value of B via the BY statement. In a variety of problems from regression to generalized linear models we will utilize the fact that the WEIGHT utility is built in to a number of SAS procedures. From a statistical theory standpoint in the case of the sample mean one can easily prove that if $E(\bar{X}) = \mu$ that $E(\bar{X}^*) = \mu$ as well. Note that

$$E(\bar{X}^*) = E(\sum_{i=1}^{n} C_i X_i / n) = \sum_{i=1}^{n} E(C_i)E(X_i) / n = \mu,$$

given $E(C_i) = 1$, that is, remarkably all bootstrap resampled estimates of the mean are unbiased estimates of μ.

Note that the number of bootstrap replications is typically recommended to be $B = 1000$ or higher for moderately sized datasets, e.g., see Booth and Sarkar (1998). However, if you can feasibly carry out a higher number of replications the precision of the bootstrap procedure can only increase, that is, from a theoretical statistical point of view you can never take too many bootstrap replications. From a practical point of view you may stretch the memory capacity and speed of your given computer. In general, one should shoot for $B = 1000$. If a value for $B > 1000$ can be practically used then by all means use it. Obviously, the memory requirements for the above algorithm can expand rapidly for moderately sized datasets and values of B around 1000. The program (SAS PROGRAM 11.1) will run very rapidly, however it is a "space hog" with respect to disk space.

In some instances we can keep the code even more simple by replacing the data-step resample in the previous approach with PROC SURVEYSELECT as seen in the following example.

```
/* SAS PROGRAM 11.2 */
proc surveyselect data=original
method=urs sampsize=4 out=resample;
by b;

proc print noobs;
var b numberhits x_i;

data rcstar;set resample;
do ii=1 to numberhits;
 output;
end;
```

The R code is as following:
```
> resamples <- lapply(1:3, function(i)
+      sample(data, replace = T))
> b1<-c(4,mean(resamples[[1]]),sd(resamples[[1]]),min(resamples[[1]]),max(res
amples[[1]]))
> names(b1)<-c("N","Mean","Std Dev", "Minimum", "Maximum")
> b2<-c(4,mean(resamples[[2]]),sd(resamples[[2]]),min(resamples[[2]]),max(res
amples[[2]]))
> names(b2)<-c("N","Mean","Std Dev", "Minimum", "Maximum")
> b3<-c(4,mean(resamples[[3]]),sd(resamples[[3]]),min(resamples[[3]]),max(res
amples[[1]]))
> names(b3)<-c("N","Mean","Std Dev", "Minimum", "Maximum")
```

The method=urs implies unrestricted random sampling with replacement and needs to be specified. Also, note that the sampsize=4 corresponds to the sample size of $n = 4$ for this example and needs to be modified manually for different sized datasets. Finally, the output from PROC SURVEYSELECT for this example will look as follows:

b	Number Hits	x_i
1	2	0.5
1	2	0.4
2	1	0.4
2	1	0.6
2	2	0.2
3	1	0.5
3	1	0.4
3	2	0.2

Therefore, the additional need to output each observation in the dataset `resample numberhits` times in `dataset restar`. The data from restar is what would then be used in order to calculate the resampled statistic of interest. This approach is slightly more inefficient than the straight generation of conditional multinomial counts but may be somewhat more straightforward for the novice user. The multinomial approach is what would be recommended if we were carrying out the bootstrap method within PROC IML.

As an alternative to outputting the dataset B number of times in the input dataset we can use SAS macros, which will carry out the same task as before albeit somewhat slower. Note however macros tend to be more efficient in terms of space requirements. You do not need to be an expert in macro programming in order to modify your own programs. The same basic macro language concepts will be used throughout the book without too much modification. We refer the reader to *SAS® 9.3 Macro Language* (SAS Institute Inc., 2011) Reference for further details. From our point of view a macro processor basically simplifies repetitive data entry and data manipulation tasks. The macro facility makes it possible to define complex input and output "subroutines." However with respect to bootstrapping we need to know only a few basic concepts:

1. All macros have a user-defined macro name, a beginning and an end.
2. Variables can be passed to macros upon the macro being called.
3. It is possible to repeat a data step over and over again via looping within a macro.
4. Macro variables can be passed to data steps and certain PROCs.

The key macro statements that we will use in the bootstrapping program below and throughout the book consist of the following:

1. %macro multiwt(brep);   The beginning of the macro is defined by the %macro statement. We have chosen to name the macro multiwt and pass it the variable named brep, which represents the number of bootstrap replications that we have chosen. For this example the number of bootstrap replications $B = 3$.
2. %do bsim=1 %to &brep;   The beginning of the macro do loop is given by the %do command. The macro variable &brep is given at the macro call. The variable bsim is the looping index variable.
3. b=∽   The macro variable &bsim is passed to the data step in order to indicate the current bootstrap resample. An ampersand indicates to the compiler that bsim is a macro variable.
4. %end;   The %end closes the macro do loop.

5. %mend;   The %mend command signifies the end of the macro multiwt.

6. %multiwt(3);   The command %multiwt(3) is the macro call which
   passes the value of 3 to the macro variable brep.

Based on these definitions we developed a macro version of the bootstrap
program contained earlier in this chapter. In addition, we "automatically"
determine the value for the sample size n in this program via the NOBS command. The macro variable brep is used to represent the number of bootstrap
replications B. All that has basically changed as compared to the previous
code is that we are generating the c's one macro iteration at a time. Later on
we will illustrate what additional calculations will be carried out within the
macro multiwt and what calculations will be carried out outside the scope of
the macro.

```
/* SAS PROGRAM 11.3 */
data original;
input x_i @@;
cards;
0.5 0.4 0.6 0.2;

data sampsize;
 set original nobs=nobs;   /*automatically obtain the sample
size*/
 n=nobs;

%macro multiwt(brep);
%do bsim=1 %to &brep;

data resample;
set sampsize;
retain sumc i;   /*need to add the previous
           count to the total */
b=&bsim;
if _n_=1 then do;
 sumc=0;
 i=1;
end;
p=1/(n-i+1);   /*p is the probability of a "success"*/

if _n_<n then do;
if n>sumc then c_i=ranbin(0,n-sumc,p);  /*generate the binomial variate*/
 else c_i=0;
 sumc=sumc+c_i;
end;
i=i+1;
if _n_=n then c_i=n-sumc;

proc append data=resample out=total;
```

```
%end;
%mend;
%multiwt(3);

proc print data=total;
var b c_i x_i;
```

The same program may be rewritten using PROC SURVEYSELECT. Note that we had to create a variable called dummy in order to automatically input the sample size into PROC SURVEYSELECT. We also no longer have the ability to weight observations. As noted earlier this may be slightly more inefficient than the previous code.

```
/* SAS PROGRAM 11.4 */
options ls=65;
data original;
input x_i @@;
dummy=1;  /*need a dummy variable for surveyselect*/
cards;
0.5 0.4 0.6 0.2
;

data sampsize;
set original nobs=nobs;
_nsize_=nobs;  /*control variable for surveyselect*/
if _n_=1 then output;

%macro multiwt(brep);

%do bsim=1 %to &brep;

proc surveyselect data=original  noprint
method=urs sampsize=sampsize out=resample;
strata dummy;


data restar;set resample;
b=&bsim;
do ii=1 to numberhits;
output;
end;

proc append data=restar out=total;

%end;
%mend;
%multiwt(3);

proc print;
var b  x_i;
```

Oftentimes for simple univariate samples it is much more efficient in terms of storage issues to use PROC IML in order to carry out the bootstrap resampling methodology. From *SAS/IML User's Guide* we have the following description: "(SAS/IML) is a multilevel, interactive programming language with dynamic capabilities. You can use commands to tune in to the finest detail or to reach out to grand operations that can process thousands of values." With respect to bootstrap methods, PROC IML is very useful through the efficient use of its array structure. We can use IML in conjunction with other PROCs, macros, or as a stand-alone programming language. Carrying out the multiwt macro from above in similar fashion using PROC IML consists of the following code.

```
/* SAS PROGRAM 11.5 */
data original;
input x_i @@;
cards;
0.5 0.4 0.6 0.2;

proc iml;
use original;
read all into data;

/*Create a n by 1 vector of data original
called data*/

n=nrow(data); /*Calculate the sample size*/
bootdata=1:n; /*Array to hold one bootstrap resample*/

brep=3;         /*Set the number of bootstrap resamples*/
do i=1 to brep;
do j=1 to n;
 index=int(ranuni(0)*n)+1;
 bootdata[j]=data[index];
end;
print i bootdata;
end;

quit;

/*********Listing File******************/
I   BOOTDATA
1      0.5   0.4   0.5   0.5
I   BOOTDATA
2      0.4   0.5   0.4   0.5
I   BOOTDATA
3      0.6   0.5   0.4   0.2
```

The USE and READ statements simply retrieve SAS datasets and import them into PROC IML. Alternatively, data may be entered directly in PROC IML with a statement such as

```
data={0.5, 0.4, 0.6, 0.2};
```

There are infinitely many possibilities with respect to utilizing this basic IML code. We may want to carry out some calculations within IML and/or outside IML. We will modify the code below for specific cases throughout the book. The main concept is the generation of a random indexing function labeled index in the IML code. Basically we are generating a random integer from 1 to n. This allows us to easily resample from the data original using a simple array structure. We see the results for three successive bootstrap resamples with $x_1^* = \{0.5, 0.4, 0.5, 0.5\}$, $x_2^* = \{0.4, 0.5, 0.5, 0.5\}$, and $x_3^* = \{0.6, 0.5, 0.4, 0.2\}$. The only real disadvantage of utilizing PROC IML is that it requires an additional SAS programming skill set.

11.10 Bootstrap Confidence Intervals

Recall from the previous section that the goal in confidence interval estimation is to find λ_1 and λ_2 such that $P(\lambda_1 < T(X; \theta) < \lambda_2) = 1 - \alpha$ given $T(X; \theta)$ is monotone in θ. In terms of statistical functions we can write $T(X; \theta) = t(\widehat{F}; \theta) - t(F; \theta)$, e.g., $\bar{X} - E(X)$, where we are essentially centering the statistic of interest about the parameter of interest to form a pivot. If the distribution function for $t(\widehat{F}; \theta)$ is known we could find a t_α such that $P(t(\widehat{F}; \theta) - t(F; \theta) \le t_\alpha) = \alpha$. Then a one-sided confidence interval for $t(F; \theta)$ is $(-\infty, t(\widehat{F}; \theta) - t_\alpha)$. In the nonparametric bootstrap setting we do not assume a form for the distribution function of $t(\widehat{F}; \theta)$. In this case we approximate the confidence interval machinery by replacing $t(\widehat{F}; \theta) - t(F; \theta)$ with the bootstrap approximation $t(\hat{F}^*; \theta) - t(\widehat{F}; \theta)$ and t_α with t_α^* estimated from bootstrap resampling. The pivotal one-sided interval is then $(-\infty, t(\widehat{F}; \theta) - t_\alpha^*)$, where t_α^* is the αth quantile of $t(\hat{F}^*; \theta) - t(\widehat{F}; \theta)$ obtained from B bootstrap resamples. As shown in Shao and Tu (1995) we then have

$$P\left(t(\widehat{F}; \theta) - t_\alpha^* > t(F; \theta)\right) = 1 - \alpha + O(n^{-1/2}).$$

The result can be proven via an Edgeworth expansion technique. Note that the nuisance parameter about scale is "built in" to the bootstrap resampling process. The two-sided $100 \times (1 - \alpha)$ confidence interval becomes $(t(\widehat{F}; \theta) - t_{1-\alpha/2}^*, t(\widehat{F}; \theta) - t_{\alpha/2}^*)$.

Returning to our coefficient of variation example with $\alpha = 0.10$ we arrive at

$$t_{\alpha/2}^* = 71.6 - 114.6 \quad \text{and} \quad t_{1-\alpha/2}^* = 146.3 - 114.6$$

such that the two-sided confidence interval is (114.6–(146.3–114.6), 114.6–(71.6–114.6)) = (82.9, 157.6). For moderate to large sample sizes this approximation works well. Also, unlike traditional confidence intervals we are not constrained that the interval is symmetric about the test statistic of interest. Improvements and modifications can be made to this approach based on various additional approximations that we will touch on. Under symmetry assumptions regarding the sampling distribution of $t\left(\widehat{F};\theta\right)$, which hold approximately when we can assume that $t\left(\widehat{F};\theta\right)$ has an asymptotic normal distribution, we can simplify the calculations above to what is known as the percentile confidence interval and given as $(b_{\alpha/2}^{*}, b_{1-\alpha/2}^{*})$, where b_{α}^{*} is the αth quantile from the resampling distribution for $t\left(\widehat{F}^{*};\theta\right)$. The percentile interval is probably the most used technique in general practice and given as (71.6, 146.3) for our coefficient of variation example.

The general lemma around percentile intervals is as follows. Suppose
$$\frac{t\left(\widehat{F};\theta\right)-t(F;\theta)}{\widehat{\sigma}_n} \xrightarrow{d} T \text{ and } \frac{t\left(\widehat{F}^{*};\theta\right)-t\left(\widehat{F};\theta\right)}{\widehat{\sigma}_n^{*}} \xrightarrow{d} T, \text{ where } Var\left(t\left(\widehat{F};\theta\right)\right)=\sigma_n. \text{ Then}$$
the random variable T does not need to follow a normal distribution, but does need to be symmetric. The percentile interval is then asymptotically correct at level $1-\alpha$. As a general rule if $t\left(\widehat{F};\theta\right)$ has an asymptotic normal distribution then bootstrap methods fit the general lemma and will be correct in the asymptotic sense.

Similar to jackknife methods bootstrap methods tend to work best for so-called smooth statistics. The "smoothness" of a statistic can be examined if we as can assume an expansion of $t\left(\widehat{F}\right)$ of the form
$$t\left(\widehat{F}\right) = t(F) + \frac{1}{n}\sum_{i=1}^{n}\phi_F(X_i) + R_n. \text{ One can examine the quadratic term in the}$$
expansion of $t\left(\widehat{F}\right)$. If the quadratic term of $\frac{1}{n}\sum_{i=1}^{n}\phi_F(X_i)$ does not "dominate" the series typically of the order $o(n^{-1})$ the statistic is "smooth." There is no set definition of smoothness. A von Mises type expansion having the form
$$t\left(\widehat{F}\right) = t(F) + \frac{1}{n}\sum_{i=1}^{n}t'\left(H(x-X_{(i)})-F\right) + R_n \text{ would be one expansion for which to}$$
examine smoothness when the derivative t' exists. The sample mean is an example of a smooth statistics whereas the sample median based on a single order statistic is not.

Let us illustrate the bootstrap percentile confidence interval method using CD4 counts obtained from newborns infected with HIV, e.g., see Sleasman et al. (1999) for a detailed description. Suppose that we are interested in calculating the 95% percentile confidence interval for the CD4 count data using a less standard measure, but more robust measure of location, say the α-trimmed mean statistic. The ***trimmed mean statistic*** is defined so as to "slice off" $\alpha \times 100$ percent of the extreme observations from both tails of the empirical distribution and takes the form of Equation (11.2) below. For symmetric distributions this statistic has the same expectation as the sample mean. For asymmetric distributions the trimmed mean will be less influenced by observations in the tail, that is, in general its expectation will be to the right or left of that of the sample mean in a direction opposite that of the tail. The median is a specific case of the trimmed mean as $\alpha \to 1/2$ in the limit of the general statistic. One may calculate the trimmed mean within SAS's PROC UNIVARIATE using the TRIMMED command along with its approximate 95% confidence interval under the assumption that the data are sampled from a symmetric population. The actual trimmed mean statistic is given as

$$t\left(\hat{F}\right) = \bar{X}_\alpha = \frac{1}{n - 2k} \sum_{i=k+1}^{n-k} X_{(i)}, \qquad (11.2)$$

where $X_{(i)}$ denotes the ith ordered observation, α denotes the trimming proportion and $k = [n\alpha]$, and the function $[.]$ again denotes the floor function. Suppose we specify for our continuing example the trimming proportion of $\alpha = 0.05$ with a sample size of $n = 44$. That implies that $k = [44 \times 0.05] = 2$ observations are trimmed from each tail. Given that this trimming strategy seems very straightforward we need to step back and ask: what is the population parameter that we are estimating? It is very important to have an understanding of what you are estimating prior to carrying out any bootstrap estimation procedure. The α-trimmed mean statistic is an estimator of the population trimmed mean:

$$t(F) = E_\alpha(X) = \frac{1}{1 - 2\alpha} \int_{F^{-1}(\alpha)}^{F^{-1}(1-\alpha)} x \, dF(x),$$

that is, the population parameter in this instance is $E_\alpha(X)$, not the expected value of X, $E(X)$. For the specific case where the distribution is symmetric about the mean $E_\alpha(X) = E(X)$. This is not the case for asymmetric distributions. Therefore, in this case our goal is to obtain a 95% confidence interval for $E_\alpha(X)$.

Within SAS PROGRAM 11.6 corresponding to our example the CD4 count data from $n = 44$ subjects is read into data original. As an alternative to what is provided in PROC UNIVARIATE we can calculate the bootstrap percentile confidence interval nonparametrically and compare the results. Note that the "guts" of the sample program is the same as what we have been utilizing throughout for simple bootstrapping. Within the simple bootstrap algorithm we can calculate the trimmed mean in PROC UNIVARIATE using the TRIMMED command and output the value via SAS's ODS system to the dataset tr, that is, there is no real additional programming to be done other than to use the already built-in calculations within PROC UNIVARIATE. The lower and upper bootstrap percentiles are then calculated and output via a separate run of PROC UNIVARIATE using the command pctlpts=2.5 97.5 pctlpre=p.

For our example dataset the trimmed mean and its standard deviation (of the trimmed mean) turned out to be $\bar{x}_{.05} = 304.9 \pm 76.8$ as compared to the sample mean $\bar{x} = 377.7 \pm 74.3$. The difference between the two statistics again illustrates the asymmetry in the data, and reinforces the fact that the built-in confidence interval procedure should probably be avoided. For this example the 95% semi-parametric confidence interval for the trimmed mean, as calculated in PROC UNIVARIATE under an asymmetry assumption, turned out to be (149.3, 460.6). For $B = 1000$ resamples the indices for the percentile interval are $\lambda_1 = 250$ and $\lambda_2 = 9750$. Therefore, the 95% bootstrap interval would be the 250th and 9750th ordered resampled values, or namely $(T^*_{(250)}(F_n(X)), T^*_{(9750)}(F_n(X)))$. After $B = 10000$ resamples the 95% bootstrap percentile interval was calculated as (181.8, 466.0). Also note that the percentile interval is not constrained to be symmetric about the statistic $\bar{x}_{.05} = 304.9$, thus making it much more flexible with respect to underlying assumptions. Given the moderately large sample size of n = 44 and the smoothness of the trimmed mean statistic we should feel fairly confident about the coverage accuracy of the bootstrap percentile confidence for this example. We will compare this interval with other more complicated bootstrap methods given later on. At the minimum the percentile method is useful for examining the assumptions of parametric or semi-parametric methods in terms of their validity. As noted earlier, in general the bootstrap-t method is what we would generally recommend. It will be described in the next section. Below is the basic SAS program used to carry out the trimmed mean percentile interval calculations for our example.

```
/* SAS PROGRAM 11.6*/
data original;
label x_i='CD4 counts';
input x_i @@;
cards;
1397 471 64 1571 663 1128 719 407
480 1147 362 2022 10 175 494 31
202 751 30 27 118 8 181 1432 31 18
105 23 8 70 12 504 252 0 100 4
545 226 390 230 28 5 0 176;

proc univariate trimmed=.05;
var x_i;
ods listing select trimmedmeans;
```

```
/**********Begin Standard Resampling Algorithm****************/
data sampsize;
 set original nobs=nobs;
 n=nobs;
do b=1 to 10000; /*output the data B times*/
 output;
end;

proc sort data=sampsize;by b;

data resample;
set sampsize;by b;
retain sumc i; /*need to add the previous
           count to the total */
if first.b then do;
 sumc=0;
 i=1;
end;
p=1/(n-i+1);  /*p is the probability of a "success"*/

if ^last.b then do;
 if n>sumc then c_i=ranbin(0,n-sumc,p); /*generate the binomial variate*/
 else c_i=0;
 sumc=sumc+c_i;
end;
i=i+1;
if last.b then c_i=n-sumc;

data main;set resample;
if c_i >0 then do;
do i=1 to c_i;
 output;
end;
end;

/*************End Standard Resampling Algorithm****************/
/******Calculate 10000 Trimmed Means************************/

proc univariate trimmed=.05;by b;
var x_i;
ods listing close;
ods output trimmedmeans=tr;


/******Calculate Percentile Interval***********************/

proc univariate data=tr noprint;
var mean;
output out=quantile pctlpts=2.5 97.5 pctlpre=p;

/******Print Results**************************/
```

```
proc print data=quantile;
title '95% Bootstrap Percentile Confidence Interval';
```

The R code is as follows:

```
> data<-c(1397, 471, 64, 1571, 663, 1128, 719, 407,
+        480, 1147, 362, 2022,  10, 175,  494, 31,
+        202, 751, 30, 27, 118, 8, 181, 1432, 31, 18,
+        105, 23, 8, 70, 12, 504, 252, 0, 100,  4,
+        545, 226, 390, 230, 28, 5,  0, 176)
> data_sort<-sort(data)
> resamples <- lapply(1:1000, function(i)
+        sample(data, replace = T))
> each_mean<-lapply(1:1000, function(i)
+        mean(resamples[[i]]))
> vector<-c()
> for (i in 1:1000){
+        vector<-c(vector,each_mean[[i]])
+        i<-i+1
+ }
> quantile(vector,c(0.025,0.975))
    2.5%     97.5%
243.0193 530.7216
```

11.11 Use of the Edgeworth Expansion to Illustrate the Accuracy of Bootstrap Intervals

We will apply the *Edgeworth expansion* technique (Hall, 1992) to illustrate the accuracy of the coverage probabilities of bootstrap confidence intervals. The Edgeworth expansion is a series that approximates a probability distribution in terms of its cumulants. The rationale for using the Edgeworth expansion over standard asymptotic normal methods is that it provides more precise statements about the error terms pertaining to the bootstrap approximations.

The version of the classic Edgeworth expansion for an approximation to the distribution function for $t(\widehat{F};\theta)$ is given as

$$F_{t(\widehat{F};\theta)}(x) = \Phi(x) - \phi(x)\left[\frac{1}{6}\gamma_1 H_2(x) + \frac{1}{24}\gamma_2 H_3(x) + \frac{1}{72}\gamma_1^2 H_5(x)\right] + o(n^{-1}),$$

where $\Phi(x)$ and $\phi(x)$ denote the standard normal cdf and pdf, $H_2(x) = x^2 - 1$, $H_3(x) = x^3 - 3x$ and $H_5(x) = x^5 - 10x^3 + 15x$ are Hermite polynomials, and γ_1 and γ_2 denote the skewness and kurtosis respectively. In general, $H_r(x) = (-1)^r e^{x^2} \dfrac{d^r}{dx^r} e^{-x^2}$ and additional series terms can be added to improve the degree of accuracy of the approximation.

A classic example for the Edgeworth approximation is as follows. Let iid observations $X_1, X_2, \ldots, X_n \sim N(0,1)$ and let $V = \sum_{i=1}^{n} X_i^2$; then it is well known that $\sim \chi_n^2$. Asymptotically we have that $T = \dfrac{V-n}{\sqrt{2n}} \sim AN(0,1)$ such that we have that the approximate distribution function for T is $F_T(x) \cong \Phi(x)$, that is, the first term in the Edgeworth expansion above. More precisely we know that in this example $\gamma_1 = \dfrac{2\sqrt{2}}{n}$ and $\gamma_2 = \dfrac{12}{n}$. Hence, a more precise approximation for the distribution function for T is given as

$$F_T(x) \cong \Phi(x) - \phi(x)\left[\frac{\sqrt{2}}{3n}(x^2-1) + \frac{1}{2n}(x^3-3x) + \frac{1}{9n}(x^5-10x^3+15x)\right]$$

with error of order $o(n^{-1})$.

To prove the bootstrap consistency of our bootstrap pivotal quantity $t(\hat{F}^*;\theta) - t(\hat{F};\theta)$ we start by examining the pivotal quantity $t(\hat{F};\theta) - t(F;\theta)$. Equivalently, we can use the pivotal quantity $\sqrt{n}(t(\hat{F};\theta) - t(F;\theta))$, which aids in the technical components of the proofs. Let $K = K(X_1, X_2, \ldots, X_n \mid F) = \sqrt{n}(t(\hat{F};\theta) - t(F;\theta))$. Denote the distribution function of K as $G_{K|F}(k) = P(K < k \mid F)$. Denote the bootstrap replication of K as $K^* = K(X_1^*, X_2^*, \ldots, X_n^* \mid F) = \sqrt{n}\left(t(\hat{F}^*;\theta) - t(\hat{F};\theta)\right)$ with distribution function $G_{K^*|\hat{F}}(k) = Pr(K^* < k \mid \hat{F})$. If the bootstrap confidence works well in a given scenario then $G_{K^*|\hat{F}}(k)$ should be "close" to $G_{K|F}(k)$.

In order to prove the consistency of the bootstrap distribution function estimator we need to show that

$$P\left(|G_{K^*|\hat{F}}(k) - G_{K|F}(k)| > \varepsilon\right) \to 0, n \to \infty.$$

For specific cases this proof can be straightforward. However the general result is technically challenging. Specific cases often require a key piece of knowledge about the given problem to complete the proof. For example, take $t(F;\theta) = E(X \mid F) = \theta$. Then $t(\hat{F};\theta) = \bar{x}$ and $t(\hat{F}^*;\theta) = \sum_{i=1}^{n} C_i X_i = \sum_{i=1}^{n} x_i^*$, where the C_i's can be considered multinomial random variables, that is, the data are fixed and the resampling counts follow a multinomial distribution. The classic proof of bootstrap consistency in this case utilizes Mallow's distance. If we have two distribution functions with $X \sim H$ and $Y \sim G$ then Mallow's distance measure is denoted as $\rho(H,G) = \underset{\tau_{xy}}{\inf} \; E\big(||X-Y||^r\big)^{1/r} = \rho(X,Y)$, where τ_{xy} is the set of all possible joint distribution functions for X and Y whose marginal distributions are H and G, respectively, where $\|x\|$ is the Euclidean norm in p-dimensional real space (Mallows, 1972).

In the bootstrap setting we apply the known Mallow's distance results

$$\rho(\hat{F},F) \xrightarrow{a.s} 0, \; \rho\left(\sum_{i=0}^{n} X_i, \sum_{i=0}^{n} Y_i\right) \le \sum_{i=0}^{n} \rho(X_i,Y_i)^2, \; \rho(H,G) = \rho(X,Y),$$

$\rho(X,Y)^2 = \rho(X-E(X),Y-E(Y))^2 + ||E(X)-E(Y)||^2$, and $\rho(aX,aY) = |a|\rho(X,Y)$ e.g., see Shao and Tu (1995). For example, using the notation from above let

$$K = K(X_1, X_2,\ldots, X_n \mid F) = \sqrt{n}\big(t(\hat{F};\theta) - t(F;\theta)\big) = \sqrt{n}(\bar{X} - \theta) \text{ and}$$

$$K^* = K(X_1^*, X_2^*, \ldots, X_n^* \mid F) = \sqrt{n}\big(t(\hat{F}^*;\theta) - t(\hat{F};\theta)\big) = \sqrt{n}(\bar{X}^* - \bar{X}). \text{ Then we have}$$

$$\begin{aligned}
\rho(G_{K^*|\hat{F}}(k), G_{K|F}(k)) &= \rho(K^*, K) \\
&= \rho(\sqrt{n}(\bar{X}^* - \bar{X}) - \sqrt{n}(\bar{X} - \theta)) \\
&= \frac{1}{\sqrt{n}}\rho\left(\sum_{i=0}^{n}(X_i - \bar{X}), \sum_{i=0}^{n}(X_i - \theta)\right) \le \sqrt{\frac{1}{n}\sum_{i=0}^{n}\rho((\bar{X}^* - \bar{X}),(\bar{X} - \theta))^2} \\
&= \rho((\bar{X}^* - \bar{X}),(\bar{X} - \theta)) \\
&= \sqrt{\rho(X^*,X)^2 - ||\theta - \bar{X}||^2} \\
&= \sqrt{\rho(\hat{F},F)^2 - ||\theta - \bar{X}||^2} = o(1),
\end{aligned}$$

given $\bar{X} \xrightarrow{a.s.} \theta$ in combination with the known Mallow's distance results outlined above. Hence, $G_{K^*|\hat{F}}(k)$ is ρ-consistent for this example, which implies it can be used to develop approximate confidence that converge to the appropriate α level for large samples. The consistency of $G_{K^*|\hat{F}}(k)$ can be shown oftentimes via the Berry–Esse'en inequality.

In the general case, why does the simple percentile interval generate a valid confidence interval with coverage that converges to $100 \times (1-\alpha)\%$ as $n \to \infty$? As before let $\hat{\theta}^* = t(\hat{F}^*;\theta)$ and $\theta = t(\hat{F};\theta)$. For the more general case we will employ Edgeworth expansion techniques, which provide less precise statements about the large sample coverage of bootstrap percentile intervals.

As in the specific case using Mallow's distance the goal is prove a large sample equivalence between $Pr(\hat{\theta} - \theta \le x \mid F)$ and $Pr(\hat{\theta}^* - \hat{\theta} \le x \mid \hat{F})$. In this regard let us first examine the Edgeworth expansions of each of these quantities such that we have

$$P\left(\hat{\theta}-\theta \le x \mid F\right)= \Phi\left(\frac{x}{\sigma}\right)+\frac{1}{\sqrt{n}}q_1\left(\frac{x}{\sigma}\mid F\right)\phi\left(\frac{x}{\sigma}\right)+\frac{1}{q_2}\left(\frac{x}{\sigma}\mid F\right)\phi\left(\frac{x}{\sigma}\right)+r,$$

and

$$P\left(\hat{\theta}^*-\hat{\theta} \le x \mid \hat{F}\right)= \Phi\left(\frac{x}{\hat{\sigma}}\right)+\frac{1}{\sqrt{n}}\ q_1\left(\frac{x}{\hat{\sigma}}\mid \hat{F}\right)\phi\left(\frac{x}{\hat{\sigma}}\right)+\frac{1}{n}q_2\left(\frac{x}{\hat{\sigma}}\mid \hat{F}\right)\phi\left(\frac{x}{\hat{\sigma}}\right)+r^*,$$

where q_1 and q_2 are a rearrangement of the H_i's from our introduction of the Edgeworth expansion above and r^* denotes the remainder term. Then we have

$$\sup_x\left|P\left(\hat{\theta}-\theta \le x \mid F\right)-P\left(\hat{\theta}^*-\hat{\theta} \le x \mid \hat{F}\right)\right|$$

$$\le \sup_x\left|\frac{1}{\sqrt{n}}\left(q_1\left(\frac{x}{\sigma}\mid F\right)-q_1\left(\frac{x}{\hat{\sigma}}\mid \hat{F}\right)\right)+\frac{1}{n}\left(q_2\left(\frac{x}{\sigma}\mid F\right)-q_2\left(\frac{x}{\hat{\sigma}}\mid \hat{F}\right)\right)\right|\phi\left(\frac{x}{\sigma}\right)+O_p(n^{-1/2})$$

given the assumption that $\hat{\sigma}-\sigma=O_p\left(n^{-\frac{1}{2}}\right)$, which yields $\phi\left(\frac{x}{\hat{\sigma}}\right)-\phi\left(\frac{x}{\sigma}\right)=O_p(n^{-1/2})$. Hence, we have that

$$\sup_x\left|P\left(\hat{\theta}-\theta \le x \mid F\right)-P\left(\hat{\theta}^*-\hat{\theta} \le x \mid \hat{F}\right)\right|=O_p(n^{-1}),$$

where $P\left(\hat{\theta}^*-\hat{\theta} \le x \mid \hat{F}\right)$ is a random quantity. It is important to note that just because the asymptotic theory is mathematically correct that there is no guarantee that the finite sample coverage will be accurate for these types of intervals. An alternative approach to the Edgeworth expansion for these problems is to use Cornish–Fisher expansions (Cornish and Fisher, 1937).

The general lemma for the percentile method is as follows. Suppose $\frac{\hat{\theta}-\theta}{\hat{\sigma}}\xrightarrow{d} T$ and $\frac{\hat{\theta}^*-\hat{\theta}}{\hat{\sigma}^*}\xrightarrow{d} T$. If we assume $\hat{\sigma} \to \sigma$ and $\hat{\sigma}^* \to \hat{\sigma}$ and T is distributed according to a symmetric distribution function then the percentile confidence interval $(b^*_{\alpha/2}, b^*_{1-\alpha/2})$ described above is asymptotically correct at level $1-\alpha$. Note that if T is asymptotically normal then we know that the distribution of T will be symmetric asymptotically. Hence, as a rule of thumb asymptotically normally distributed T's will provide valid large sample percentile bootstrap confidence intervals for the statistical functional $t(F;\theta)$.

Warning. A common mistake of practitioners is to start with the statistic and not consider exactly what the function it links to is. Hence, they are interpreting their confidence intervals about the wrong parameter, e.g., Suppose $t(F;\theta) = E(X_{(n)} \mid F)$. Then the T of interest is not the sample maximum $X_{(n)}$ but is $E(X_{(n)} \mid \hat{F})$, which is a weighted average of a linear combination of order statistics. We can refine the percentile method to have better accuracy in finite samples using the approaches below.

11.12 Bootstrap-t Percentile Intervals

The ***bootstrap-t percentile interval*** is a slight modification of the percentile method used in order to get better finite sample coverage probabilities. The key idea is to add a correction by replacing the quantity $t(\hat{F}^*;\theta) - t(\hat{F};\theta)$ with

$\dfrac{\sigma_{t(\hat{F})}}{\sigma_{t(\hat{F}^*)}}\left(t(\hat{F}^*;\theta) - t(\hat{F};\theta)\right)$, where $\sigma^2_{t(\hat{F};\theta)}$ is the variance estimate for $t(\hat{F};\theta)$, e.g., $\dfrac{S^2}{n}$

for $\bar{X}$, and $\sigma^2_{t(\hat{F}^*;\theta)} = \sum_{i=1}^{B}\left(t(\hat{F}^*;\theta)_i - \overline{t(\hat{F}^*;\theta)}\right)^2$, where $\overline{t(\hat{F}^*;\theta)}$ is the average of the

bootstrap resampled values. If an analytical expression for $\sigma^2_{t(\hat{F};\theta)}$ is unavailable or not easily calculated a double bootstrap approach is necessary, e.g., see SAS PROGRAM 11.9. The heuristic idea is that percentile intervals tend to suffer undercoverage in small samples; the scalar correction $\dfrac{\sigma_{t(\hat{F})}}{\sigma_{t(\hat{F}^*)}}$ provides slightly wider intervals and hence better coverage probabilities. Similar to the percentile interval proofs let $\hat{\theta}^* = t(\hat{F}^*;\theta)$ and $\theta = t(\hat{F};\theta)$. Then one can use an Edgeworth expansion technique to show that

$$\sup_x \left| P\left(\frac{\hat{\theta} - \theta}{\sigma_{t(\hat{F})}} \le x \mid F\right) - P\left(\frac{\hat{\theta}^* - \hat{\theta}}{\sigma_{t(\hat{F}^*)}} \le x \mid \hat{F}\right) \right| = O_p(n^{-1})$$

as compared to $O_p(n^{-1/2})$ for the percentile interval. There is no guarantee that the bootstrap-t percentile approach will work better than the percentile method, but it has been our experience that it is worth the additional effort in the small sample setting. The tricky issue here is that there are oftentimes not closed form solutions for the correction factor $\dfrac{\sigma_{t(\hat{F})}}{\sigma_{t(\hat{F}^*)}}$. In this case a double bootstrap method resampling method is used to approximate $\dfrac{\sigma_{t(\hat{F})}}{\sigma_{t(\hat{F}^*)}}$ with $\dfrac{\sigma_{t(\hat{F}^*)}}{\sigma_{t(\hat{F}^{**})}}$, where $\sigma_{t(\hat{F}^{**})}$ is obtained from subsamples of the original resamples.

Example. Let us revisit our example from the percentile interval section involving the trimmed mean $\bar{x}_\alpha$. As you recall we were interested in measures of location for CD4 count data. Previously we calculated 95% bootstrap percentile confidence intervals for $E_{.05}(X)$ and $E_{.25}(X)$ based upon the trimmed means $T(F_n(X)) - \bar{x}_{.05}$ and $T(F_n(X)) - \bar{x}_{.25}$, respectively. In order to recalculate these intervals for the same dataset using the bootstrap-t method, as compared to the percentile interval approach, we need some additional programming steps. These are given in the example SAS PROGRAM 11.7.

The first step in modifying the existing programs is to create a dummy variable used to merge bootstrap quantities labeled dummy. For this example dummy = 1 for every data and resample value. To calculate the trimmed mean and its standard deviation we employed the SAS ODS system with the command ods output trimmedmeans=trbase in conjunction with PROC UNIVARIATE. This allows us to output the trimmed mean and standard deviation to the dataset trbase within our sample program. It is important to note that the standard deviation estimate is labeled as the standard error in SAS, that is, what is calculated is the standard error estimate for X and the standard deviation for the statistic $\bar{X}_\alpha$.

After outputting the trimmed mean and its standard deviation from PROC UNIVARIATE we reassigned them new variable names within the dataset rename. This was necessary so that values were not overwritten when merged with the bootstrap resampled trimmed means and standard deviations of the same name. As with the original trimmed mean calculation the bootstrap resampled statistics were also calculated using PROC UNIVARIATE and output using ODS to dataset combine. In addition, within dataset combine we calculated the $\frac{\sigma_{t(\hat{F})}}{\sigma_{t(\hat{F}^*)}}\left(t\left(\hat{F}^*;\theta\right) - t\left(\widehat{F};\theta\right)\right)$'s needed in order to calculate the interval. The bootstrap-t interval based on the ordered $\frac{\sigma_{t(\hat{F})}}{\sigma_{t(\hat{F}^*)}}\left(t\left(\hat{F}^*;\theta\right) - t\left(\widehat{F};\theta\right)\right)$'s was then processed via PROC UNIVARIATE. We also recalculated the percentile interval within this program for comparison. The intervals were distinguished by the percentile prefixes pp and pt, for the percentile and bootstrap-t methods, respectively.

For our example run $B = 10000$ resamples were used. The 95% percentile interval turned out to be (179.9, 471.1) as compared to the previous run given in the earlier section of (181.8, 466.0). This gives you an idea of how much the intervals might change from successive runs, even with $B = 10000$ resamples. The bootstrap-t 95% confidence interval turned out to be $(S_{(250)}^*(\cdot), S_{(9750)}^*(\cdot)) = (170.5, 537.1)$. Recall also that the semi-parametric interval built in to SAS, calculated under the assumption of symmetry, yielded the interval (149.3, 460.6). Given the apparent skewness in our example CD4 count dataset the bootstrap-t interval may be shown to be theoretically preferable to the semi-parametric interval calculated by SAS in this instance. The bootstrap-t interval for this example is reflective of the skewness of the original dataset, and is wider than the percentile method since it was scaled more appropriately. Also, notice how the bootstrap-t interval is shifted slightly to the right as compared to the semi-parametric interval, again due to the asymmetry of the original dataset.

Note that the symmetry assumption may be relaxed somewhat if the trimming proportion is increased. Let us examine the effect of the choice of trimming proportion as well, e.g., say we wished to use a more robust measure of location. We can rerun the example with a trimming proportion of $\alpha = .25$, as compared to $\alpha = .05$ above, that is, in this case we will eliminate 25% of the extreme observations from either tail of the distribution prior to estimating the mean. For our CD4 count data $\bar{x}_{25} = 210.1 \pm 61.5$ as compared to $\bar{x}_{.05} = 304.9 \pm 76.8$, and $\bar{x} = 377.7 \pm 74.3$. The confidence intervals in turn for $\bar{x}_{25}$ were (108.0, 351.1), (99.3, 397.2), and (82.3, 338.0) for the percentile, bootstrap-t, and semi-parametric method, respectively. The intervals are not too dissimilar. In general, the more trimming that takes place the more we can relax the assumption of an underlying symmetrical distribution.

```
/* SAS PROGRAM 11.7 */
data original;
label x_i='CD4 counts';
input x_i @@;
 dummy=1; /*define a dummy variable to merge on*/
cards;

1397 471 64 1571 663 1128 719 407
480 1147 362 2022  10 175  494   31
202 751 30 27 118 8 181 1432 31 18
105 23 8 70 12 504 252 0 100   4
545 226 390 230 28 5   0 176
;

proc univariate trimmed=.05;by dummy;
var x_i;
ods listing select trimmedmeans;
ods output trimmedmeans=trbase; /*output trimmed mean and standard deviation*/

data rename;set trbase;       /*re-label the variables*/
keep dummy tbase stdbase;
tbase=mean;
stdbase=stdmean;

/***********Begin Standard Resampling Algorithm*****************/

data sampsize;
 set original nobs=nobs;
 n=nobs;
do b=1 to 10000;  /*output the data B times*/
 output;
end;

proc sort data=sampsize;by b;

data resample;
```

```
set sampsize;by b;
retain sumc i;   /*need to add the previous
           count to the total */
if first.b then do;
 sumc=0;
 i=1;
end;


p=1/(n-i+1);   /*p is the probability of a "success"*/

if ^last.b then do;
 if n>sumc then c_i=ranbin(0,n-sumc,p); /*generate the binomial variate*/
 else c_i=0;
 sumc=sumc+c_i;
end;
i=i+1;
if last.b then c_i=n-sumc;

data main;set resample;
if c_i >0 then do;
do i=1 to c_i;
 output;
end;
end;

/*************End Standard Resampling Algorithm*****************/
proc univariate trimmed=.05;by dummy b;
var x_i;
ods output trimmedmeans=tr;

data combine;merge tr rename;by dummy;
s=tbase-stdbase*(mean-tbase)/stdmean;

proc gplot data=combine;
plot stdmean*mean;

proc gchart;
vbar s;

proc univariate data=combine noprint;
var mean s;
output out=quantile pctlpts=2.5 97.5 pctlpre=pp pt;

proc print data= quantile;
title '95% Bootstrap Percentile and t Confidence Intervals';
```

11.13 Further Refinement of Bootstrap Confidence Intervals

The two key features that tend to drive bootstrap confidence interval accuracy in finite samples are symmetry and scale adjustments, particularly as they pertain to the percentile interval. The bootstrap-t interval provides a scale adjustment, but does not overcome potential asymmetry of the test statistic distribution in finite samples. In general, if some monotone function exists such that

$$P\left(\phi\left(t\left(\hat{F};\theta\right)\right) - \phi(t(F;\theta)) < x\right) = \psi(x)$$

holds for all possible F's where $\psi(x)$ is a continuous and symmetric function, that is $\psi(x) = 1 - \psi(-x)$ is assumed continuous, then the lower bound $= \phi^{-1}\left(\phi\left(t\left(\hat{F};\theta\right)\right) - z_{\alpha/2}\right)$, where $z_{\alpha/2} = \psi^{-1}(\alpha/2)$ and $\phi(x)$ is a monotone increasing transformation. As a simple example let $\phi(x) = x$, $t\left(\hat{F};\theta\right) = \bar{X}$, $t(F;\theta) = \theta$ with $\psi(x) = \Phi(\sqrt{n}x/\sigma)$, where σ is a scale parameter. So, for the relationship above to hold the big assumption is symmetry. The bootstrap percentile interval version of this framework is

$$P\left(\phi\left(t\left(\hat{F}^{*};\theta\right)\right) - \phi\left(t(\hat{F};\theta)\right) < x\right) = \psi^{*}(x),$$

where the key assumption is that $\phi\left(t(\hat{F};\theta)\right)$ is symmetric given large samples, such that the percentile interval holds approximately to a first-order approximation.

Using this framework second-order finite sample corrections can be developed. Now consider

$$P\left(\phi\left(t\left(\hat{F};\theta\right)\right) - \phi\left(t(F;\theta)\right) + z_0 < x\right) = \psi(x),$$

where z_0 is a constant. In order to illustrate the concept we start with a nonbootstrap example around Fisher's z-transformation, e.g., see Fisher (1921). In this case $\phi(x) = \sqrt{n}\tanh^{-1}(x)$, $t\left(\hat{F};\theta\right) = r$, and $\phi(t(F;\theta)) = \rho$, where r is Pearson's sample correlation and ρ is the population correlation. Then $\sqrt{n}\left(\tanh^{-1}(r) - \tanh^{-1}(\rho)\right)$ has a more symmetric variance-stabilized distribution than $\sqrt{n}(r - \rho)$. However, in finite samples $\sqrt{n}\left(\tanh^{-1}(r) - \tanh^{-1}(\rho)\right) - \rho/\sqrt{2}n$ is an even better approximation to that of $\sqrt{n}\left(\tanh^{-1}(r) - \tanh^{-1}(\rho)\right)$ in general if ϕ, ρ, and z_0 are known, e.g., see Konish (1978). Then the lower bound for the confidence interval for ρ in the case can be written in the form $\phi^{-1}\left(\phi\left(t\left(\hat{F};\theta\right)\right) - z_{\alpha/2} + z_0\right)$.

The bootstrap variant of this approach, termed the bootstrap *bias-corrected* approach, starts with a calibration step where we write

$$P\left(\phi\!\left(t\!\left(\hat{F}^*;\theta\right)\right)-\phi\!\left(t\!\left(\hat{F};\theta\right)\right)+z_0<x\right)=\psi^*(x),$$

where $z_0=\psi^{-1}\!\left(K^*\!\left(t\!\left(\hat{F}^*;\theta\right)\right)\right)$ and $K^*(t(\hat{F}^*;\theta))$ is the distribution function of $\phi\!\left(t\!\left(\hat{F}^*;\theta\right)\right)-\phi(t(\hat{F};\theta))$. If the distribution of $t\!\left(\hat{F}^*;\theta\right)$ is symmetric about $\phi\!\left(t(\hat{F};\theta)\right)$ then $z_0=0$, and we have the same result as the standard percentile interval. Calculating z_0 in practice is difficult since in general we do not know the form of $\psi(x)$. In applications we can consider approximating $\psi(x)$ with $\Phi(x)$, the standard normal distribution function. Then the estimator $\hat{z}_0=\Phi^{-1}\!\left(K^*\!\left(t\!\left(\hat{F}^*;\theta\right)\right)\right)$. If the distribution of $t\!\left(\hat{F}^*;\theta\right)$ is symmetric about $\phi\!\left(t(\hat{F};\theta)\right)$ then $\hat{z}_0\approx0$, that is, $K^*\!\left(t\!\left(\hat{F}^*;\theta\right)\right)\approx1/2$. The confidence bounds for $t(F;\theta)$ then become

$$\text{lower}=\hat{F}^{*-1}_{t\left(\hat{F}^*;\theta\right)}\left[\Phi(2\hat{z}_0+\Phi^{-1}(\alpha/2))\right],$$

$$\text{upper}=\hat{F}^{*-1}_{t\left(\hat{F}^*;\theta\right)}\left[\Phi(2\hat{z}_0+\Phi^{-1}(1-\alpha/2))\right].$$

The example below is to calculate the 95% confidence interval for Tukey's trimean:

```
/* SAS PROGRAM 11.8 */
**********************************;
** Bias Corrected Percentile Method****;
**********************************;
* The program below estimates the trimean and its confidence interval;

data counts;
label pl_ct='platelet count';
input pl_ct @@;
cards;
1397 471 64   1571 663 1128 719 407
480 1147 362 2022 10   175 494 31
202 751 30   27   118 8 181 1432 31   18
105 23   8 70   12   504 252 0 100 4
545 226 390 230 28   5 0 176
;

proc iml;
 use counts;
 read all into data;

 *reset print;

 n=nrow(data);
 brep=5000;          * Number of bootstrap replications;
```

```
total=n*brep;
bootdata=j(total,3, 0);


* Create bootstrap replications;
do i=1 to total;
index=int(ranuni(0)*n)+1;
bootdata[i,1]=data[index]; bootdata[i,2]=int((i-1)/n)+1;   * This is
the number of replications;
end;

call sortndx(ndx, bootdata, {2, 1});
          * Sort data by replication number and values;
bootdata=bootdata[ndx,];

do i=1 to total;
bootdata[i,3]=mod(i,n) + (mod(i,n)=0)*n;
        * This is the order of each replicated data;
end;

* Find trimmed mean;

subset=bootdata[loc(bootdata[,3]=int(n/4)+1|bootdata[,3]=int(n/2)+1
          |bootdata[,3]=int(3*n/4)+1),1];
matrix1=I(brep);
matrix2={0.25 0.5 0.25};
matrix3=matrix1 @ matrix2;
tukey = matrix3 * subset;

call sort(tukey, {1});
tukey=tukey;

* Find trimmed mean for the original data;
call sortndx(ndx, data, {1});
data=data[ndx,;
trimmean=1/4 * data[int(n/4)+1,1]+1/2 * data[int(n/2)+1,1]
          + 1/4 * data[int(n*3/4)+1,1];

*Calculate b;
subset = tukey[loc(tukey[,1] <= trimmean),];
p=nrow(subset)/brep;
b=quantile('NORMAL', p); * b=z_0;

* Calculate confidence interval;
alpha=0.05;
z_alpha_2 = quantile('NORMAL', alpha/2);
Q_l=int(brep*probnorm(2*b + z_alpha_2));
Q_u=int(brep*probnorm(2*b - z_alpha_2));

if Q_l=0 then Lower=0;
 else Lower=tukey[Q_l];
 Upper=tukey[Q_u];

CI=trimmean||p||b||Lower||Upper;
```

```
colname={'trimmean' 'P' 'b' 'lower' 'upper'};
print CI[colname=colname];


quit;
```

The results of SAS program 11.8 are given in Table 11.1.

If the statistic $t(\hat{F}^*;\theta)$ cannot be estimated directly, a double-bootstrap strategy may be needed.

TABLE 11.1

The Estimated Confidence Interval for the Population Trimean Based on 5000 Replications

Trimean	P	b	lower	upper
223.5	0.4388	−0.154012	112.25	386.75

The corresponding macro version of the SAS program is:

```
/* SAS PROGRAM 11.9 */
data original;
label x_i='CD4 counts';
input x_i @@;
 dummy=1; /*define a dummy variable to merge on*/
cards;
1397 471 64 1571 663 1128 719 407
480 1147 362 2022  10 175  494   31
202 751 30 27 118 8 181 1432 31 18
105 23 8 70 12 504 252 0 100   4
545 226 390 230 28 5   0 176
;


ods listing close;


proc univariate trimmed=.05;by dummy;
var x_i;
ods listing select trimmedmeans;
ods output trimmedmeans=trbase;


data rename;set trbase;
keep dummy tbase ;
tbase=mean;


ods printer ps file='trim_BC.ps';
```

```
data sampsize;
 set original nobs=nobs;
 n=nobs;
do b=1 to 10000;   /*output the data B times*/
 output;
end;


proc sort data=sampsize;by b;


data resample;
set sampsize;by b;
retain sumc i;    /*need to add the previous
            count to the total */
if first.b then do;
 sumc=0;
 i=1;
end;
p=1/(n-i+1);   /*p is the probability of a "success"*/

if ^last.b then do;
 if n>sumc then c_i=ranbin(0,n-sumc,p);  /*generate the binomial variate*/
 else c_i=0;
 sumc=sumc+c_i;
end;
i=i+1;
if last.b then c_i=n-sumc;


data main;set resample;
if c_i >0 then do;
do i=1 to c_i;
 output;
end;
end;

proc univariate trimmed=.05;by dummy b;
var x_i;
ods output trimmedmeans=tr;

data combine;merge tr rename;by dummy;
ind=0;
if mean<tbase then ind=1;

proc means mean noprint;
var ind;
output out=bias mean=phat;

%macro bc;

data percents;set bias;
alpha=0.05;
z0=probit(phat);
lower=100*probnorm(2*z0+probit(alpha/2));
upper=100*probnorm(2*z0+probit(1-alpha/2));   /*need percentiles*/
```

```
call symput ('lll', lower);
call symput ('uuu', upper);

proc univariate noprint pctldef=4 data=combine;
var mean;
output out=quantile pctlpts= &lll &uuu pctlpre=p;

%mend;
%bc;

proc print;


ods listing;
```

The 95% bias corrected confidence interval is (179.92, 471.49).

The next extension for finite samples involves two correction factors and is known as the bias-corrected and accelerated (BCa) interval; whereas above bias refers to the first-order term in the bias of $E\left(t\left(\hat{F};\theta\right)\right)$, in this case we write our corrected distribution function as

$$P\left(\frac{\phi\left(t\left(\hat{F}^*;\theta\right)\right)-\phi\left(t\left(\hat{F};\theta\right)\right)}{1+a\phi\left(t\left(\hat{F};\theta\right)\right)}+z_0<x\right)=\psi^*(x),$$

where a is what is known as the acceleration constant, which adjusts for finite sample skewness for the distribution of $\phi\left(t\left(\hat{F}^*;\theta\right)\right)-\phi\left(t\left(\hat{F};\theta\right)\right)$. In this case we again approximate z_0 and a such that are approximate upper and lower bounds become

$$\text{lower}=\hat{F}^{*-1}_{t\left(\hat{F}^*;\theta\right)}\left[\Phi\left(\hat{z}_0+\frac{\hat{z}_0+\Phi^{-1}(\alpha/2)}{1-\hat{a}(\hat{z}_0+\Phi^{-1}(\alpha/2))}\right)\right],$$

$$\text{upper}=\hat{F}^{*-1}_{t\left(\hat{F}^*;\theta\right)}\left[\Phi\left(\hat{z}_0+\frac{\hat{z}_0+\Phi^{-1}(1-\alpha/2)}{1-\hat{a}(\hat{z}_0+K^{-1}(1-\alpha/2))}\right)\right],$$

where $\hat{z}_0=\Phi^{-1}\left(K^*\left(t\left(\hat{F}^*;\theta\right)\right)\right)$, $\hat{a}=\dfrac{\frac{1}{6}\sum_{i=1}^{B}w_i^3}{\left(\sum_{i=1}^{B}w_i^2\right)^{3/2}}$, and $w_i=t_i\left(\hat{F}^*;\theta\right)-\bar{t}\left(\hat{F}^*;\theta\right)$. In

general, the bias-corrected and bias-accelerated intervals may not perform as expected due to the fact that we are estimating z_0 and a.

```
/* SAS PROGRAM 11.10*/
*********************************;
** Bias-Corrected and Accelerated Method****;
*********************************;
* The program below estimates the trimean and its confidence
interval;

data counts;
 label pl_ct='platelet count';
 input pl_ct @@;
 cards;
 1397 471 64   1571 663 1128 719 407
 480 1147 362 2022 10   175 494 31
 202 751 30   27   118 8 181 1432 31   18
 105 23   8 70   12   504 252 0 100 4
 545 226 390 230 28   5 0 176
 ;
/*
 data counts;
 label pl_ct='platelet count';
 input pl_ct @@;
 cards;
 230 222 179 191 103 293 316 520 143 226
 225 255 169 204   99 107 280 226 143 259
 ;
*/
proc iml;
 use counts;
 read all into data;

*reset print;

 n=nrow(data);
 brep=500;          * Number of bootstrap replications;

 total=n*brep;
 bootdata=j(total,3, 0);

* Create bootstrap replications;
 do i=1 to total;
 index=int(ranuni(0)*n)+1;
 bootdata[i,1]=data[index]; bootdata[i,2]=int((i-1)/n)+1;   *
 This is the number of replications;
 end;

call sortndx(ndx, bootdata, {2, 1});
         * Sort data by replication number and values;
 bootdata=bootdata[ndx,];

do i=1 to total;
 bootdata[i,3]=mod(i,n) + (mod(i,n)=0)*n;
         * This is the order of each replicated data;
end;

* Calculate a;
call sort(data, {1});
```

```
col=(1:n)`;
data_perm=data||col;

do i=1 to n;
 permut=data_perm[loc(data_perm[,2] ^= i),];
 col2=(1:n-1)`;
 permut=permut||col2;

 trim_perm=1/4 * permut[int((n-1)/4)+1,1] + 1/2 *
 permut[int((n-1)/2)+1, 1]
               + 1/4 * permut[int((n-1)*3/4) +1,1];
 perm_a=perm_a//trim_perm;
end;
print perm_a;

a_vector=perm_a||col||col||col;
a_vector[,4] = a_vector[+,1]/n;
a_vector[,2] = (a_vector[,1] - a_vector[,4])##3;
a_vector[,3] =  (a_vector[,1] - a_vector[,4])##2;
a=a_vector[+,2] /6/a_vector[+,3]##1.5;                       *a;

* Find trimmed mean;
subset=bootdata[loc(bootdata[,3]=int(n/4)+1|bootdata[,3]=int(n/2)+1
                   |bootdata[,3]=int(3*n/4)+1),1];
matrix1=I(brep);
matrix2={0.25 0.5 0.25};
matrix3=matrix1 @ matrix2;
tukey = matrix3 * subset;

call sort(tukey, {1});
tukey=tukey;

* Find trimmed mean for the original data;
call sortndx(ndx, data, {1});
data=data[ndx,];
trimmean=1/4 * data[int(n/4)+1,1] + 1/2 * data[int(n/2)+1, 1]
         + 1/4 * data[int(n*3/4) +1,1];

*Calculate b;
subset = tukey[loc(tukey[,1] <= trimmean),];
p=nrow(subset)/brep;
b=fuzz(quantile('NORMAL', p)); * b=z_0;

* Calculate confidence interval;
alpha=0.05;
z_alpha_2=quantile('NORMAL', alpha/2);
Q_l=int(brep *probnorm(b + (z_alpha_2 + b)/(1 - a * (z_alpha_2 + b))));
Q_u=int(brep*probnorm(b + (- z_alpha_2 + b)/(1 - a * (- z_alpha_2 + b))));

if Q_l=0 then Lower=0;
 else Lower=tukey[Q_l];
Upper=tukey[Q_u];

CI=trimmean||p||a||b||Lower||Upper;
colname={'trimmean' 'P' 'a' 'b' 'lower' 'upper'};
 print CI[colname=colname];
quit;
```

The results are shown in Table 11.2

TABLE 11.2

The Estimated Confidence Interval for the Trimmed Mean Based on 5000
Replications

Trimean	P	a	b	lower	upper
223.5	0.4348	−0.011665	−0.164167	116	376.25

The BCa method produces a narrower confidence interval than BC method.
A corresponding macro version of SAS PROGRAM 11.10 follows:

```
/* SAS PROGRAM 11.11 */
data original;
 label x_i='platelet count';
 input x_i@@;
 dummy=1;
 cards;
1397 471 64 1571 663 1128 719 407
480 1147 362 2022 10 175 494 31
202 751 30 27 118 8 181 1432 31 18
105 23 8 70 12 504 252 0 100 4
545 226 390 230 28 5 0 176
;

* The trimmed mean of the original data;
proc univariate data=original trimmed=.05;by dummy;
var x_i;
ods listing select trimmedmeans;
ods output trimmedmeans=trbase;
quit;

data rename;set trbase;
keep dummy tbase ;
tbase=mean;

ods printer ps file='trim_BC.ps';


data sampsize;
 set original nobs=nobs;
 n=nobs;
do b=1 to 10000;   /*output the data B times*/
 output;
end;

proc sort data=sampsize;by b;

*Bootstrap sampling;
data resample;
set sampsize;by b;
retain sumc i;   /*need to add the previous
                 count to the total */
```

```
if first.b then do;
 sumc=0;
 i=1;
end;
p=1/(n-i+1);  /*p is the probability of a "success"*/

if ^last.b then do;
 if n>sumc then c_i=ranbin(0,n-sumc,p); /*generate the binomial variate*/
 else c_i=0;
 sumc=sumc+c_i;
end;
i=i+1;
if last.b then c_i=n-sumc;

data main;set resample;
if c_i >0 then do;
do i=1 to c_i;
output;
end;
end;
run;

* The estimated trimmed mean of the bootstrap samples;
proc univariate data=main trimmed=.05;by dummy b;
var x_i;
ods output trimmedmeans=tr;
run;

data combine;merge tr rename;by dummy;
ind=0;
if mean<tbase then ind=1;
run;

* Calculating z0, the bias;
proc means data=combine mean noprint;
var ind;
output out=bias mean=phat;
run;

* Calculating a, the acceleration;
data temp;
 set original;
 id=_n_;
run;

%macro jackknife();
%do i=1 %to 44;
dm "log;clear;output;clear";
proc univariate data=temp trimmed=.05;by dummy;
var x_i;
where id ne &i;
ods output trimmedmeans=jack;
run;

proc append data=jack out=jackknife;
```

```
run;
%end;
%mend;
%jackknife;

proc means data=jackknife noprint;
 var mean;
 by dummy;
 output out=summary mean=mean_trimean;
run;

data jk;
 merge jackknife summary;
 by dummy;
 num=( mean_trimean - mean )**3;
 den=(  mean_trimean - mean )**2;
 keep mean mean_trimean num den;
run;

proc means data=jk;
 var num den;
 output out=summary sum=sum_num sum_den;
run;

data bias;
 merge bias summary;
 ahat=sum_num/6/sum_den**1.5;
run;

%macro bc;

data percents;set bias;
alpha=0.05;
z0=probit(phat);
lower=100*probnorm(z0 + (z0 + probit(alpha/2))
    /(1 - ahat*(z0 +probit(alpha/2) )));
upper=100*probnorm(z0 + (z0 + probit(1-alpha/2))
    /(1 - ahat*(z0 +probit(1-alpha/2) )));
/*need percentiles*/
call symput('lll',lower);
call symput('uuu',upper);

proc univariate noprint pctldef=4 data=combine;
var mean;
output out=quantile pctlpts= &lll &uuu pctlpre=p;
run;
%mend;
%bc;

proc print;
run;

ods listing;
```

The 95% confidence interval is (186.09, 482.38).

The R code is as follows:

```
> data<-c(1397,  471,  64, 1571,  663, 1128,  719,  407,
>            480, 1147, 362, 2022,   10,  175,   494,  31,
>            202,  751,  30,   27,  118,    8,  181, 1432, 31, 18,
>            105,   23,   8,   70,   12,  504,  252,    0, 100,  4,
>            545,  226, 390,  230,   28,    5,    0,  176)
> library(boot)
> my.mean = function(x, indices) {
+     return( mean( x[indices] ) )
+ }
> time.boot = boot(data, my.mean, 5000)
> boot.ci(time.boot,type="bca")
BOOTSTRAP CONFIDENCE INTERVAL CALCULATIONS
Based on 5000 bootstrap replicates

CALL :
boot.ci(boot.out = time.boot, type = "bca")

Intervals :
Level        BCa
95%    (253.1, 550.7 )
Calculations and Intervals on Original Scale
```

11.14 Bootstrap Tilting

The direct linkage between *empirical likelihood* (EL) methods outlined in Chapter 10 and bootstrap methodologies is through a specific technique developed by Efron (1981) who coined the term *nonparametric tilting,* which now is referred to as *bootstrap tilting*. In fact one could make the case that bootstrap tilting is essentially one of the forerunners to nonparametric EL methods. As we outline the procedure for bootstrap tilting we note that this is an approach developed by Efron (1981) for hypothesis testing via bootstrap methodology with an eye towards improved Type I error control of test procedures as compared to more straightforward bootstrap resampling schemes.

The general bootstrap tilting approach as given as follows: Suppose we are interested in testing $H_0 : \theta = \theta_0$, equivalently written in terms of the notation of statistical functionals as $H_0 : t(F) = t(F_0)$ versus $H_0 : t(F) > t(F_0)$, as opposed to confidence interval generation. The idea behind tilting is to use a nonparametric estimate of F_0 relative to maintaining the Type I error control, that is, minimize statistical functional-based distances such as $\left| Pr\left(t\left(\hat{F}_0 \right) > t(F_0) \mid H_0 \right) - \alpha \right|$ under H_0 for a desired α-level such as 0.05. This approach implies using a form of the empirical estimator constrained under

H_0 of the form $F_{0,n}(x) = \sum_{i=1}^{n} w_{0,i} I\{X_i \leq x\}$. The $w_{0,i}$'s are chosen to minimize the distance from $w_i = 1/n$, $i = 1, 2, \ldots, n$, under the null hypothesis constraint $t(\hat{F}_0) = \theta_0$ and constraints on the weights of $\sum_{i=1}^{n} w_{0,i} = 1$ given all $w_{0,i} > 0$, $i = 1, 2, \ldots.n$. One approach for determining the weights is via the Kullback–Leibler distance, e.g., see Efron (1981). Other distance measures such as those based on entropy concepts may also be used. The weights obtained using the Kullback–Leibler distance-based approach are identical to those obtained via the EL method described in this entry. Once the $w_{0,i}$'s are determined the null distribution can be estimated via Monte Carlo resampling B times from $\hat{F}_0$. In rare cases the null distribution may be obtained directly, e.g. when the parameter of interest is the population quantile given as $\theta = F^{-1}(u)$. The approximate bootstrap p-value estimated via Monte Carlo resampling is given as $\#(\hat{\theta}_0^* s > \theta_0)/B$, where $\hat{\theta}_0^*$ denotes the estimator obtained from a bootstrap resample from $\hat{F}_0$. For the specific example $\theta = t(F) = \int x dF$ is the mean, the weights $w_{0,i}$ are chosen that minimize the Kullback–Leibler distance $D(w, w_0) = \sum_{i=1}^{n} w_{0,i} \log(n w_{0,i})$ subject to the constraints $\sum_{i=1}^{n} w_{0,i} x_i = \theta_0$, $\sum_{i=1}^{n} w_{0,i} = 1$, and all $w_{0,i} > 0$, $i = 1, 2, \ldots.n$. Parametric alternatives follow similarly to those described relative to confidence interval generation given above, that is, resample from $F_{\hat{\mu}_0}$, where $\hat{\mu}_0$ is estimated under H_0. An interesting example of use of the bootstrap tilting approach in clinical trials is illustrated in Chuang and Lai (2000) relative to estimating confidence intervals for trials with group sequential stopping rules where a natural pivot does not exist. The R package tilt.boot (R package version 1.1–1.3) provides a straightforward approach for carrying out these calculations.

12

Examples of Homework Questions

In this chapter we demonstrate examples of homework questions related to our course. In order to solve several tasks shown below, students will be encouraged to read additional relevant literature. It is suggested to start each lecture class by answering students' inquiries regarding the previously assigned homework problems. In this manner, the material of the course can be extended. In the following sections, in certain cases, we provide comments regarding selected homework questions.

12.1 Homework 1

1. Provide an example when the random sequence $\xi_n \xrightarrow{p} \xi$, but ξ_n not $\xrightarrow{a.s.} \xi$.

2. Using Taylor's theorem, show that $\exp(\hat{i}t) = \cos(t) + \hat{i}\,\sin(t)$, where $\hat{i} = \sqrt{-1}$ satisfies $\hat{i}^2 = -1$.

3. Find $\hat{i}^{\hat{i}}$.

4. Find $\displaystyle\int_0^\infty \exp(-|s|x)\sin(x)dx$. (Hint: Use the rule $\int v\,du = vu - \int u\,dv$.)

5. Obtain the value of the integral $\displaystyle\int_0^\infty \frac{\sin(t)}{t}dt$.

6. Let the stopping time $N(H)$ have the form $N(H) = \inf\left\{n : \sum_{i=1}^n X_i \geq H\right\}$, where $X_1, X_2, \dots$ are iid random variables with $E(X_1) > 0$. Show that

   $$EN(H) = \sum_{j=1}^\infty P\{N(H) \geq j\}. \text{ Is the equation } EN(H) = \sum_{j=1}^\infty P\left\{\sum_{i=1}^j X_i < H\right\}$$

   correct? If not what do we require to correct this equation?

7. Download and install the R software. Try to perform simple R procedures, e.g., *hist, mean*, etc.

12.2 Homework 2

1. Fisher information $\iota(.)$:

   Let $X \sim N(\mu, 1)$, where μ is unknown. Calculate $\iota(\mu)$.

   Let $X \sim N(0, \sigma^2)$, where σ^2 is unknown. Calculate $\iota(\sigma^2)$.

   Let $X \sim Exp(\lambda)$, where λ is unknown. Calculate $\iota(\lambda)$.

2. Let $X_i, i \geq 1$, be iid with $EX_1 = 0$. Show an example of a stopping

   rule N such that $E\left(\sum_{i=1}^{N} X_i\right) \neq 0$.

3. Assume $X_1, ..., X_n$ are independent, $E(X_i) = 0$, $\text{var}(X_i) = \sigma_i^2 < \infty$,
   $E|X_i|^3 < \infty, i = 1, ..., n$. Prove the central limit theorem (CLT) based

   result regarding $\dfrac{1}{\sqrt{B_n}} \sum_{i=1}^{n} X_i, B_n = \sum_{i=1}^{n} \sigma_i^2$ as $n \to \infty$. In this context,

   what are conditions on σ_i^2 that we need to assume in order for the
   result to hold?

4. Suggest a method for using **R** to evaluate numerically (experimentally) the theoretical result related to Question 3 above, employing the Monte Carlo concept. Provide intuitive ideas and the relevant R code.

12.3 Homework 3

1. Let the random variables $X_1, ..., X_n$ be dependent and denote the
   sigma algebra as $\Im_n = \sigma\{X_1, ..., X_n\}$. Assume that $E(X_1) = \mu$ and

   $E(X_i | \Im_{i-1}) = \mu, i = 2, .., n$, where μ is a constant. Please find $E\left(\prod_{i=1}^{n} X_i\right)$.

2. The likelihood ratio (LR) with a corresponding sigma algebra is
   an H_0-martingale and an H_1-submartingale. Please evaluate in
   this context the statistic $\log(LR_n)$ based on dependent data points
   $X_1, ..., X_n$, when the hypothesis H_0 says $X_1, ..., X_n \sim f_0$ versus H_1 :
   $X_1, ..., X_n \sim f_1$, where f_0 and f_1 are joint density functions.

3. Assume $(X_n, \Im_n)$ is a martingale. What are $\left(|X_n|, \Im_n\right)$ and $\left(|X_n|^2, \Im_n\right)$?

4. Using the Monte Carlo method calculate numerically the value of

   $J = \int_{-\infty}^{\infty} \exp(-|u|^{1.7}) u^3 \sin(u) du$. Compare the obtained result with a

   result that can be conducted using the R function *integrate*. Find approximately the sample size N such that the Monte Carlo estimator J_N of J satisfies $\Pr\{|J_N - J| > 0.001\} \cong 0.05$.

5. Using the Monte Carlo method, calculate numerically

$$J = \int_{-4}^{5} \int_{-\infty}^{\infty} \exp(-|u|^{1.7} - t^2)u^3 \sin(u\cos(t))dtdu, \text{ approximating this inte-}$$

gral via the Monte Carlo estimator J_N. Plot values of $|J_N - J|$ against ten different values of N (e.g., $N = 100, 250, 350, 500, 600$, etc.), where N is the size of a generated sample that you employ to compute J_N in the Monte Carlo manner.

12.4 Homework 4

The Wald martingale.

1. Let observations $X_1, \ldots, X_n$ be iid. Denote $\phi(t)$ to be a characteristic function of X_1. Show that $W_j = \exp((-1)^{1/2}t \sum_{k=1}^{j} X_k)\phi(t)^{-j}$ is a martingale (here define an appropriate σ–algebra).

Goodness-of-fit tests:

2. Let observations $X_1, \ldots, X_n$ be iid with a density function f. We would like to test for $H_0: f = f_0$ versus $H_1: f \neq f_0$, where a form of f_0 is known.

   2.1 Show that in this statement of the problem there are no most powerful tests.

   2.2 Assume f_0 is completely known; prove that to test for H_0 is equivalent to testing the uniformity of f.

   2.3 Research one test for normality and explain a principle on which the test is based.

Measurement model with autoregressive errors:

3. Assume we observe $X_1, \ldots, X_n$ from the model $X_i = \mu + e_i$, $e_i = \beta e_{i-1} + \varepsilon_i$, $e_0 = 0$, $i = 1, \ldots, n$, where ε_i, $i = 1, \ldots, n$, are iid random variables with a density function f and μ is a constant.

   3.1 Derive the likelihood function based on the observations $X_1, \ldots, X_n$.

   3.2 Assuming $\varepsilon_i \sim N(0,1)$, derive the most powerful test for $H_0: \mu = 0$, $\beta = 0.5$ verus $H_1: \mu = 0.5$, $\beta = 0.7$ (the proof should be presented).

   3.3 Assuming $\varepsilon_i \sim N(0,1)$, find the maximum likelihood estimators of μ, β in analytical closed (as possible) forms.

3.4 Using Monte Carlo generated data (setup the true $\mu = 0.5, \beta = 0.7$), test for the normality of distributions of the maximum likelihood estimators obtained above, for $n = 5,7,10,12,25,50$. Show your conclusions regarding this Monte Carlo type study.

Comments. Regarding Question 2.2, we can note that if $X_1,\ldots,X_n \sim F_0$ then $F_0(X_1),\ldots,F_0(X_n) \sim U(0,1)$. Regarding Question 2.3, it can be suggested to read the Introduction in Vexler and Gurevich (2010). As an example, the following test strategy based on characterization of normality can be demonstrated. Assume we observe $X_1,\ldots,X_n$ that are iid. In order to construct a test for normality, Lin and Mudholkar (1980) used the fact that $X_1,\ldots,X_n \sim N(\mu,\sigma^2)$ if and only if the sample mean and the sample variance based on $X_1,\ldots,X_n$ are independently distributed. In this case one can define

$$Y_i = n^{-1}\left(\sum_{j=1:j\neq i}^{n} X_j^2 - (n-1)^{-1}\left(\sum_{j=1:j\neq i}^{n} X_j\right)^2\right) \text{ and consider the sample correlation between}$$

$$X_i - (n-1)^{-1}\left(\sum_{j=1:j\neq i}^{n} X_j\right) \text{ and } Y_i \text{ or between } X_i - (n-1)^{-1}\left(\sum_{j=1:j\neq i}^{n} X_j\right) \text{ and } Y_i^{1/3}.$$

The H_0-distribution of the test statistic proposed by Lin and Mudholkar (1980) does not depend on (μ,σ^2). Then the corresponding critical values of the test can be tabulated using the Monte Carlo method.

12.5 Homework 5

Two-sample nonparametric testing.

1. Assume we have iid observations $X_1,\ldots,X_n \sim F_X$ that are independent of iid observations $Y_1,\ldots,Y_m \sim F_Y$, where the distribution functions F_X, F_Y are unknown. We would like to test for $F_X = F_Y$, using the ranks-based test statistic $G_{nm} = \left|\dfrac{1}{nm}\sum_{i=1}^{n}\sum_{j=1}^{m} I\{X_i \geq Y_j\} - \dfrac{1}{2}\right|$. For large values of this statistic, we reject the null hypothesis.

   1.1. What is a simple method that can be used to obtain critical values of the test? (Hint: Use the Monte Carlo method, generating samples of $X_1,\ldots,X_n \sim F_X$ and $Y_1,\ldots,Y_m \sim F_Y$ to calculate approximate values of $C_{0.05} : \Pr_{F_X = F_Y}\{G_{nm} \geq C_{0.05}\} = 0.05$ based on $X,Y \sim N(0,1); X,Y \sim Unif(-1,1); X,Y \sim N(100,7)$ with, e.g., $n = m = 20$. Make a conclusion and try to prove theoretically your guess.)

1.2. Conduct simulations to obtain the Monte Carlo powers of the test via the following scenarios:

$n = m = 10, X \sim N(0,1), Y \sim Unif[-1,1]; n = m = 15, X \sim N(0,1), Y \sim Unif[-1,1];$

$n = m = 40, X \sim N(0,1), Y \sim Unif[-1,1]; n = 10, m = 30, X \sim N(0,1), Y \sim Unif[-1,1];$

$n = 30, m = 10, X \sim N(0,1), Y \sim Unif[-1,1]; n = m = 10, X \sim Gamma(1,2), Y \sim Unif[0,5]$

at $\alpha = Pr_{F_X = F_Y} \{G_{nm} \geq C_{0.05}\} = 0.05$ (please formulate your results in the form of a table).

Power calculations:

2. Consider the simple linear regression model

$$Y_i = \beta X_i + \varepsilon_i, \varepsilon_i \; iid \sim N(0,1), i = 1,\ldots,n.$$

Assume that in a future study we plan to test for $\beta = 0$ versu $\beta \neq 0$, applying the corresponding maximum likelihood ratio test MLR_n based on $(Y|X)$ (here, the symbol "|" means "given"). X's are expected to be close to be from the $Unif(-1,1)$ distribution. To design the future study, please fix the Type I error rate as 0.05 and fill out the following table, presenting the Monte Carlo powers of the test with respect to the situations shown in the table below.

	Expected Effect β		
	$\beta = 0.1$	$\beta = 0.5$	$\beta = 1$
$n = 10$			
$n = 20$			
$n = 50$			
$n = 100$			

Sequential Probability Ratio Test (SPRT):

3. Assume that we survey sequentially iid observations $Y_1, Y_2 \ldots$. Then answer the following:

3.1 Write the SPRT for $H_0 : Y \sim N(0,1)$ versus $H_1 : Y \sim N(0.5,1)$.

3.2 Calculate values of the corresponding thresholds to use in the SPRT, provided that we want to preserve the Type I and II errors rates as $\alpha = 0.05, \beta = 0.15$, respectively.

3.3 Using Monte Carlo techniques evaluate the expectation of the corresponding stopping time under the null hypothesis H_0 as well as under the alternative hypothesis H_1.

3.4 Suppose that we observe retrospectively iid data points $X_1, \ldots, X_n$ and the likelihood ratio (LR) based on $X_1, \ldots, X_n$ is applied to test for $H_0 : Y \sim N(0,1)$ versus $H_1 : Y \sim N(0.5,1)$ at $\alpha = 0.05$. What should the sample size n be to obtain the power $1 - \beta = 1 - 0.15$? (Hint: You can use the CLT to obtain the critical value of the log(LR) test statistic as well as to evaluate the needed n under H_1.)

3.5   Compare the results of 3.4 with 3.3.

Comments. Regarding Question 1.1, one can note that

$$\mathrm{Pr}_{F_X = F_Y} \{ G_{nm} \geq C_{0.05} \} = \int I \left\{ \left| \frac{1}{nm} \sum_{i=1}^{n} \sum_{j=1}^{m} I\{ X_i \geq Y_j \} - \frac{1}{2} \right| \geq C_{0.05} \right\} d\Psi_{nm},$$

where Ψ_{nm} is the joint distribution function of the random variables $I\{ X_i \geq Y_j \}$, $i = 1,..,n, j = 1,...,m$. Under the hypothesis $F_X = F_Y$, we have $I\{ X_i \geq Y_j \} = I\{ F_X(X_i) \geq F_Y(Y_j) \}$, $i = 1,...,n, j = 1,...,m$ and then their joint distribution does not depend on $F_X = F_Y$. Then the test statistic is exact, meaning that its distribution is independent of the underlying data distribution, under the hypothesis $F_X = F_Y$. Regarding Question 3.4, we suggest application of the Monte Carlo approach. One can also use the distribution function of the log-likelihood ratio $\sum_{i=1}^{n} \xi_i$, where $\xi_i = \log \left(\dfrac{f_{H_1}(X_i)}{f_{H_0}(X_i)} \right)$, $i = 1,...,n$ with f_{H_1} and f_{H_0}, which are the density functions related to $N(0,1)$ and $N(0.5,1)$, respectively. Alternatively, defining the test threshold as C, we note that

$$\mathrm{Pr}_{H_0} \left\{ \frac{\sum_{i=1}^{n} \xi_i - n E_{H_0}(\xi_1)}{n^{1/2} \left(Var_{H_0}(\xi_1) \right)^{1/2}} \geq \frac{C - n E_{H_0}(\xi_1)}{n^{1/2} \left(Var_{H_0}(\xi_1) \right)^{1/2}} \right\} = 0.05 \quad \text{and}$$

$$\mathrm{Pr}_{H_1} \left\{ \frac{\sum_{i=1}^{n} \xi_i - n E_{H_1}(\xi_1)}{n^{1/2} \left(Var_{H_1}(\xi_1) \right)^{1/2}} \geq \frac{C - n E_{H_1}(\xi_1)}{n^{1/2} \left(Var_{H_1}(\xi_1) \right)^{1/2}} \right\} = 0.85.$$

Then, using the CLT, we can derive n and C, solving the equations

$$1 - \Phi \left(\frac{C - n E_{H_0}(\xi_1)}{n^{1/2} \left(Var_{H_0}(\xi_1) \right)^{1/2}} \right) = 0.05, \quad 1 - \Phi \left(\frac{C - n E_{H_1}(\xi_1)}{n^{1/2} \left(Var_{H_1}(\xi_1) \right)^{1/2}} \right) = 0.85,$$

where $\Phi(u) = (2\pi)^{-1/2} \int_{-\infty}^{u} e^{-z^2/2} dz$. It can be suggested to compare these three approaches.

12.6 Homeworks 6 and 7

In order to work on the tasks presented in this section, students should use real-world data. In our course, we consider data from a study evaluating bio-markers related to atherosclerotic coronary heart disease. In this study, free radicals have been implicated in the atherosclerotic coronary heart disease process. Well-developed laboratory methods may grant an ample number of biomarkers of individual oxidative stress and antioxidant status. These markers quantify different phases of the oxidative stress and antioxidant status process of an individual. A population-based sample of randomly selected residents of Erie and Niagara counties of the state of New York, USA., 35–79 years of age, was the focus of this investigation. The New York State Department of Motor Vehicles driver's license rolls were utilized as the sampling frame for adults between the ages of 35 and 65; the elderly sample (age 65–79) was randomly selected from the Health Care Financing Administration database. A cohort of 939 men and women were selected for the analyses yielding 143 cases (individuals with myocardial infarction, **MI=1**) and 796 controls (**MI=0**). Participants provided a 12-hour fasting blood specimen for biochemical analysis at baseline, and a number of parameters were examined from fresh blood samples.

We evaluate measurements related to the biomarker TBARS (see for details Schisterman et al., 2001).

Homework 6

1. Using the nonparametric test defined in Section 12.5, Question 1, test the hypothesis that a distribution function of TBARS measurements related to MI=0 is equal to a distribution function of TBARS measurements related to MI=1.

2. Please provide a test for normality based on measurements of TBARS that correspond to MI=0, MI=1, and the full data, respectively. Plot relevant histograms and Q-Q plots.

3. Consider the power (Box–Cox) transformation of TBARS measurements, that is,

$$h(X,\lambda) = \begin{cases} \dfrac{sign(X)|X|^{\lambda} - 1}{\lambda}, & \lambda \neq 0 \\ sign(X)\log|X|, & \lambda = 0, \end{cases}$$

where $X_1,...,X_n$ are observations and $\{h(X_1,\lambda),...,h(X_n,\lambda)\}$ is the transformed data.

Assume $h(X,\lambda) \sim N(\mu,\sigma^2)$, where the parameters λ, μ, σ^2 are unknown.

3.1 Calculate values of the maximum likelihood estimators $\hat{\lambda}_0, \hat{\lambda}_1, \hat{\lambda}_f$ of λ based on the data with MI=0, MI=1, and the full data, respectively (using numerical calculations).

3.2 Calculate the asymptotic 95% confidence intervals for $\hat{\lambda}_0, \hat{\lambda}_1, \hat{\lambda}_f$.

3.3 Test transformed observations $h(TBARS, \hat{\lambda}_0)$ (on data with MI=0), $h(TBARS, \hat{\lambda}_1)$ (on data with MI=1), and $h(TBARS, \hat{\lambda}_f)$ (on the full data) for normality, e.g., applying the Shapiro–Wilk test.

4. Calculate a value of the 2log maximum likelihood ratio

$$2\log\left(\prod_{MI=0} f(h(TBARS,\hat{\lambda}_0)) \prod_{MI=1} f(h(TBARS,\hat{\lambda}_1)) \Bigg/ \prod_{MI=0,1} f(h(TBARS,\hat{\lambda}_f))\right)$$

to test for the hypothesis from Question 1. Compare results related to Questions 1 and 4.

Comments. Regarding Question 3.1, we suggest obtaining the estimators of μ and σ^2 in explicit forms, whereas the estimator of λ can be derived by using a numerical method, e.g., via the R built-in operator *uniroot* or *optimize*. The corresponding schematic R code can have the form

G<-function(λ){

$$\hat{\mu} = \sum_{i=1}^{n} h(X_i,\lambda)/n$$

$$\hat{\sigma}^2 = \sum_{i=1}^{n} \left(h(X_i,\lambda)-\hat{\mu}\right)^2/n$$

return $\left(\log\left(\left(2\pi\hat{\sigma}^2\right)^{-n/2}\exp(-1/2)\right)\right)$
}
GV<-Vectorize(G)
$\hat{\lambda}$ =optimize (GV,maximum = TRUE)\$maximum

Homework 7
Let us perform the following Jackknife-type procedure.

Denote TBARS measurements related to MI=1 as Data A with the sample size N_A and TBARS measurements related to MI=0 as Data B with the sample size N_B.

Consider the next algorithm:
Define $n = 0$.

Step 1: Randomly select $N_A - n$ observations from Data A; and $N_B - n$ observations from Data B. (The R operator *sample* can be used in this step.)

Step 2: Use the selected observations in Step 1 to calculate values of the maximum likelihood estimators $\hat{\lambda}_0, \hat{\lambda}_1$ of λ (see Homework 6, Question 3) and then test transformed observations $h(TBARS, \hat{\lambda}_0)$ (based on the selected sample from Data A) and $h(TBARS, \hat{\lambda}_1)$ (based on the selected sample from Data B) for normality, e.g., applying the Shapiro–Wilk test. Record the corresponding p-values as p_0 and p_1, respectively.

Step 3: Repeat Steps 1–2 5000 times, obtaining average values based on p_0's and p_1's, say $P^A_{N_A - n} = \bar{p}_0$ and $P^B_{N_B - n} = \bar{p}_1$.

Redefine $n = n + 10$ and perform Steps 1–3.

The outputs of the procedure above are the average p-values $P^A_{N_A}, P^A_{N_A - 10}, P^A_{N_A - 20}, P^A_{N_A - 30}, \dots$ and $P^B_{N_B}, P^B_{N_B - 10}, P^B_{N_B - 20}, P^B_{N_B - 30}, \dots$ that can be plotted against the sample sizes $N_A, N_A - 10, N_A - 20, N_A - 30, \dots$. This can be used to evaluate models of functional dependencies between P^k_u and u, where $k = A, B$.

For example, we can estimate the models $P^k_u = \dfrac{\exp(a_k + b_k u)}{1 + \exp(a_k + b_k u)}$, where a_k and b_k are coefficients, $k = A, B$.

One can employ the obtained models to extrapolate values of P^k_u for $u > N_k$, $k = A, B$. In this case, assume that α' denotes a fixed level. Then we can consider the scheme below.

If $P^k_{N_k} > \alpha'$ and the extrapolated values of P^k_u increase, we can conclude that probably while increasing the sample size we could not reject the corresponding null hypothesis.

If $P^k_{N_k} > \alpha'$ and the extrapolated values of P^k_u decrease, we can forecast the sample size u_0: $\{1 + \exp(-a_k - b_k u_0)\}^{-1} = \alpha'$, when we could expect to reject the corresponding null hypothesis.

The procedure demonstrated above can be easily modified for application as an experimental data-driven sample size calculation method in various practical situations.

13

Examples of Exams

In this chapter we demonstrate examples of midterm, final, and qualifying exams. In the following sections, in certain cases, we provide comments regarding a subset of selected exam questions.

13.1 Midterm Exams

Example 1:

This exam has 4 questions, some of which have subparts. Each question has an indicated point value. The total points for the exam are 100 points.

Show all your work. Justify all answers.
Good luck!

Question 1 (30 points) Characteristic functions

Provide a proof about the one-to-one mapping proposition related to the result: "For every characteristic function there is a corresponding unique distribution function." (Hint: Show that for all random variables its characteristic function ϕ **exists.** Formulate and prove the inversion theorem that shows $F(y) - F(x)$ is equal to a functional of $\phi(t)$, where F and ϕ are the distribution and characteristic functions, respectively. Consider cases when we can operate with $dF(u)/du$ and when we cannot use $dF(u)/du$. If you need, derive the characteristic function of a normally distributed random variable.)

Question 2 (30 points)

Assume data points $X_1, \ldots, X_n$ are from a joint density function $f(x_1, \ldots, x_n; \theta)$, where θ is an unknown parameter. Suppose we want to test for $H_0 : \theta = 0$ versus $H_1 : \theta \neq 0$ then complete the following:

2.1 Write the maximum likelihood ratio ML_n and formulate the maximum likelihood ratio test. Write the corresponding Bayes factor type likelihood ratio, BL_n, test statistic. Show an optimality of BL_n in the context of "most powerful decision rules" and interpret the optimality.

2.2 Derive the asymptotic distribution function of the statistic ML_n, under H_0. How can this asymptotic result about the MLR test be used in practice?

Question 3 (20 points)

Consider the test statistics ML_n and BL_n from Question 2. Under H_0, are they a martingale, submartingale, or supermartingale? Can you provide relevant conclusions regarding the expected performance of the tests based on ML_n and BL_n test statistics?

Question 4 (20 points)

Formulate the SPRT (Wald sequential test), evaluating the Type I and II errors rates of the test.

Example 2:

11 AM–12:20 PM

This exam has 4 questions, some of which have subparts. Each question has an indicated point value. The total points for the exam are 100 points.

Show all your work. Justify all answers.
Good luck!

Question 1 (20 points) Characteristic functions

1.1 Define the characteristic function $\phi(t)$ of a random variable X. Show $\phi(t)$ exists, for all X and t. Assume X has a normal density function $f(u) = \left(2\pi\sigma^2\right)^{-1/2} \exp(-u^2 / (2\sigma^2))$. What is a form of $\phi(t)$? Assume X has a density function $f(u) = \exp(-u)I(u > 0)$. What is a form of $\phi(t)$?

1.2 Let $X_1, \ldots, X_n$ be iid with $EX_1 = \mu$ $(E|X_1|^{1+\varepsilon} < \infty, \varepsilon > 0$ is not required). Prove that $(X_1 + \ldots + X_n)/n \to \mu$ as $n \to \infty$.

Question 2 (30 points)

See Question 2, Section 13.1, Example 1.

Question 3 (15 points)

3.1 Provide the definition of a stopping time, presenting an example of a stopping time (prove formally that your statistic is a stopping time).

3.2 Let v and u be stopping times. Are $\min(v-1, u), \max(v, u), u+1$ stopping times? (Relevant proofs should be shown.)

Question 4 (35 points)

4.1 Formulate and prove the optional stopping theorem for martingales (provide formal definitions of objects that you use in this theorem).

4.2 Prove the Dub theorem (inequality) based on nonnegative martingales.

4.3 Sequential change point detection. Suppose we observe sequentially iid measurements $X_1, X_2 \ldots$. To detect a change point in the data distribution (i.e., to test for $H_0 : X_1, X_2 \ldots \sim f_0$ vs. $H_1 : X_1, X_2, \ldots,$ $X_{v-1} \sim f_0; X_v, X_{v+1}, \ldots \sim f_1$, where the densities f_0, f_1 are known, the change point v is unknown) we use the stopping time

$$N(H) = \inf\left\{ n : SR_n = \sum_{k=1}^{n} \prod_{i=k}^{n} \frac{f_1(X_i)}{f_0(X_i)} > H \right\} \text{ (we stop and reject } H_0). \text{ Derive}$$

the lower bound for the expression $E_{N(H)}\{N(H)\}$. Why do we need this inequality in practice?

Example 3:

11 AM–12:20 PM

This exam has 4 questions, some of which have subparts. Each question indicates its point value. The total is 100 points.

Show all your work. Justify all answers.
Good luck!

Question 1 (37 points) Characteristic functions

See Question 1, Section 13.1, Example 1.

Question 2 (19 points)

Assume data points $X_1, \ldots, X_n$ are iid with a density function $f(x \mid \theta)$, where θ is an unknown parameter. Define the maximum likelihood estimator of θ to be $\hat{\theta}_n$, which is based on $X_1, \ldots, X_n$. Derive the asymptotic distribution of $n^{0.5} \left(\hat{\theta}_n - \theta \right)$ as $n \to \infty$. Show the relevant conditions and the corresponding proof.

Question 3 (25 points)

Assume data points $X_1, \ldots, X_n$ are from a joint density function $f(x_1, \ldots, x_n; \theta)$, where θ is an unknown parameter. Suppose we want to test $H_0 : \theta = 0$ versus $H_1 : \theta \neq 0$. Complete the following:

3.1 Write the Bayes factor type likelihood ratio BLR_n; Show the optimality of BLR_n in the context of "most powerful decision rules."

3.2 Find the asymptotic $(n \to \infty)$ distribution function of the statistic MLR_n, the maximum likelihood ratio, under H_0.

Question 4 (19 points)

See Question 4.1, Section 13.1, Example 2.

Example 4:

11 AM–12:20 PM

This exam has 3 questions, some of which have subparts. Each question indicates its point value. The total is 100 points.

Show all your work. Justify all answers.
Good luck!

Question 1 (41 points) Characteristic functions

See Question 1, Section 13.1, Example 1.

Question 2 (36 points)

Let $\varepsilon_1, \ldots, \varepsilon_d$ be iid random variables from $N(0,1)$. Assume we have data points $X_1, \ldots, X_n$ that are iid observations and X_1 has a density function f that has a form of the density function of $\sum_{i=1}^{d} (\varepsilon_i)^2$, where the **integer** parameter d is unknown and $d \le 10$.

2.1 Write the maximum likelihood ratio (MLR) statistic, MLR_n, and formulate the MLR test for $H_0 : EX_1 = \theta_0$ versus $H_1 : EX_1 \ne \theta_0$, where θ_0 is known. (Hint: Use characteristic functions to derive the form of f.)

2.2 Propose an integrated most powerful test for $H_0 : EX_1 = \theta_0$ versus $H_1 : EX_1 \ne \theta_0$ (θ_0 is known), provided that we are interested in obtaining the maximum integrated power of the test when values of the alternative parameter can have all possible values with no preference. (Hint: Use a Bayes factor type procedure.). Formally prove that your test is integrated most powerful.

Question 3 (23 points)

(Here provide formal definitions of objects that you use to answer the following questions, e.g., the definition of a martingale.)
See Questions 4.1–4.2, Section 13.1, Example 2.

Example 5:

11 AM–12:20 PM

This exam has 4 questions, some of which have subparts. Each question indicates its point value. The total is 100 points.

Show all your work. Justify all answers.
Good luck!

Question 1 (17 points) Characteristic functions

See Question 1, Section 13.1, Example 2.

Question 2 (19 points)

See Question 2, Section 13.1, Example 3.

Question 3 (27 points)

Assume data points $X_1, \ldots, X_n$ are from a joint density function $f(x_1, \ldots, x_n; \theta)$, where θ is an unknown parameter. Suppose we want to test for $H_0 : \theta = 0$ versus $H_1 : \theta \neq 0$ then answer the following:

3.1 See Question 3.1, Section 13.1, Example 3.

3.2 Assume the observations are iid random variables with an unknown distribution. Define the corresponding empirical likelihood ratio test for $H_0 : \theta = 0$ versus $H_1 : \theta \neq 0$, where $\theta = EX_1$. Show (and prove) the asymptotic H_0-distribution of the 2log of the empirical likelihood ratio.

Question 4 (37 points)

4.1 Let v and u be stopping times. Are $\min(v-1, u), \max(v, u), u+1$, $u/10, 10u$ stopping times?

4.2–4.3 See Questions 4.1, 4.3, Section 13.1, Example 2.

4.4 Assume iid random variables $X_1 > 0, X_2 > 0, \ldots$ Defining the integer random variable $N(H) = \inf \left\{ n : \sum_{i=1}^{n} X_i > H \right\}$, show: (1) $N(H)$ is a stopping time; (2) the non-asymptotic upper bound for $EN(H)$.

Example 6:

11 AM–12:20 PM

This exam has 5 questions, some of which have subparts. Each question indicates its point value. The total is 100 points.

Show all your work. Justify all answers.
Good luck!

Question 1 (35 points) Characteristic functions

See Question 1, Section 13.1, Example 1.

Question 2 (8 points)

Let the statistic LR_n define the likelihood ratio to be applied to test for H_0 versus H_1. Prove that $f_{H_1}^{LR}(u) / f_{H_0}^{LR}(u) = u$, where f_H^{LR} denotes the density function of LR_n under $H = H_0$ or $H = H_1$, respectively.

Question 3 (21 points)

Let $\xi_1,\ldots,\xi_d$ be iid random variables from $N(0,1)$, $\eta_1,\ldots,\eta_d$ denote iid random variables from $N(0,1)$, and $\omega_1,\ldots,\omega_d$ be iid random variables that just have the two values 0 and 1 with $\Pr\{\omega_1 = 0\} = 0.5$. Let the random variables $\xi_1,\ldots,\xi_d$, $\eta_1,\ldots,\eta_d$ and $\omega_1,\ldots,\omega_d$ be independent and $\varepsilon_i = \omega_i\xi_i + (1-\omega_i)\eta_i$, $i = 1,\ldots,d$.

Assume we have data points $X_1,\ldots,X_n$ that are iid observations and X_1 has a density function f that has a form of the density function of $\sum_{i=1}^{d}(\varepsilon_i)^2$, where the **integer** parameter d is unknown and $d \leq 10$.

3.1 Write the maximum likelihood ratio (MLR) statistic, MLR_n, and formulate the MLR test for $H_0 : EX_1 = \theta_0$ versus $H_1 : EX_1 \neq \theta_0$, where θ_0 is known. (Hint: Use characteristic functions to derive the form of f.)

3.2 Propose, giving the corresponding proof, the integrated most powerful test for $H_0 : EX_1 = \theta_0$ versus $H_1 : EX_1 \neq \theta_0$ (here θ_0 is known), provided that we are interested to obtain the maximum integrated power of the test when values of the alternative parameter can have all possible values with no preference.

Question 4 (27 points)

(Here provide the formal definitions of objects that you use to answer the following questions, e.g., the definition of a martingale.)

4.1–4.2 See Questions 4.1–4.2, Section 13.1, Example 2.

4.3 Suppose iid random variables $X_1 > 0,\ldots,X_n > 0,\ldots$ have $EX_1 = Var(X_1) = 1$. Define

$$\tau = \inf\left\{n > 0 : \sum_{i=1}^{n} X_i \geq n - n^{0.7}\right\}.$$

Is τ a stopping time? (Hints: consider the event $\{\tau \geq N\}$ via an event based on $\sum_{i=1}^{N} X_i$, use the Chebyshev inequality to analyze the needed probability, and let $N \to \infty$.)

Question 5 (9 points)

Define $\tau(H) = \inf\left\{n > 0 : \sum_{i=1}^{n} X_i \geq H\right\}$, where iid random variables $X_1 > 0,\ldots,X_n > 0,\ldots$ have $EX_1 = a$. Show how to obtain a non-asymptotic upper bound for $E\{\tau(H)\}$ that is linear with respect to H as $H \to \infty$.

Comments. Regarding Question 4.3, we have

$$\Pr(\tau \geq N) = \Pr\left(\max_{n \leq N}\left(\sum_{i=1}^{n} X_i - n + n^{0.7}\right) < 0\right) \leq \Pr\left(\sum_{i=1}^{N}(1 - X_i) > N^{0.7}\right)$$

$$\leq \frac{E\left(\sum_{i=1}^{N}(1 - X_i)\right)^2}{N^{1.4}} = \frac{N}{N^{1.4}} \xrightarrow[N \to \infty]{} 0.$$

Example 7:

11 AM–12:20 PM

This exam has 4 questions, some of which have subparts. Each question indicates its point value. The total is 100 points.

Show all your work. Justify all answers.
Good luck!

Questions 1 (42 points) Characteristic functions

1.1 See Question 1, Section 13.1, Example 1.

1.2 Assume $f(x)$ and $\phi(t)$ are the density and characteristic functions of a random variable, respectively. Let $\phi(t)$ be a real function ($\phi(t)$ has real values for real values of t). Using a proposition that you should show with the proof to answer Question 1.1, prove that

$$f(x) = \frac{1}{2\pi}\int_{-\infty}^{\infty} \cos(tx)\phi(t)\,dt,$$

provided that $\phi(t)$ is an integrable function.

Question 2 (17 points)

2.1 See Question 2, Section 13.1, Example 6.

2.2 See Question 2, Section 13.1, Example 3.

Question 3 (17 points)

3.1. Let $X_1, \ldots, X_n$ be iid observations. Suppose we are interested in testing for $H_0 : X_1 \sim f_0$ versus $H_1 : X_1 \sim f_0(u)\exp(\theta_1 u + \theta_2)$, where $f_0(u)$ is a density function, and the H_1-parameters $\theta_1 > 0, \theta_2$ are unknown. In this case, propose the appropriate most powerful test, justifying the proposed test's properties.

3.2. See Question 3.2, Section 13.1, Example 3.

Question 4 (24 points)

4.1 Formulate and prove the optional stopping theorem.

4.2 Suppose we observe sequentially $X_1, X_2, X_3 \ldots$ that are iid data points from the exponential distribution $F(u) = 1 - \exp(-u/\lambda), u \geq 0; F(u) = 0, u < 0$. To observe one X we should pay A dollars depending on values of λ. Suppose we want to estimate λ using the maximum likelihood estimator $\hat{\lambda}_n$ based on n observations.

4.2.1 Propose an optimal procedure to minimize the risk function

$$L(n) = A\lambda^4 n + E\left(\hat{\lambda}_n - \lambda\right)^2.$$

4.2.2 Show a non-asymptotic upper bound of $E\left(\sum_{i=1}^{N} X_i\right)$, where N is a length (a number of needed observations) of the procedure defined in in the context of Question 4.2.1. The obtained form of the upper bound should be a direct function of A and λ. Should you use propositions, these propositions must be proven.

Comments. Regarding Question 1.2, we have $\phi(t) = E\left(e^{it\xi}\right) = E\{\cos(t\xi)\}$. Then

$$f(x) = \frac{1}{2\pi} \int_{-\infty}^{\infty} e^{-itx}\phi(t)dt = \frac{1}{2\pi} E \int_{-\infty}^{\infty} \left(\cos(tx) - i\sin(tx)\right)\cos(t\xi)dt,$$

where $\int_{-\infty}^{\infty} \sin(tx)\cos(t\xi)dt = 0$, since $\sin(-tx)\cos(-t\xi) = -\sin(tx)\cos(t\xi)$.

Example 8:

11 AM–12:20 PM

This exam has 5 questions, some of which have subparts. Each question indicates its point value. The total is 100 points.

Show all your work. Justify all answers.
Good luck!

Question 1 (29 points) Characteristic functions

1.1 See Question 1, Section 13.1, Example 1.

1.2 Let X and Y be independent random variables. Assume $X - Y$ and $X + Y$ are identically distributed. Show that the characteristic function of Y is a real-valued function.

Question 2 (21 points)

See Question 4.2, Section 13.1, Example 7.

Question 3 (18 points)

Assume we observe iid data points $X_1, \ldots, X_n$ and X_1 is from a density function $f(x)$. Suppose we want to test $H_0 : f = f_0$ versus $H_1 : f(x) = f_0(u)\exp(\theta u + \phi)$, where $\theta > 0$.

If the alternative parameters θ and ϕ are known, write the corresponding most powerful test statistic, providing a relevant proof.

Question 4 (15 points)

4.1 Let iid observations $X_1, \ldots, X_n$ be from a $N(\theta, 1)$ distribution. Suppose we want to test for $H_0 : \theta = \theta_0$ versus $H_1 : \theta = \theta_1$, using the most powerful test statistic. Provide an explicit formula to calculate the expected p-value related to the corresponding test, showing the corresponding proof.

4.2 Let TS_n define a likelihood ratio. Obtain the likelihood ratio based on TS_n, showing a needed proof.

Question 5 (17 points)

5.1 Write the definition of a stopping time and provide an example. Write the definition of a martingale and provide an example.

5.2 Formulate and prove the optional stopping theorem.

Comments. Regarding Question 1.2, we have $E\exp(\mathrm{i}t(X-Y)) = E\exp(\mathrm{i}t(X+Y))$. Then $E\exp(\mathrm{i}t(-Y)) = E\exp(\mathrm{i}t(Y))$. Thus $E(\cos(tY) - \mathrm{i}\sin(tY)) = E(\cos(tY) + \mathrm{i}\sin(tY))$. This implies $E(\sin(tY)) = 0$.

Example 9:

11 AM–12:20 PM

This exam has 6 questions, some of which have subparts. Each question indicates its point value. The total is 100 points.

Show all your work. Justify all answers.
Good luck!

Question 1 (33 points)

See Question 1, Section 13.1, Example 1.

Question 2 (7 points)

See Question 2, Section 13.1, Example 6.

Question 3 (9 points)

Assume that a random variable ξ has a gamma distribution with density function given as

$$f(u;\alpha,\gamma) = \begin{cases} \alpha^{\gamma} u^{\gamma-1} e^{-\alpha u} / \Gamma(\gamma), u \geq 0 \\ 0, \qquad u < 0, \end{cases}$$

where $\alpha > 0$, γ are parameters, and $\Gamma(\gamma)$ is the Euler gamma function $\int_0^{\infty} u^{\gamma-1} e^{-u} du$. Derive an explicit form of the characteristic function of ξ (Hint: The approach follows similar to that of normally distributed random variables).

Question 4 (15 points)

See Question 3.1, Section 13.1, Example 6.

(Hint: To give a complete answer, you can use the characteristic function based method to derive the form of f, a density function of the observations.)

Question 5 (27 points)

See Question 4, Section 13.1, Example 6.

Question 6 (9 points)

See Question 5, Section 13.1, Example 6.

13.2 Final Exams

Example 1:

11:45 AM–02:45 PM

This exam has 5 questions, some of which have subparts. Each question indicates its point value. The total is 100 points.

Show all your work. Justify all answers.
Good luck!

Question 1 (25 points)

1.1 Describe the basic components of receiver operating characteristic curve analyses based on continuous measurements of biomarkers.

1.2 Assume a measurement model with autoregressive error terms of the form

$$X_i = \mu + \varepsilon_i, \quad \varepsilon_i = \beta \varepsilon_{i-1} + \xi_i, \quad \xi_0 = 0, \quad i = 1,\ldots,n,$$

where $\xi_i, i = 1,\ldots,n$, are independent identically distributed (iid) random variables with the distribution function $\left(2\pi\sigma^2\right)^{-1/2} \int_{-\infty}^{u} \exp(-u^2/(2\sigma^2))du$; μ, β, σ are parameters. Suppose we are interested in the maximum likelihood ratio test for $H_0 : \mu = 0, \beta = 0, \sigma = 1$ versus $H_1 : \mu \neq 0, \beta \neq 0, \sigma = 1$. Write the maximum likelihood ratio test in an analytical closed (as possible) form. Provide a schematic algorithm to evaluate the power of the test based on a Monte Carlo study, when n is fixed, and we focus on the test power, when $\mu = 0.1, \beta = 0.5$.

Question 2 (25 points). Formulate and prove the following propositions

2.1 The optional stopping theorem for martingales;

2.2 The Dub theorem (inequality) based on nonnegative martingales;

2.3 The Ville and Wald inequality.

Question 3 (20 points)

3.1 Write a definition of a stopping time, providing an example of a statistical inference based on a stopping time.

3.2 Let v and u be stopping times. Are $\min(v-1,u), \max(v,u), u+2$ stopping times (provide relevant proofs)?

3.3 Prove the Wald theorem regarding the expectation of a random sum of iid random variables. Can you use the Wald theorem to calculate

$$E\left(\sum_{i=1}^{\tau-1} X_i\right), \text{ where } X_1,\ldots,X_n \text{ are iid with } EX_1 = 1 \text{ and } \tau \text{ is a stopping}$$

time with $E\tau = 25$?

Question 4 (15 points)

Prove the following propositions.

4.1 Let $X_1,\ldots,X_n$ be iid with $EX_1 = \mu$, $Var(X_1) = \sigma^2$, $E|X_1|^3 < \infty$. Then the statistic $(X_1 + \ldots + X_n - a_n)/b_n$ has asymptotically (as $n \to \infty$) a standard normal distribution, where please define the forms of a_n and b_n.

4.2 See Question 1.2, Section 13.1, Example 2.

Question 5 (15 points)

Let $X_1,\ldots,X_n$ be iid observations with $EX_1 = \mu$. Suppose that we are interested in testing $H_0 : \mu = 0$ vs. $H_1 : \mu \neq 0$. In this case, provide the corresponding empirical likelihood ratio test. Derive a relevant asymptotic proposition about this test that can be used in order to control the Type I error rate of the test.

Example 2:

03:30 PM–05:00 PM

This exam has 4 questions, some of which have subparts. Each question indicates its point value. The total is 100 points.

Show all your work. Justify all answers.
Good luck!

Question 1 (40 points)

See Question 1, Section 13.1, Example 1.

Question 2 (35 points)

Assume data points $X_1, \ldots, X_n$ are iid. Suppose we are interested in testing the hypothesis $H_0 : EX_1 = \theta_0$ versus $H_1 : EX_1 \neq \theta_0$, where θ_0 is known.

2.1 Let $X \sim Gamma(\alpha, \beta)$. Derive the maximum likelihood ratio (MLR) test statistic ML_n and formulate the MLR test for $H_0 : E(X_1) = \theta_0, \beta = \beta_0$ versus $H_1 : E(X_1) \neq \theta_0, \beta \neq \beta_0$, where θ_0, β_0 are known. Find the asymptotic distribution function of the test statistic $2\log(ML_n)$ under H_0 (Wilks' theorem).

2.2 See Question 3.2, Section 13.1, Example 5. Show (and prove) the asymptotic distribution of the empirical likelihood ratio test statistic under H_0 (the nonparametric version of Wilks' theorem).

Question 3 (10 points)

Formulate and prove the Ville and Wald inequality.

Question 4 (15 points)

Assume the measurement model with autoregressive error terms of the form

$$X_i = \mu + \varepsilon_i, \quad \varepsilon_i = \beta \varepsilon_{i-1} + \xi_i, \quad \varepsilon_0 = 0, \quad i = 1, \ldots, n,$$

where ξ_i, $i = 1, \ldots, n$, are independent identically distributed (iid) random variables with the distribution function

$$\Pr\{\xi_1 < u\} = (2\pi)^{-1/2} \int_{-\infty}^{u} \exp(-u^2/2) du; \mu, \beta \text{ are parameters.}$$

Show how to obtain the likelihood function based on $\{X_i \quad i=1,\ldots,n\}$, in a general case. Derive the likelihood function based on observed $X_1,\ldots X_n$.

Example 3:

04:30 PM–07:30 PM

This exam has 7 questions, some of which have subparts. Each question indicates its point value. The total is 100 points.

Show all your work. Justify all answers.
Good luck!

Question 1 (29 points) Characteristic functions

1.1 Define the characteristic function $\phi(t)$ of a random variable X. Show $\phi(t)$ exists, for all X and t. Assume X has the density function $f(u) = (2\pi\sigma^2)^{-1/2} \exp(-(u-\mu)^2/(2\sigma^2))$ with parameters μ and σ^2. Write out the expression for $\phi(t)$.

1.2 See Question 1, Section 13.1, Example 1.

1.3 See Question 1.2, Section 13.1, Example 2.

Question 2 (8 points)

Formulate and prove the central limit theorem related to the stopping time

$$N(H) = \inf\left\{n: \sum_{i=1}^{n} X_i \geq H\right\}, \text{ where } X_1 > 0, X_2 > 0,\ldots \text{ are iid, } EX_1 = a, Var(X_1) = \sigma^2 < \infty$$

and $H \to \infty$. (Here an asymptotic distribution of $N(H)$ should be shown.)

Question 3 (21 points)

Assume data points $X_1,\ldots,X_n$ are from a joint density function $f(x_1,\ldots,x_n;\theta)$, where θ is an unknown parameter. Suppose we want to test $H_0: \theta = 0$ versus $H_1: \theta \neq 0$. Complete the following:

3.1 Write the maximum likelihood ratio MLR_n and formulate the MLR test. Write the Bayes factor type likelihood ratio BLR_n. Show an optimality of BLR_n in the context of "most powerful decision rules" and interpret the optimality.

3.2 Find the asymptotic $(n \to \infty)$ distribution function of the statistic $2\log(MLR_n)$, under H_0.

3.3 Assume $X_1, \ldots, X_n$ are iid and the parameter $\theta = EX_1$. Let $f(x_1, \ldots, x_n; \theta)$ be unknown. To test for $H_0 : \theta = 0$ versus $H_1 : \theta \neq 0$, formulate the empirical likelihood ratio test statistic ELR_n. Find the asymptotic $(n \to \infty)$ distribution function of the statistic $2\log(ELR_n)$, under H_0, provided that $E|X_1|^3 < \infty$.

Question 4 (5 points)

What are Martingale, Submartingale and Supermartingale? Consider the test statistics MLR_n and BLR_n from Question 3. Under H_0, are these statistics Martingale, Submartingale, or Supermartingale? Justify your response.

Question 5 (11 points)

5.1 Formulate and prove: the Dub theorem (inequality) based on non-negative martingales and the Ville and Wald inequality

5.2 See Question 4.3, Section 13.1, Example 2.

Question 6 (10 points)

See Question 4, Section 13.1, Example 1.

Question 7 (16 points)

7.1 Show (in detail with all needed proofs) that

$$P\left\{\sum_{i=1}^{n} X_i \geq \frac{an}{m^{0.5}} + dm^{0.5}, \text{ for some } n \geq 1\right\} \leq \exp\{-2ad\}, d = \frac{\log(\varepsilon)}{2a},$$

for all $\varepsilon > 0$ and $a > 0$,

where $X_1, \ldots, X_n$ are iid and $X_1 \sim N(0,1)$. Here a proof of the general inequality

$$P\left\{\sum_{i=1}^{n} X_i \geq m^{0.5} A(\frac{n}{m}, \varepsilon) \text{ for some } n \geq 1\right\} \leq \frac{1}{\varepsilon} \quad (A(.,.) \text{ is a function that you}$$

should define) is required to be presented.

7.2 Suppose we are interested in confidence sequences with uniformly small error probability for the mean of a normal distribution $N(\theta, 1)$. Carry out the following:

7.2.1 Define the relevant confidence sequences.

7.2.2 Show the corresponding proofs.

7.2.3 Show how to operate with the required result.

7.2.4 Compare this approach with the conventional non-uniform confidence interval estimation.

Example 4:

11 AM–12:20 PM

This exam has 5 questions, some of which have subparts. Each question indicates its point value. The total is 100 points.

Show all your work. Justify all answers.
Good luck!

Question 1 (25 points)

Prove the following theorem (the inversion formula). Let f define a density function of a random variable X. Then

$$f(x) = \frac{1}{2\pi} \int_{-\infty}^{\infty} e^{-\mathrm{i}tx} E\left(e^{\mathrm{i}tX}\right) dt, \mathrm{i}^2 = -1, \mathrm{i} = \sqrt{-1}.$$

Question 2 (19 points)

Assume we have data points $X_1, \ldots, X_n$ that are iid observations from a density function f and $EX_1 = \theta$. We would like to test for $H_0 : \theta = \theta_0$ versus $H_1 : \theta = \theta_1$. Let f and θ_1 be unknown. Write the empirical likelihood ratio test statistic ELR_n. Find the asymptotic $(n \to \infty)$ distribution function of the statistic $2 \log ELR_n$, under H_0.

How can one use this asymptotic result to carry forth the ELR test in practice?

Question 3 (19 points)

See Question 2, Section 13.2, Example 3.

Question 4 (17 points)

4.1 Prove the Wald lemma regarding the expectation of a random sum of iid random variables. Can you use the Wald lemma to calculate

$$E\left(\sum_{i=1}^{\tau-1} X_i\right),$$ where $X_1,\ldots,X_n$ are iid with $EX_1 = 1$ and τ is a stopping

time with $E\tau = 25$? Relevant formal definitions of objects that you use (e.g., of a σ-algebra) should be presented.

4.2 See Question 4.3, Section 13.1, Example 2.

Question 5 (20 points)

Define statistics a_n and A_n based on a sample $z_1,\ldots,z_n$ of iid observations with the median M, such that the probability $\Pr\{a_n \le M \le A_n$ for every $n \ge m\}$ can be monitored (m is an integer number). The relevant proof should be present.

Example 5:

11:45 AM–1:05 PM

This exam has 6 questions, some of which have subparts. Each question indicates its point value. The total is 100 points.

Show all your work. Justify all answers.
Good luck!

Question 1 (12 points)

See Question 2, Section 13.2, Example 3.

Question 2 (16 points)

Assume that data points $X_1,\ldots,X_n$ are from a joint density function $f(x_1,\ldots,x_n;\theta)$, where θ is an unknown parameter. Suppose we want to test for $H_0 : \theta = 0$ versus $H_1 : \theta \ne 0$ then answer the following:

2.1 Write the maximum likelihood ratio MLR_n and formulate the MLR test. Find the asymptotic ($n \to \infty$) distribution function of the statistic $2\log MLR_n$, under H_0. Show how this asymptotic result can be used for the MLR test application.

2.2 Assume we would like to show how the asymptotic distribution obtained in Question 2.1 above is appropriate to the actual (real) distribution of the statistic $2logMLR_n$, when the sample size n is fixed. In this case, suggest an algorithm to compare the actual distribution of the test statistic with the asymptotic approximation to the actual distribution, when n is, say, 10, 20, 30.

Question 3 (19 points)

Relevant formal definitions of objects that you use to answer the question below (e.g., of a stopping time) should be presented. Formulate and prove:

3.1 The Dub theorem (inequality).

3.2 The Ville and Wald inequality.

Question 4 (13 points)

See Question 4, Section 13.1, Example 1.

Question 5 (14 points)

Confidence sequences for the median. See Question 5, Section 13.2, Example 4.

Question 6 (26 points)

See Question 3.3, Section 13.2, Example 3.

Example 6:

11.45 AM–1:05 PM

This exam has 7 questions, some of which have subparts. Each question indicates its point value. The total is 100 points.

Show all your work. Justify all answers.
Good luck!

Question 1 (19 points)

Assume we observe iid data points $X_1, \ldots, X_n$ and iid data points $Y_1, \ldots, Y_n$. It is known that $\operatorname{var}(X_1) = \sigma_X^2 < \infty$, $\operatorname{var}(Y_1) = \sigma_Y^2 < \infty$, $\Pr\{X_i \le u, Y_j \le v\} = \Pr\{X_i \le u\}\Pr\{Y_j \le v\}$ for $i \ne j$, and $\operatorname{cov}(X_i, Y_i) = \sigma_{XY}$, where σ_X^2, σ_Y^2 and σ_{XY} are known. An investigator wants to use the test statistic $G_n = \sqrt{n}\left(\dfrac{1}{n}\sum_{i=1}^{n} X_i - \dfrac{1}{n}\sum_{i=1}^{n} Y_i\right)$ to test for the hypothesis $H_0 : EX_1 = EY_1$. Using the method based on characteristic functions, propose an approach to control asymptotically, as $n \to 0$, the Type I error rate of the test: reject H_0 for large values of G_n. The corresponding proof should be shown. Do we need additional assumptions on the data distributions?

Question 2 (15 points)

See Question 2, Section 13.1, Example 3.

Question 3 (29 points)

Assume we have data points $X_1, \ldots, X_n$ that are iid observations and $EX_1 = \theta$. Suppose we would like to test $H_0 : \theta = \theta_0$ versus $H_1 : \theta = \theta_1$. Complete the following:

3.1 Let X_1 have a density function f with a known form that depends on θ. When θ_1 is assumed to be known, write the most powerful test statistic (the relevant proof should be shown).

3.2 Assuming θ_1 is unknown, write the maximum likelihood ratio MLR_n and formulate the MLR test based on $X_1, \ldots, X_n$. Find the asymptotic $(n \to \infty)$ distribution function of the statistic $2\log MLR_n$, under H_0.

3.3 Assume f and θ_1 are unknown. Write the empirical likelihood ratio test statistic ELR_n. Find the asymptotic $(n \to \infty)$ distribution function of the statistic $2\log ELR_n$, under H_0, provided that $E|X_1|^3 < \infty$.

Question 4 (10 points)

See Question 4, Section 13.1, Example 1.

Question 5 (9 points)

See Question 4.3, Section 13.1, Example 2.

Question 6 (9 points)

If it is possible, formulate a test with power 1. Relevant proofs should be shown.

Question 7 (9 points)

See Question 4, Section 13.2, Example 2.

Example 7:

This exam has 7 questions, some of which have subparts. Each question indicates its point value. The total is 100 points.

Show all your work. Justify all answers.
Good luck!

Question 1 (15 points)

1.1 Let $X_1, \ldots, X_n$ be independent identically Cauchy-distributed random variables with the characteristic function $\exp(-|t|)$ of X_1. What is a distribution function of $(X_1 + \ldots + X_n)/n$?

1.2 See Question 1.2, Section 13.1, Example 2.

Question 2 (14 points)

See Question 2, Section 13.3, Example 3.

Question 3 (14 points)

Let $\xi_1, \ldots, \xi_d$ be iid random variables from $N(0,1)$, $\eta_1, \ldots, \eta_d$ denote iid random variables from $N(0,1)$, and $\omega_1, \ldots, \omega_d$ be iid random variables that have only the two values 0 and 1 with $\Pr\{\omega_1 = 0\} = 0.5$. The random variables $\xi_1, \ldots, \xi_d$, $\eta_1, \ldots, \eta_d$, and $\omega_1, \ldots, \omega_d$ are independent and $\varepsilon_i = \omega_i \xi_i + (1 - \omega_i)\eta_i, i = 1, \ldots, d$.

Assume we have data points $X_1, \ldots, X_n$ that are iid observations and X_1 has a density function f that has a form of the density function of $\sum_{i=1}^{d} (\varepsilon_i)^2$, where the **integer** parameter d is unknown and $d \le 10$. Propose, giving the corresponding proof, the integrated most powerful test for $H_0 : EX_1 = \theta_0$ versus $H_1 : EX_1 \neq \theta_0$ (here θ_0 is known), provided that we are interested to obtain the maximum integrated power of the test when values of the alternative parameter can have all possible values with no preference. Should you need to use f, the analytical form of f should be derived. (Hint: Use characteristic functions to derive the form of f.)

Question 4 (19 points)

4.1 Define a martingale, submartingale, and supermartingale.

4.2 See Question 4.1, Section 13.1, Example 5.

4.3 Let $(X_n > 0, \Im_n)$ denote a martingale with $EX_1 = 1$. Is $\tau(H) = \min\{n > 0 : X_n > H\}$, where $H > 1$, a stopping time? (Corresponding proof should be shown.)

Question 5 (9 points)

Formulate and prove the Dub theorem (inequality).

Question 6 (14 points)

See Question 4.3, Section 13.1, Example 2.

Question 7 (15 points)

Confidence sequences for the median. See Question 5, Section 13.2, Example 4.

Example 8:

11:00 AM–12:20 PM

This exam has 9 questions, some of which have subparts. Each question indicates its point value. The total is 100 points.

Show all your work. Justify all answers.
Good luck!

Question 1 (18 points)

1.1 See Question 1.2, Section 13.1, Example 2.

1.2 Prove that the characteristic function of a symmetric (around 0) random variable is real-valued and even.

Question 2 (9 points)

Assume that $X_1, \ldots, X_n$ are iid random variables and
$X_1 \sim Exp(1)$, $S_n = (X_1 + \ldots + X_n)$. Let N define an integer random variable
that satisfies $\Pr\{N < \infty\} = 1, \{N \ge n\} \in \sigma(X_1, \ldots, X_n)$, where $\sigma(X_1, \ldots, X_n)$
is the σ-algebra based on $(X_1, \ldots, X_n)$. Calculate a value of
$E\exp(\hat{\imath} t S_N + N\log(1 - \hat{\imath} t))$, $\hat{\imath}^2 = -1$, where t is a real number. Proofs of the
theorems you use to solve this problem do not need to be shown.

Question 3 (9 points)

Biomarker levels were measured from disease and healthy populations, providing the iid observations $X_1 = 0.39, X_2 = 1.97, X_3 = 1.03, X_4 = 0.16$ that are assumed to be from a normal distribution as well as iid observations $Y_1 = 0.42, Y_2 = 0.29, Y_3 = 0.56, Y_4 = -0.68, Y_5 = -0.54$ that are assumed to be from a normal distribution, respectively.

Define the receiver operating characteristic (ROC) curve and the area under the curve (AUC).

Obtain a formal notation of the AUC.

Estimate the AUC.

What can you conclude regarding the discriminating ability of the biomarker with respect to the disease?

(Values that may help you to approximate the estimated AUC:
$\Pr\{\xi < x\} \approx 0.56, when\ x = 1, \xi \sim N(0.7, 4); \ \Pr\{\xi < x\} \approx 0.21, when\ x = 0, \xi \sim N(0.8, 1)$;
$\Pr\{\xi < x\} \approx 0.18, when\ x = 1, \xi \sim N(0.9, 1) \ \Pr\{\xi < x\} \approx 0.18, when\ x = 0, \xi \sim N(0.9, 1)$.)

Question 4 (11 points)

See Question 2, Section 13.1, Example 3.

Question 5 (14 points)

See Question 2, Section 13.2, Example 4.

Question 6 (11 points)

See Question 3, Section 13.2, Example 4.

Question 7 (10 points)

See Question 4, Section 13.1, Example 1.

Question 8 (9 points)

See Question 4.3, Section 13.1, Example 2.

Question 9 (9 points)

Confidence sequences for the median. See Question 5, Section 13.2, Example 4.

Comments. Regarding Question 1.2, we have $F(u) = 1 - F(-u)$. Then

$$\phi(t) = E\left(e^{it\xi}\right) = \int_{-\infty}^{\infty} e^{itu}\, dF(u) = \int_{\infty}^{-\infty} e^{-itu}\, dF(-u) = \int_{\infty}^{-\infty} e^{-itu} d\left(1 - F(u)\right) = \int_{-\infty}^{\infty} e^{-itu} d\left(F(u)\right)$$

$$= E\left(e^{-it\xi}\right).$$

Thus

$$\int_{-\infty}^{\infty} \left(\cos(tu) + i\sin(tu)\right) dF(u) = \int_{-\infty}^{\infty} \left(\cos(-tu) + i\sin(-tu)\right) dF(u),$$

where $\cos(tu) = \cos(-tu)$ and $\sin(-tx) = -\sin(tx)$. This leads to $E\left\{\sin(t\xi)\right\} = 0$ and then

$$\phi(t) = E\left(e^{it\xi}\right) = E\left\{\cos(t\xi)\right\}.$$

Regarding Question 2, we consider

$$E\left\{\exp\left(itS_n + n\log(1 - it)\right) \mid \sigma(X_1, \ldots, X_{n-1})\right\}.$$

for a fixed n. It is clear that

$$E\left\{\exp\left(itS_n + n\log(1 - it)\right) \mid \sigma(X_1, \ldots, X_{n-1})\right\} = \exp\left(itS_{n-1} + n\log(1 - it)\right)\varphi(t),$$

where $\varphi(t)$ is the characteristic function of X_1. This implies

$$E\left\{\exp\left(itS_n + n\log(1 - it)\right) \mid \sigma(X_1, \ldots, X_{n-1})\right\} = \exp\left(itS_{n-1} + (n-1)\log(1 - it)\right).$$

Then $\left\{\exp\left(itS_n + n\log(1 - it)\right), \sigma(X_1, \ldots, X_n)\right\}$ is a martingale and we can apply the optional stopping theorem.

Example 9:

This exam has 8 questions, some of which have subparts. Each question indicates its point value. The total is 100 points.

Show all your work. Justify all answers.
Good luck!

Question 1 (12 points)

Assume a receiver operating characteristic (ROC) curve corresponds to values of a biomarker measured with respect to a disease population, say X, and a healthy population, say Y. Let X and Y be independent and log-normally distributed, such that $X \sim \exp(\xi_1), Y \sim \exp(\xi_2)$, where $\xi_1 \sim N(\mu_1, \sigma_1^2), \xi_2 \sim N(\mu_2, \sigma_2^2)$ with known σ_1^2, σ_2^2 and unknown μ_1, μ_2. In order to estimate the area under the ROC curve (AUC), we observe iid data points $X_1, \ldots, X_n$ and iid data points $Y_1, \ldots, Y_m$ corresponding to X and Y, respectively.

Propose an estimator of the corresponding AUC. Using the δ-method, evaluate the asymptotic variance of the proposed estimator.

Question 2 (15 points)

See Question 2, Section 13.1, Example 3.

Question 3 (21 points)

See Question 3, Section 13.2, Example 6.

Question 4 (10 points)

See Question 4, Section 13.1, Example 1.

Question 5 (8 points)

See Question 4.3, Section 13.1, Example 2.

Question 6 (9 points)

If it is possible, formulate a test with power one. Relevant proofs should be shown.

Question 7 (10 points)

See Question 4, Section 13.2, Example 2.

Question 8 (15 points)

Assume iid random variables $X_1, X_2 \ldots$ are from the Uniform[0,1] distribution. Define the random variable $\tau = \inf\{n \geq 1 : X_n > a_n\}$.

Is τ a stopping time with respect to the σ-algebra $\mathfrak{I}_n = \sigma(X_1, \ldots, X_n)$, when $a_i = \left(1 - 1/(i+1)^2\right), i \geq 1$?

Is τ a stopping time with respect to $\mathfrak{I}_n = \sigma(X_1, \ldots, X_n)$, when $a_i = \left(1 - 1/(i+1)\right), i \geq 1$? Corresponding proofs should be shown.

13.3 Qualifying Exams

Example 1:

The PhD theory qualifying exam, Part I

8:30 AM–12:30 PM

This exam has 4 questions, some of which have subparts. Each question indicates its point value. The total is 100 points.

Show all your work. Justify all answers.
Good luck!

Question 1 (20 points) Characteristic functions

1.1 Define the characteristic function $\phi(t)$ of a random variable X. Show (and prove) that $\phi(t)$ exists, for all probability distributions of X and all real t. Assume X has the density function $f(u) = \left(2\pi\sigma^2\right)^{-1/2} \exp(-u^2/(2\sigma^2))$. What is a form of $\phi(t)$? Assume X has the density function $f(u) = \exp(-u), u > 0$. What is a form of $\phi(t)$?

1.2 Using characteristic functions, derive the analytical form of the distribution function of a χ_d^2-distributed random variable ξ, where d is the degree of freedom. (Hint: Use Gamma distributions.)

1.3 See Question 1.2, Section 13.1, Example 2.

Question 2 (30 points) Asymptotic results

2.1 Let $X_1,\ldots,X_n$ be iid observations. Suppose X_1 has a density function f that can be presented in a known parametric form depending on an unknown parameter θ. Define the maximum likelihood estimator of θ. Formulate and prove the theorem regarding an asymptotic distribution of the maximum likelihood estimator. (Please do not forget the assumptions of the theorem.)

2.2 Suppose we want to test for $H_0 : \theta = 0$ versus $H_1 : \theta \neq 0$ based on observations from Question 2.1 above.

    2.2.1 Towards this end, define the maximum likelihood ratio statistic ML_n and formulate the maximum likelihood ratio (MLR) test.

    2.2.2 Using the theorem from Question 2.1, derive the asymptotic distribution function of the statistic $2\log ML_n$, under H_0.

    2.2.3 Assume the sample size n is not large. Can you suggest a computational algorithm as an alternative to the asymptotic result from Question 2.2.2? If yes, provide the algorithm.

Question 3 (35 points) Testing

3.1 Let $X_1,\ldots,X_n$ be observations that have a joint density function $f.f$ can be presented in a known parametric form depending on an unknown parameter θ.

    3.1.1 Propose (and prove) the most powerful test for $H_0 : \theta = 0$ versus $H_1 : \theta = 1$.

    3.1.2 Propose (and prove) the integrated most powerful test for $H_0 : \theta = 0$ versus $H_1 : \theta \neq 0$ with respect to that we are interested in obtaining the maximum integrated power of the test when values of the alternative parameter belong to the uniform function

$$\pi(\theta) = \begin{cases} 1, \theta \in [0,1] \\ 0, \theta < 0 \qquad \text{(Hint: Use a Bayes factor type procedure.)} \\ 0, \theta > 1. \end{cases}$$

    3.1.3 Consider the test statistics from Wuestions 2.2.1, 3.1.1 and 3.1.2, say ML, L, and BL, respectively. Are the ML, L, and BL test statistics a martingale, submartingale or supermartingale under H_0? Are the log-transformed values, $log(ML)$, $log(L)$, and $log(BL)$ a martingale, submartingale or supermartingale under H_0? How about under H_1? Can you draw conclusions regarding the test statistics?

3.2 Assume a measurement model with autoregressive errors in the form of

$$X_i = \mu + \varepsilon_i, \quad \varepsilon_i = \beta\varepsilon_{i-1} + \xi_i, \ \xi_0 = 0, \quad i = 1,\ldots,n,$$

where ξ_i, $i = 1,\ldots,n$, are independent identically distributed (iid) with the distribution function $(2\pi)^{-1/2}\int_{-\infty}^{u}\exp(-u^2/2)du$. Suppose we are interested in the maximum likelihood ratio test for $H_0 : \mu = -1$ and $\varepsilon_i, i = 1,\ldots n$, are independent versus $H_1 : \mu = 0$ and $\varepsilon_i, i = 1,\ldots n$, are dependent. Then complete the following:

Write the relevant test in an analytical closed form.

Provide a schematic algorithm to evaluate the power of the test based on a Monte Carlo study.

3.3 See Question 4, Section 13.1, Example 1.

Question 4 (15 points)

4.1 Formulate and prove the optional stopping theorem for martingales (here provide formal definitions of objects that you use in this theorem, e.g., the definition of a stopping time).

4.2 Prove the Dub theorem (inequality) based on a nonnegative martingale.

4.3 Prove the Ville and Wald inequality.

Example 2:

The PhD theory qualifying exam, Part I

8:30 AM–12:30 PM

This exam has 8 questions, some of which have subparts. Each question indicates its point value. The total is 100 points.

Show all your work. Justify all answers.
Good luck!

Question 1 (31 points)

1.1 Let x, y denote real variables and $i^2 = -1, i = \sqrt{-1}$.
Show (prove) that $\exp(ix) = \cos(x) + i\sin(x)$.
Compute $(i)^i$ in the form of a real variable.

1.2 Define the characteristic function $\phi(t)$ of a random variable X. Prove that $\phi(t)$ exists for all probability distributions and all real t.

1.3 Prove the following theorem (the inversion formula). Let $y > x$ be real arguments of the distribution function $F(u) = \Pr\{X \le u\}$, where $F(.)$ is a continuous function at the points x and y. Then

$$F(y) - F(x) = \frac{1}{2\pi} \lim_{\sigma \to 0} \int_{-\infty}^{\infty} \frac{\exp(-itx) - \exp(-ity)}{it} \phi(t) \exp\left(-\frac{t^2 \sigma^2}{2}\right) dt.$$

1.4 See Question 1.2, Section 13.1, Example 2.

Question 2 (16 points)

Let $\varepsilon_1, \ldots, \varepsilon_d$ be iid random variables from $N(0,1)$. Assume we have data points $X_1, \ldots, X_n$ that are iid observations and X_1 has the density function f in a form of the density function of $\sum_{i=1}^{d} (\varepsilon_i)^2$, where the **integer** parameter d is unknown and $d \le 10$.

2.1 Write the maximum likelihood ratio (MLR) statistic, ML_n, and formulate the MLR test for $H_0 : EX_1 = \theta_0$ versus $H_1 : EX_1 \ne \theta_0$, where θ_0 is known. (Hint: Use characteristic functions to derive the form of f.)

2.2 Propose, providing a proof, the integrated most powerful test for $H_0 : EX_1 = \theta_0$ versus $H_1 : EX_1 \ne \theta_0$ (here θ_0 is known), provided that we are interested in obtaining the maximum integrated power of the test when values of the alternative parameter can have all possible values with no preference. (Hint: Use a Bayes factor type procedure.)

2.3 Assume the sample size n is not large. How can we apply the tests from Questions 2.1 and 2.2, in practice, without analytical evaluations of distribution functions of the test statistics? (i.e., assuming that you have a data set, how do you execute the tests?) Can you suggest computational algorithms? If yes, write the relevant algorithms. (Justify all answers.)

Question 3 (8 points)

Assume we observe iid data points $X_1, \ldots, X_n$ that follow a joint density function $f(x_1, \ldots, x_n; \theta)$, where θ is an unknown parameter. Suppose we want to test for the hypothesis $H_0 : \theta = \theta_0$ versus $H_1 : \theta = \theta_1$, where θ_0, θ_1 are known. In this case, propose (and give the relevant prove) the most powerful test. Examine theoretically asymptotic distributions of $\log(LR_n)/\sqrt{n}$ (here LR_n is the test statistic proposed by you) under H_0 and H_1, respectively. Show that $\log(LR_n)/n \xrightarrow[n \to \infty]{p} a$, where the constant $a \le 0$, under H_0 and $a \ge 0$, under H_1. (Hint: Use the central limit theorem, the proof of which **should be present**.)

Question 4 (14 points)

4.1 Formulate and prove the optional stopping theorem for martingales (here provide formal definitions of objects that you use, e.g., the definition of a martingale).

4.2 Prove the Wald theorem regarding the expectation of a random sum of iid random variables. Can you use the Wald theorem to calculate

$$E\left(\sum_{i=1}^{\tau-1} X_i\right), \ E\left(\sum_{i=1}^{\tau+1} X_i\right) \text{ and } E\left(\sum_{1\le i\le \tau/2} X_i\right), \text{ where } X_1,\dots,X_n \text{ are iid with}$$

$EX_1 = -1$ and τ is a stopping time with $E\tau = 4.5$? If yes, calculate the expectations.

4.3 Formulate and prove the following inequalities:
Dub theorem (Inequality) based on nonnegative martingales.
The Ville and Wald inequality.

Question 5 (7 points)

See Question 4, Section 13.1, Example 1.

Question 6 (8 points)

Assume the measurement model with autoregressive errors in the form of

$$X_i = \mu + \varepsilon_i, \quad \varepsilon_i = \beta\,\varepsilon_{i-1} + \xi_i, \quad \xi_0 = 0, \quad i = 1,\dots,n,$$

where ξ_i, $i = 1,\dots,n$, are independent identically distributed (iid) with the distribution function $(2\pi)^{-1/2}\int_{-\infty}^{u} \exp(-u^2/2)du$. We are interested in the maximum likelihood ratio test for

$H_0 : \mu = -1$ and $\varepsilon_i, i = 1,\dots n$, are independent

versus

$H_1 : \mu = 0$ and $\varepsilon_i, i = 1,\dots n$, are dependent.

Write the relevant test in an analytical closed form (here needed operations with joint densities and obtained forms of the relevant likelihoods should be explained).
Is the obtained test statistic, say L, a martingale/submartingale/supermartingale, under H_0 / H_1?
Is $log(L)$ a martingale/submartingale/supermartingale, under H_0?
(The proofs should be shown.)

Question 7 (8 points)

See Question 3.3, Section 13.2, Example 3.

Question 8 (7 points)

Let the stopping time have the form of $N(H) = \inf\left\{n : \sum_{i=1}^{n} x_i \geq H\right\}$, where x_i are iid random variables with $Ex_1 > 0$.

8.1 Show that $EN(H) = \sum_{j=1}^{\infty} P\{N(H) \geq j\}$. Is $EN(H) = \sum_{j=1}^{\infty} P\left\{\sum_{i=1}^{j} x_i < H\right\}$? If not what do we need to correct this equation?

8.2 Formulate (no proof is required) the central limit theorem related to the stopping time $N(H) = \inf\left\{n : \sum_{i=1}^{n} X_i \geq H\right\}$, where $X_i > 0, i > 0$, $EX_1 = a > 0, Var(X_1) = \sigma^2 < \infty$, and $H \to \infty$. (Here the asymptotic distribution of $N(H)$ should be shown.)

Example 3:

The PhD theory qualifying exam, Part I

8:30AM–12:30PM

This exam has 5 questions, some of which have subparts. Each question indicates its point value. The total is 100 points.

Show all your work. Justify all answers.
Good luck!

Question 1 (19 points)

1.1 Let x, y denote real variables and $i^2 = -1$, where i denotes an imaginary number. Compare $i^{(2i)}$ with $|\exp(-\pi) + i \exp(-\pi)|$ (i.e., "=", "<", ">"). (Here the proof and needed definitions should be provided.)

1.2 Obtain the characteristic function $\phi(t)$ of a random variable X that has a normal distribution $N(\mu, \sigma^2)$, where $EX = \mu$, $var(X) = \sigma^2$. (Justify your answer.)

1.3 See Question 1.3, Section 13.3, Example 2.

Question 2 (32 points)

2.1 Find, showing the proof, the asymptotic distribution of $\sum_{i=1}^{n} X_i / n^{1/2}$ as $n \to \infty$, where the random variables $X_1, \ldots, X_n$ are iid (independent identically distributed) with $EX_1 = 0$, $\mathrm{var}(X_1) = \sigma^2$.

2.2 See Question 2, Section 13.1, Example 3.

2.3 Consider the stopping time $N(H) = \inf\left\{ n : \sum_{i=1}^{n} X_i \geq H \right\}$, where $X_1 > 0, \ldots, X_n > 0$ are iid, $EX_1 = a < \infty$, $Var(X_1) = \sigma^2 < \infty$. Find, showing a proof, an asymptotic $(H \to \infty)$ distribution of $N(H)$.

2.4 Assume we observe iid data points $X_1, \ldots, X_n$ that are from a known joint density function $f(x_1, \ldots, x_n; \theta)$, where θ is an unknown parameter. We want to test for the hypothesis $H_0 : \theta = \theta_0$ versus $H_1 : \theta = \theta_1$, where θ_0, θ_1 are known. In this case, propose (and give the relevant proof) the most powerful test statistic, say, LR_n. Prove the asymptotic consistency of the proposed test: $\log(LR_n) / n \xrightarrow[n \to \infty]{p} a$, where the constant $a \leq 0$, under H_0 and $a \geq 0$, under H_1, just using that

$$\left| \int_{-\infty}^{\infty} \log\left(\frac{f_{H_1}(u)}{f_{H_0}(u)} \right) f_{H_0}(u) du \right| < \infty \text{ and } \left| \int_{-\infty}^{\infty} \log\left(\frac{f_{H_1}(u)}{f_{H_0}(u)} \right) f_{H_1}(u) du \right| < \infty \text{ (but}$$

without the constraint $\int_{-\infty}^{\infty} \left| \log\left(\frac{f_{H_1}(u)}{f_{H_0}(u)} \right) \right|^{1+\varepsilon} f_{H_j}(u) du < \infty$, $j = 0, 1, \varepsilon > 0$),

where f_{H_0} and f_{H_1} are the density functions of X_1 under H_0 and H_1, respectively. (You should define the limit value a and show $a \leq 0$, under H_0 and $a \geq 0$, under H_1.)

Question 3 (21 points)

3.1 See Question 4, Section 13.2, Example 2.

3.2 Assume you save your money in a bank and each day, i, you obtain a random benefit $r_i > 5.5$ that is independent of $r_1, \ldots, r_{i-1}$; you also can obtain money via a risky game having each day $Z_i = \begin{cases} 10, & \Pr\{Z_i = 10\} = 1/3 \\ -5, & \Pr\{Z_i = -5\} = 2/3 \end{cases}$

dollars, $i = 0, 1, \ldots$ (random variables Z_i are iid and independent of $r_1, \ldots, r_i$). You decide to stop the game when you collect \$100, that is, when $\sum_{i=1}^{} (Z_i + r_i) \geq 100$ the first time. When you stop, what will be your total expected benefit from the game (i.e., $E \sum_{i=1} (Z_i)$)? In general, formulate and prove the needed theorems to illustrate this result. Relevant formal definitions of objects that you use (e.g., of a stopping time) should be presented. When you apply a theorem the corresponding conditions should be checked.

3.3 See Question 4.3, Section 13.3, Example 2.

Question 4 (7 points)

See Question 4, Section 13.1, Example 1.

Question 5 (21 points)

5.1 See Question 7.1, Section 13.2, Example 3.

5.2 See Question 7.2, Section 13.2, Example 3.

5.3 Assume we survey $X_1, \ldots, X_n, \ldots$ iid observations and $X_1 \sim N(\theta, 1)$. Can we test for $\theta \leq 0$ versus $\theta > 0$ with power 1? If yes, propose the test and formal arguments (proofs).

Comments. Regarding Question 3.2, we note that, defining the random variable $\tau = \inf \left\{ n \geq 1 : \sum_{i=1}^{n} (Z_i + r_i) \geq 100 \right\}$, since $(Z_i + r_i) > 0$, we have, for a fixed N,

$$\Pr\{\tau > N\} = \Pr \left\{ \sum_{i=1}^{N} (Z_i + r_i) < 100 \right\} = \Pr \left\{ \exp \left(-\frac{1}{100} \sum_{i=1}^{N} (Z_i + r_i) \right) > e^{-1} \right\}$$

$$\leq e E \exp \left(-\frac{1}{100} \sum_{i=1}^{N} (Z_i + r_i) \right)$$

$$= e \left(E \exp \left(-\frac{1}{100} (Z_1 + r_1) \right) \right)^N \xrightarrow[N \to \infty]{} 0. \quad \Pr\{\tau < \infty\} = 1.$$

Then τ is a stopping time.

Example 4:

The PhD theory qualifying exam, Part I

8:30 AM–12:30 PM

This exam has 5 questions, some of which have subparts. Each question indicates its point value. The total is 100 points.

Show all your work. Justify all answers.
Good luck!

Question 1 (23 points)

1.1 See Question 1.1, Section 13.3, Example 1.

1.2 Assume independent random variables ξ_1 and ξ_2 are identically distributed with

$$\Pr\{\xi_1 < u\} = \begin{cases} 1, & u > 1 \\ (u)^{0.5}, & 0 \leq u \leq 1 \\ 0, & u < 0. \end{cases}$$

Derive the characteristic function $\phi(t)$ of $\eta = \max(\xi_1, \xi_2)$.

1.3 Using characteristic functions, derive the analytical form of the distribution function of a χ_d^2-distributed random variable ξ, where d is the degree of freedom. (Hint: Use Gamma distributions.)

1.4 See Question 1.2, Section 13.1, Example 2.

1.5 See Question 1, Section 13.2, Example 4.

Question 2 (23 points)

Assume we have data points $X_1, \ldots, X_n$ that are iid observations and $EX_1 = \theta$. We would like to test for the hypothesis $H_0 : \theta = \theta_0$ versus $H_1 : \theta = \theta_1$.

2.1 Let X_1 have a density function f with a known form that depends on θ. When θ_1 is assumed to be known, propose the most powerful test statistic (a relevant proof should be shown).
Is the couple (the corresponding test statistic and the sigma algebra $\sigma\{X_1, \ldots, X_n\}$) a martingale, submartingale, or supermartingale, under H_0/under H_1? (Justify your answer.)
Show (prove) that asymptotic distributions of $(n)^{-1/2} \times \log$ of the test statistic, under H_0 and H_1, respectively. (Should you use a theorem, show a relevant proof of the theorem.)

How can one use the asymptotic result obtained under H_0 to perform the test in practice? If possible, suggest an alternative method to evaluate the H_0-distribution of the test statistic.

2.2 Write the maximum likelihood ratio MLR_n and formulate the MLR test based on $X_1, \ldots, X_n$. Find the asymptotic ($n \to \infty$) distribution function of the statistic $2\log(MLR_n)$, under H_0.

Is the couple (the corresponding test statistic and sigma algebra $\sigma\{X_1, \ldots, X_n\}$) a martingale, submartingale or supermartingale under H_0? (Justify your answer.)

Illustrate how one can use this asymptotic result to perform the test in practice? Propose (if it is possible) an alternative to this use of the H_0-asymptotic distribution of the test statistic.

2.3 Assume f, the density function of $X_1, \ldots, X_n$, and θ_1 are unknown. Formulate the empirical likelihood ratio test statistic ELR_n. Find the asymptotic ($n \to \infty$) distribution function of the statistic $2\log(ELR_n)$, under H_0, provided that $E|X_1|^3 < \infty$. How can one use this asymptotic result to perform the corresponding test, in practice? Propose (if it is possible) an alternative to this use of the H_0-asymptotic distribution of the test statistic.

Question 3 (11 points)

Assume a measurement model with autoregressive error terms in the form

$$X_i = \mu + \varepsilon_i, \quad \varepsilon_i = \beta\varepsilon_{i-1} + \xi_i, \quad \varepsilon_0 = 0, X_0 = 0, \quad i = 1, \ldots, n,$$

where ξ_i, $i = 1, \ldots, n$ are independent identically distributed (iid) with a known density function $f_\varepsilon(u)$. Our data is based on observed $X_1, \ldots, X_n$.

3.1 Obtain the likelihood function (the joint density function) $f(X_1, \ldots, X_n)$, providing relevant formal arguments. The target likelihood should be presented in terms based on f_ε. (Suggestion: Show that $f(X_1, \ldots, X_n) = \prod f(X \cdots).$)

3.2 Let $\mu = 1$ and suppose that we would like to test that ε_i, $i = 1, \ldots, n$, are independent identically distributed random variables. Propose an integrated most powerful test, showing the relevant proof, when our interest is for $\beta \in (0, 1]$ uniformly under the alternative hypothesis.

Is the couple, the corresponding test statistic and the sigma algebra $\sigma\{X_1, \ldots, X_n\}$, a martingale, submartingale, or supermartingale under H_0? (Justify your answer.)

Can you suggest a method for obtaining critical values of the test statistic?

Question 4 (31 points)

4.1 Formulate and prove the optional stopping theorem. Relevant formal definitions of objects that you use (e.g., of martingales, a stopping time) should be presented.

4.2 Prove the Wald theorem regarding the expectation of a random sum of iid random variables.

4.3 Suppose $X_1 > 0, \ldots, X_n > 0$ are iid with $EX_1 = 1$ and τ is a stopping time with $E\tau = 25$. Can you use the Wald theorem to calculate

$$E\left(\sum_{i=1}^{\tau+1} X_i\right), E\left(\sum_{i=1}^{\tau/3} X_i\right), E\left(\sum_{i:i\le X_1+X_{25}} X_i\right), E\left(\sum_{i=1}^{v_1} X_i\right), E\left(\sum_{i=1}^{v_2+\tau} X_i\right), E\left(\sum_{i=1}^{v_2-\tau} X_i\right),$$

where $v_1 = \min\{n : X_n > 2n\}$, $v_2 = \min\left\{n : \sum_{i=1}^{n}(X_i) > 10000\right\}$? Justify your answers.

4.4 See Question 4.3, Section 13.3, Example 2.

4.5 See Question 2, Section 13.2, Example 3.

4.6 See Question 4, Section 13.1, Example 1.

Question 5 (12 points)

5.1 See Question 7.1, Section 13.2, Example 3.

5.2 See Question 5.3, Section 13.3, Example 3.

Example 5:

The PhD theory qualifying exam, Part I

8:30 AM–12:30 PM

This exam has 5 questions, some of which have subparts. Each question indicates its point value. The total is 100 points.

Show all your work. Justify all answers.
Good luck!

Question 1 (8 points)

1.1 Assume we observe $X_1, X_2, X_3 \ldots$, which are independent identically distributed (iid) data points with $EX_1 = \mu$ and an unknown variance.

To observe one X we should pay A dollars. We want to estimate μ using $\bar{X}_N = \sum_{i=1}^{N} X_i / N$. Propose a procedure to estimate μ minimizing the risk function $L(n) = An + E(\bar{X}_n - \mu)^2$ with respect to n.

1.2 Biomarker levels were measured from disease and healthy populations, providing iid observations $X_1 = 0.39, X_2 = 1.97, X_3 = 1.03, X_4 = 0.16$ that are assumed to be from a continuous distribution as well as iid observations $Y_1 = 0.42, Y_2 = 0.29, Y_3 = 0.56, Y_4 = -0.68, Y_5 = -0.54$ that are assumed to be from a continuous distribution, respectively. Define the receiver operating characteristic (ROC) curve and the area under the curve (AUC). Estimate nonparametrically the AUC. What can you conclude regarding the discriminating ability of the biomarker with respect to the disease?

Question 2 (28 points)

Define $i^2 = -1$, where i is an imaginary number, $i = \sqrt{-1}$.

2.1 See Questions 1.1–1.3, Section 13.3, Example 2.

2.2 Suppose the random variable η has a continuous density function and the characteristic function $\phi(t) = (\exp(it - t^2 / 2) - \exp(-t^2 / 2)) / (it)$, $i^2 = -1$. We know that $\eta = \eta_1 + \eta_2$, where $\eta_1 \sim N(0, 1)$ and η_2 has a continuous density function. Derive the density function of η_2. Show how to formally calculate the density function using the inversion formula. (Suggestion: Use the Dirichlet integrals that are employed to prove the inversion formula.)

2.3 Using characteristic functions, derive an analytical form of the distribution function of a χ_d^2-distributed random variable ξ, where d is the degree of freedom. (Hint: Use Gamma distributions.)

2.4 See Question 1.2, Section 13.1, Example 2.

Question 3 (20 points)

3.1 Assume we have two independent samples with data points $X_1, \ldots, X_n$ and $Y_1, \ldots, Y_m$, respectively. Let $X_1, \ldots, X_n$ be iid random observations with density function $f_x(x \mid \theta_X)$ and let $Y_1, \ldots, Y_m$ denote iid random observations with density function $f_y(x \mid \theta_Y)$, where θ_X and θ_Y are unknown parameters. Define $\hat{\theta}_n^X$ and $\hat{\theta}_m^Y$ to be the maximum likelihood estimators of θ_X and θ_Y based on $X_1, \ldots, X_n$ and $Y_1, \ldots, Y_m$, respectively. Given that $\theta_X = \theta_Y$, derive the asymptotic distribution of $(n + m)^{0.5}(\hat{\theta}_n^X - \hat{\theta}_m^Y)$, when $m / n \to \gamma$, for a known fixed γ, as $n \to \infty$. Show the relevant conditions and the proof. (Hint: Use that $a - b = (a - c) + (c - b)$.)

3.2 Assume we have data points $X_1,\ldots,X_n$ that are iid observations and $EX_1 = \theta$. Suppose we would like to test for the hypothesis $H_0 : \theta = \theta_0$. Write the maximum likelihood ratio test statistic MLR_n and formulate the MLR test based on $X_1,\ldots,X_n$. Find the asymptotic $(n \to \infty)$ distribution function of the statistic $2\log(MLR_n)$, under H_0.

Is the couple (the test statistic and sigma algebra $\sigma\{X_1,\ldots,X_n\}$) a martingale, submartingale, or supermartingale, under H_0? (Justify your answer.) Illustrate how to apply this asymptotic result in practice.

3.3 Suppose that we would like to test that iid observations $X_1,\ldots,X_n$ are from the density function $f_0(x)$ versus $X_1,\ldots,X_n \sim f_1(x\,|\,\theta)$, where the parameter $\theta > 0$ is unknown. Assume that $f_1(x\,|\,\theta) = f_0(x)\exp(\theta x - \phi(\theta))$, where ϕ is an unknown function. Write the most powerful test statistic and provide the corresponding proof.

Question 4 (28 points)

4.1 Formulate and prove the optional stopping theorem. Relevant formal definitions of objects that you use (e.g., martingales, a stopping time) should be presented.

4.2 Prove the Wald theorem regarding the expectation of a random sum of iid random variables.

4.3 Suppose $X_1 > 0,\ldots,X_n > 0,\ldots$ are iid random variable with $EX_1 = 1$ and τ is a stopping time with $E\tau = 25$. Can you use the Wald theorem to calculate

$$E\left(\sum_{i=1}^{\tau+1} X_i\right), E\left(\sum_{i=1}^{\tau/3} X_i\right), E\left(\sum_{i:i\le X_1+X_{25}} X_i\right), E\left(\sum_{i=1}^{v_1} X_i\right), E\left(\sum_{i=1}^{v_2+\tau} X_i\right), E\left(\sum_{i=1}^{v_2-\tau} X_i\right),$$

where $v_1 = \min\left\{n \ge 1 : \sum_{i=1}^{n} X_i > 2n^2(n+1)\right\}$ and $v_2 = \min\left\{n : \sum_{i=1}^{n} X_i > 10000\right\}$?

Justify your answers. (Suggestion: While analyzing v_1, you can use Chebyshev's inequality and that $\lim_{n\to\infty} \sum_{k=1}^{n} \frac{1}{k(k+1)} = \lim_{n\to\infty} \frac{n}{(n+1)} = 1$.)

4.4 Show the non-asymptotic inequality

$$E\left(\sum_{i=1}^{N(t)} X_i\right) \le \exp(1)(EX_1)\frac{E(\exp(-X_1/t))}{(1-E(\exp(-X_1/t)))},$$

where $X_1 > 0, \ldots, X_n > 0, \ldots$ are iid random variables with $EX_1 < \infty$ and

$$N(t) = \min\left\{n : \sum_{i=1}^{n} X_i > t\right\}.$$

4.5 See Question 4.3, Section 13.3, Example 2.

4.6 See Question 2, Section 13.2, Example 3.

4.7 See Question 4, Section 13.1, Example 1.

Question 5 (16 points)

5.1 See Question 7.1, Section 13.2, Example 3.

5.2 See Question 5.3, Section 13.3, Example 3.

5.3 See Question 7.2, Section 13.2, Example 3.

Comments. Regarding Question 2.2, we can use that $\exp(itx) = \cos(tx) + i\sin(tx)$ and the proof scheme related to the inversion theorem

$$F(y) - F(x) = \frac{1}{2\pi} \lim_{\sigma \to 0} \int_{-\infty}^{\infty} \frac{\exp(-itx) - \exp(-ity)}{it} \phi(t) \exp(-t^2\sigma^2) dt$$

in order to obtain the integrals $\int \cos(it(1-x))/(it)$, $\int \sin(it(1-x))/(it)$. Regarding Question 4.3, one can note that

$$\Pr(v_1 < \infty) = \sum_{j=1}^{\infty} \Pr(v_1 = j) = \sum_{j=1}^{\infty} \Pr\left(\max_{n<j} \sum_{i=1}^{n}(X_i) - 2n^2(n+1) < 0, \sum_{i=1}^{j}(X_i) > 2j^2(j+1)\right)$$

$$\leq \sum_{j=1}^{\infty} \Pr\left(\sum_{i=1}^{j}(X_i) > 2j^2(j+1)\right) \leq \sum_{j=1}^{\infty} \frac{E\left(\sum_{i=1}^{j} X_i\right)}{2j^2(j+1)} = \frac{1}{2}\sum_{j=1}^{\infty} \frac{1}{j(j+1)} = \frac{1}{2}.$$

Example 6:

The PhD theory qualifying exam, Part I

8:30 AM–12:30 PM

This exam has 5 questions, some of which have subparts. Each question indicates its point value. The total is 100 points.

Show all your work. Justify all answers.
Good luck!

Question 1 (10 points)

1.1 See Question 3, Section 13.2, Example 8.

1.2 See Question 4,2, Section 13.1, Example 7.

Question 2 (29 points)

2.1 Let X and Y be iid random variables with the characteristic function $\phi(t)$. Show that $|\phi(t)|^2$ is a characteristic function of $X-Y$.

2.2 Assume the random variables $X_1, X_2, X_3 \ldots$ are iid. The function $\phi(t)$ is a characteristic function of X_1. Define the characteristic function of $X_1 + X_2 + X_3 + \ldots + X_v$, where v is an integer random variable independent of $X_1, X_2, X_3 \ldots$ with $\Pr\{v = k\} = p_k, k = 1, 2, \ldots$

2.3 See Questions 1.1–1.3, Section 13.3, Example 2.

2.4 Suppose the random variable η has a continuous density function and the characteristic function $f(t) = \left(\exp(it - t^2/2) - \exp(-t^2/2)\right)/(it)$, $i^2 = -1$. We know that $\eta = \eta_1 + \eta_2$, where $\eta_1 \sim N(0,1)$ and η_2 has a continuous density function and η_1, η_2 are independent random variables. Derive the density function of η_2.
Show how to formally calculate the density function of η_2 using the inversion formula. (Suggestion: Use the Dirichlet integrals that are employed to prove the inversion formula.)

2.5 Let $X_1, \ldots, X_n$ be independent random variables with $EX_i = 0$, $EX_i^2 = \sigma_i^2 < \infty, i = 1, \ldots, n$. Use the method based on characteristic functions to define the asymptotic distribution of $\sum_{i=1}^{n} X_i / \left(\sum_{i=1}^{n} \sigma_i^2\right)^{0.5}$

as $n \to \infty$. What are the conditions on σ_i^2 and the moments of $X_1, \ldots, X_n$ you need, in order to show the result regarding the asymptotic distribution of $\sum_{i=1}^{n} X_i / \left(\sum_{i=1}^{n} \sigma_i^2\right)^{0.5}$?

Question 3 (31 points)

3.1 Suppose we observe iid data points $X_1,\ldots,X_n$ that are from a known joint density function $f(x_1,\ldots,x_n;\theta)$, where θ is an unknown parameter and we want to test the hypothesis $H_0:\theta=\theta_0$ versus $H_1:\theta=\theta_1$, where θ_0,θ_1 are known. Complete the following:

   3.1.1 Derive (and give the relevant proof) the most powerful test statistic, say, LR_n for H_0.

   3.1.2 See Question 2.4, Section 13.3, Example 3.

3.2 See Question 2, Section 13.1, Example 3.

3.3 Let $X_1,\ldots,X_n$ be observations that have joint density function f. f can be presented in a known parametric form depending on an unknown parameter θ.

   3.3.1 Propose (and prove) the integrated most powerful test for $H_0:\theta=0$ versus $H_1:\theta\neq 0$ with respect to obtaining the maximum integrated power of the test when values of the alternative parameter satisfy the uniform distribution with the density $\pi(\theta)=\begin{cases}1,\theta\in[0,1]\\0,\theta<0\\0,\theta>1.\end{cases}$

   3.3.2 Write the maximum likelihood ratio MLR_n and formulate the MLR test for $H_0:\theta=0$ versus $H_1:\theta\neq 0$ based on $X_1,\ldots,X_n$. Find the asymptotic $(n\to\infty)$ distribution function of the statistic $2\log MLR_n$, under H_0.
Illustrate how one can use this asymptotic result in practice.

   3.3.3 Is the couple (MLR_n and sigma algebra $\sigma\{X_1,\ldots,X_n\}$) a martingale, submartingale, or supermartingale under H_0? (Justify your answer.)

3.4 Assume f, the density function of $X_1,\ldots,X_n$, is unknown, $X_1,\ldots,X_n$ are iid, and $\theta=EX_1$. Complete the following:

   3.4.1 Formulate the empirical likelihood ratio test statistic ELR_n.

   3.4.2 Find the asymptotic $(n\to\infty)$ distribution function of the statistic $2\log(ELR_n)2\log(ELR_n)$, under H_0, provided that $E|X_1|^3<\infty$.

   3.4.3 How does one use this asymptotic result to perform the corresponding test, in practice?

3.5 See Question 3.3, Section 13.3, Example 5.

Question 4 (25 points)

4.1 Assume you save your money in a bank each day, i, and you obtain a random benefit $r_i>5.5$, where $r_1,\ldots,r_i,\ldots$ are iid. You also can obtain money via a risky game having each day $Z_i = \begin{cases} 10, & \Pr\{Z_i = 10\} = 1/3 \\ -5, & \Pr\{Z_i = -5\} = 2/3 \end{cases}$

dollars, $i = 0,1,\ldots$ (random variables Z_i are iid and independent of $r_1,\ldots,r_i$).

You decide to stop the game when you will collect \$100, that is, when

$$\sum_{i=1} (Z_i + r_i) \geq 100 \text{ the first time.}$$

It is known that $E\exp(-sr_i) = 0.5\left[\exp(-s10)/3 + 2\exp(s5)/3\right]^{-1}$ with $s = 1/100$.

4.1.1 When you stop, what will be your expected benefit from the risky game (i.e., $E\sum_{i=1}(Z_i)$)? When you apply the needed theorem, corresponding conditions should be checked. (Here the equation $\Pr\{\xi < u\} = \Pr\{\exp(-\xi/u) > \exp(-1)\}$ and Chebyshev's inequality can be applied.)

4.1.2 Formulate and prove the needed theorems in general. Relevant formal definitions of objects that you use (e.g., of a stopping time) should be presented.

4.2 Prove the Wald lemma regarding the expectation of a random sum of iid random variables.

4.3 See Question 4.3, Section 13.3, Example 2.

4.4 See Question 2, Section 13.2, Example 3.

4.5 See Question 4, Section 13.1, Example 1.

Question 5 (5 points)

Confidence sequences for the median. See Question 5, Section 13.2, Example 4. Compare this result with the corresponding well-known non-uniform confidence interval estimation.

Comments. Regarding Question 4.1, we note that, defining the random variable $\tau = \inf\left\{ n \geq 1 : \sum_{i=1}^{n} (Z_i + r_i) \geq 100 \right\}$, since $(Z_i + r_i) > 0$, we have, for a fixed N,

$$\Pr\{\tau > N\} = \Pr\left\{ \sum_{i=1}^{N}(Z_i + r_i) < 100 \right\} = \Pr\left\{ \exp\left(-\frac{1}{100}\sum_{i=1}^{N}(Z_i + r_i) \right) > e^{-1} \right\}$$

$$\leq eE\exp\left(-\frac{1}{100}\sum_{i=1}^{N}(Z_i + r_i) \right) = e\left(E\exp\left(-\frac{1}{100}(Z_1 + r_1) \right) \right)^{N} \underset{N\to\infty}{\to} 0. \quad \Pr\{\tau < \infty\} = 1.$$

Then τ is a stopping time.

Example 7:

The PhD theory qualifying exam, Part I

8:30–12:30

This exam has 10 questions, some of which have subparts. Each question indicates its point value. The total is 100 points.

Show all your work. Justify all answers.
Good luck!

Question 1 (9 points)

Assume a statistician has observed data points $X_1,\ldots,X_n$ and developed a test statistic T_n to test the hypothesis H_0 versus $H_1 = $ not H_0 based on $X_1,\ldots,X_n$. We do not survey $X_1,\ldots,X_n$, but we know the value of T_n and that T_n is distributed accordingly to the known density functions $f_0(u)$ and $f_1(u)$ under H_0 and H_1, respectively.

1.1 Can you propose a transformation of T_n (i.e., say, a function $G(T_n)$) that will improve the power of the test, when any other transformations, e.g., $K(T_n)$ based on a function $K(u)$, could provide less powerful tests, compared with the test based on $G(T_n)$? If you can construct such function G, you should provide a corresponding proof.

1.2 What is a form of T_n that satisfies $G(T_n) = T_n$? The corresponding proof must be shown here.
(Hint: The concept of the most powerful testing can be applied here.)

Question 2 (5 points)

Assume that $X_1,\ldots,X_n$ are independent and identically distributed (iid) random variables and $X_1 \sim N(0,1)$, $S_n = (X_1 + \ldots + X_n)$. N, an integer random variable, defines a stopping time. Calculate a value of $E\exp(itS_N + t^2 N / 2)$, where $i^2 = -1$ and t is a real number. Proofs of the theorems you use in this question are not required to be shown.

Question 3 (4 points)

See Question 3, Section 13.2, Example 8.

Question 4 (7 points)

See Question 4,2, Section 13.1, Example 7.

Question 5 (14 points)

5.1 Assume independent random variables ξ_1 and ξ_2 are identically Exp(1)-distributed. Derive the characteristic function $\phi(t)$ of $\eta = \min(\xi_1, \xi_2)$.

5.2 See Question 1.2, Section 13.1, Example 2.

5.3 See Question 1, Section 13.2, Example 4.

Question 6 (3 points)

Let the observations $X_1, \ldots, X_n$ be distributed with parameters (θ, σ), where σ is unknown. We want to test parametrically for the parameter θ ($\theta = 0$ under H_0). Define the Type I error rate of the test. Justify your answer.

Question 7 (20 points)

See Question 2, Section 13.3, Example 4.

Question 8 (10 points)

See Question 3, Section 13.3, Example 4.

Question 9 (23 points)

9.1 Formulate and prove the optional stopping theorem. Relevant formal definitions of objects that you use (e.g., martingales, a stopping time) should be present.

9.2 See Question 4.3, Section 13.3, Example 2.

9.3 See Question 2, Section 13.2, Example 3.

9.4 See Question 4, Section 13.1, Example 1.

Question 10 (5 points)

See Question 5.3, Section 13.3, Example 3.

Comments. Regarding Question 2, we consider $E\{\exp(itS_n + t^2n/2)\,|\,\sigma(X_1, \ldots, X_{n-1})\}$, for a fixed n. It is clear that $E\{\exp(itS_n + t^2n/2)\,|\,\sigma(X_1, \ldots, X_{n-1})\} = \exp(itS_{n-1} + t^2n/2)\varphi(t)$, where $\varphi(t)$ is the characteristic function of X_1. This implies

$$E\{\exp(itS_n + t^2n/2)\,|\,\sigma(X_1, \ldots, X_{n-1})\} = \exp(itS_{n-1} + t^2(n-1)/2).$$

Then $\left\{\exp\left(itS_n + t^2n/2\right), \sigma(X_1,...,X_n)\right\}$ is a martingale and we can apply the optional stopping theorem.

Example 8:

The PhD theory qualifying exam, Part I

8:30AM–12:30PM

This exam has 5 questions, some of which have subparts. Each question indicates its point value. The total is 100 points.

Show all your work. Justify all answers.
Good luck!

Question 1 (17 points)

1.1 Assume we have a test statistic, T, that is distributed as $N(1, \sigma^2 = 4)$ and $N(2, \sigma^2 = 5)$ under the null and alternative hypothesis, respectively. Define the expected p-value of the test statistic. Obtain the simple formal notation of the corresponding expected p-value, approximating it numerically via the use of the standard normal distribution curve below:

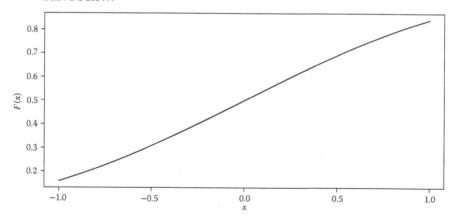

1.2 Suppose we observe values of the likelihood ratio test statistics $LR_i, i = 1,...,m$. The ratio LR_i was calculated corresponding to the hypotheses H_{0i} versus $H_{1i}, i = 1,...,m$. It is assumed that $LR_i, i = 1,...,m$, are independent and, for all $i = 1,...,m$, H_{ki} is a component of the hypothesis $H_k, k = 0,1$. Let the density functions $f^{LR_i}(u)$ of $LR_i, i = 1,...,m$, satisfy $f^{LR_i}(u \mid H_k) = f^{LR_i}(u \mid H_{ki}), k = 0,1, i = 1,...,m$.

Derive a likelihood ratio test statistic based on the observations $LR_1, ..., LR_m$ to test for H_0 versus H_1, providing relevant proofs of used propositions.

1.3 Biomarker levels were measured from disease and healthy populations, providing the independent and identically distributed (iid) observations $X_1 = 0.39, X_2 = 1.97, X_3 = 1.03, X_4 = 0.16$ that are assumed to be from a continuous distribution F_X as well as iid observations $Y_1 = 0.42, Y_2 = 0.29, Y_3 = 0.56, Y_4 = -0.68, Y_5 = -0.54$ that are assumed to be from a continuous distribution F_Y, respectively. Define the receiver operating characteristic (ROC) curve and an area under the curve (AUC). Estimate the AUC nonparametrically.
Estimate the AUC, assuming F_X and F_Y are normal distribution functions (the graph in Question 1.1 can help you).
What can you conclude regarding the discriminating ability of the biomarker with respect to the disease?

1.4 See Question 4,2, Section 13.1, Example 7.

Question 2 (29 points)

2.1 See Question 2.1, Section 13.3, Example 6.

2.2 Let X and Y be independent random variables. Assume $X - Y$ and $X + Y$ are identically distributed. Show the characteristic function of Y is a real value function.

2.3 See Question 2, Section 13.2, Example 8.

2.4 What is $|\ln(i)|, i^2 = -1$?

2.5 See Question 1.3, Section 13.3, Example 2.

2.6 Suppose the random variable η has a continuous density function and the characteristic function $\phi(t) = \left(\exp(it - t^2 / 2) - \exp(-t^2 / 2)\right) / (it), i^2 = -1$.
We know that $\eta = \eta_1 + \eta_2$, where $\eta_1 \sim N(0,1)$ and η_2 has a continuous density function. Derive the density function of η_2. Show formally how to obtain (calculate) the density function, using the inversion formula. (Suggestion: Use the Dirichlet integrals that are employed to prove the inversion formula.)

2.7 See Question 2.5, Section 13.3, Example 6.

Question 3 (23 points)

3.1 We observe iid data points $X_1, ..., X_n$ that are from a known joint density function $f(x_1, ..., x_n; \theta)$, where θ is an unknown parameter. We want to test for the hypothesis $H_0 : \theta = \theta_0$ versus $H_1 : \theta = \theta_1$, where θ_0, θ_1 are known.

3.1.1 Propose (and give a relevant prove) the most powerful test statistic, say, LR_n for H_0 versus H_1.

3.1.2 See Question 2.4, Section 13.3, Example 3.

3.2. Let $X_1,\ldots,X_n$ be observations that have a joint density function f that can be presented in a known parametric form, depending on an unknown parameter θ.

3.2.1 Propose (and prove) an integrated most powerful test for $H_0 : \theta = 0$ versus $H_1 : \theta \neq 0$ with respect to obtaining the maximum integrated power of the test when values of the alternative parameter satisfy the uniform distribution function with the density

$$\pi(\theta) = \begin{cases} 1, \theta \in [0,1] \\ 0, \theta < 0 \\ 0, \theta > 1. \end{cases}$$

3.2.2 Write the maximum likelihood ratio MLR_n and formulate the MLR test for $H_0 : \theta = 0$ versu $H_1 : \theta \neq 0$ based on $X_1,\ldots,X_n$. Find the asymptotic $(n \to \infty)$ distribution function of the statistic $2\log(MLR_n)$, under H_0.

3.2.3 Is the couple (MLR_n and sigma algebra $\sigma\{X_1,\ldots,X_n\}$) a martingale, submartingale, or supermartingale, under H_0? (Justify your answer.)

3.3 Assume f, the density function of $X_1,\ldots,X_n$, is unknown, $X_1,\ldots,X_n$ are iid and $\theta = EX_1$.

3.3.1 Define the empirical likelihood ratio test statistic ELR_n.

3.3.2 Find the asymptotic $(n \to \infty)$ distribution function of the statistic $2\log(ELR_n)$, under H_0, provided that $E|X_1|^3 < \infty$.

3.4 See Question 3.3, Section 13.3, Example 5.

Question 4 (26 points)

4.1. Assume you save your money in a bank account each day, i, and you obtain a random benefit $r_i > 5.5$, $r_1,\ldots,r_i,\ldots$ are iid. You also can obtain

money via a risky game having each day $Z_i = \begin{cases} 11, & \Pr\{Z_i = 10\} = 1/3 \\ -5, & \Pr\{Z_i = -5\} = 2/3 \end{cases}$

dollars, $i = 0,1,\ldots$ (random variables Z_i are iid and independent of $r_1,\ldots,r_i$).

You decide to stop the game when you will collect \$100, that is, when at a first time n: $\displaystyle\sum_{i=1}^{n}(Z_i + r_i) \geq 100$.

It is known that, for all $t > 0$ and $j > 0$, $\Pr\left\{\sum_{i=1}^{j}(Z_i + r_i) \le t\right\} = t/(j(j+1))$, when

$t/(j(j+1)) \le 1$, and $\Pr\left\{\sum_{i=1}^{j}(Z_i + r_i) \le t\right\} = 1$, when $t/(j(j+1)) \ge 1$.

4.1.1 What will be your expected benefit from the risky game stopped

at a first time n: $\sum_{i=1}^{n}(Z_i + r_i) \ge 100$, that is, $E\left(\sum_{i=1}^{n}Z_i\right)$? When you

apply a needed theorem, corresponding conditions should be

checked. (Suggestion: Use that $\sum_{i=1}^{\infty}1/(j(j+1)) = 1$.)

4.1.2 Formulate and prove needed theorems in general. Relevant formal definitions of objects that you use (e.g., of a stopping time) should be presented.

4.2 Prove the optional stopping theorem.

4.3 Formulate and prove the Dub theorem (inequality) based on non-negative martingales.

4.4 See Question 3, Section 13.2, Example 4.

4.5 See Question 4, Section 13.1, Example 1.

4.6 See Question 4.3, Section 13.1, Example 2.

Question 5 (5 points)

See Question 5.3, Section 13.3, Example 3.

Comments. Several relevant comments can be found with respect to the examples shown in the sections above. Regarding Question 4.1, we note that,

defining the random variable $\tau = \inf\left\{n \ge 1 : \sum_{i=1}^{n}(Z_i + r_i) \ge 100\right\}$, since $(Z_i + r_i) > 0$, we have, for a fixed N,

$$\Pr\{\tau > N\} = \Pr\left\{\sum_{i=1}^{N}(Z_i + r_i) < 100\right\} = \Pr\left\{\exp\left(-\frac{1}{100}\sum_{i=1}^{N}(Z_i + r_i)\right) > e^{-1}\right\}$$

$$\le eE\exp\left(-\frac{1}{100}\sum_{i=1}^{N}(Z_i + r_i)\right) = e\left(E\exp\left(-\frac{1}{100}(Z_1 + r_1)\right)\right)^{N} \underset{N\to\infty}{\to} 0. \quad \Pr\{\tau < \infty\} = 1.$$

Then τ is a stopping time with $E(\tau) = \sum_{j=1}^{\infty}\Pr\left\{\sum_{i=1}^{j}(Z_i + r_i) < 100\right\}$.

14

Examples of Course Projects

In this chapter we outline examples of projects that can be proposed for individuals or groups of students relative to the course material contained in this textbook. In order to work on the projects, students will be encouraged to state correctly the corresponding problems, read the relevant literature and provide a research result. The minimal expectation is that a Monte Carlo study is performed in the context of the corresponding project. We believe that interesting solutions related to the proposed projects have the potential to be published in statistical journals. This can motivate students to try to develop methodological approaches regarding the course projects.

14.1 Change Point Problems in the Model of Logistic Regression Subject to Measurement Errors

Assume we observe independent data points $\{Y_i = (0,1), i = 1,...,n\}$ that satisfy the model

$$\Pr(Y_i = 1 \mid X_i) = (1 + \exp(-\alpha_0 - \beta_0 X_i))^{-1} I(v < i) + (1 + \exp(-\alpha_1 - \beta_1 X_i))^{-1} I(v \geq i),$$

where $\alpha_0, \alpha_1, \beta_0, \beta_1$ and v are parameters. The issue examined in this study is a change point problem of hypothesis testing, where $H_0 : v \notin [1,n]$ versus $H_1 : 1 \leq v \leq n$, $v > 0$ is unknown. In this statement we consider scenarios when $\{X_i, i = 1,...,n\}$ are unobserved, whereas the change point detection schemes should be based on $\{Y_i, Z_i = X_i + \varepsilon_i, i = 1,...,n\}$, where $\varepsilon_1,...,\varepsilon_n$ denote the measurement error terms.

14.2 Bayesian Inference for Best Combinations Based on Values of Multiple Biomarkers

In Section 7.5, we considered the best combinations of multiple biomarkers in the context of the ROC analysis. The proposed method extends the Su and

Liu (1993) concept to cases when prior information related to the parameters of biomarker distributions is assumed to be specified.

14.3 Empirical Bayesian Inference for Best Combinations Based on Values of Multiple Biomarkers

In the case of multivariate normally distributed data, Stein (1956) proved that when the dimension of the observed vectors is greater than or equal to three, the maximum likelihood estimators (MLEs) are inadmissible estimators of the corresponding parameters. James and Stein (1961) provided another estimator that yields a frequentist risk (MSE) smaller than that of the MLEs. Efron and Morris (1972) showed that the James–Stein estimator belongs to a class of *posterior empirical Bayes* (PEB) point estimators in the Gaussian/Gaussian model (Carlin and Louis, 2011). Su and Liu (1993) proposed the MLEs of best combinations based on multivariate normally distributed values of biomarkers. In this project, we evaluate an improvement of Su and Liu's estimation scheme, using the PEB concept instead of the MLE.

14.4 Best Combinations Based on Log Normally Distributed Values of Multiple Biomarkers

Oftentimes measurements related to biological processes follow a log-normal distribution (see for details Limpert, et al., 2001; Vexler et al., 2016a, pp. 13–14). In this context, we assume, without the loss of generality, that two biomarkers are measured presenting log-normally distributed values of (X_1, X_2) and (Y_1, Y_2) corresponding to the case and control populations. In general, X_1 and X_2 can be dependent, and Y_1 can be dependent on Y_2. In order to apply the ROC curve analysis, one can use the following approaches: (1) the Su and Liu (1993) method, obtaining the best linear combination based on normally distributed $(\log(X_1), \log(X_2))$ and $(\log(Y_1), \log(Y_2))$ variables; (2) we can construct the best combination of the biomarker values using the distribution of (X_1, X_2) and (Y_1, Y_2) (e.g., Pepe and Thompson, 2000); (3) the best linear combination based on log-normally distributed (X_1, X_2) and (Y_1, Y_2) variables; (4) a technique that approximates the distribution function of a sum of log-normally distributed random variables via a log-normal distribution. The research question in this project is to compare these techniques, making suggestions when to employ method (1), (2), (3), or (4) with respect to different values of the data distribution parameters, taking into account relative complexities of the methods.

14.5 Empirical Likelihood Ratio Tests for Parameters of Linear Regressions

Consider, for example, the following relatively simple scenario. Observe independent data points $(Y_1, X_1), ..., (Y_n, X_n)$ that satisfy the linear regression model $E(Y_i \mid X_i) = \beta X_i, i = 1, ..., n$, where β is a parameter. Assume we are interested in the empirical likelihood ratio test of $H_0 : \beta = \beta_0$ versus $H_1 : \beta \neq \beta_0$. Following the empirical likelihood methodology (Chapter 10), under the null hypothesis, the empirical likelihood can be presented as

$$
\max_{0 < p_1, ..., p_n < 1} \left(\prod_{i=1}^{n} p_i : \sum_{i=1}^{n} p_i = 1, \sum_{i=1}^{n} p_i (Y_i - \beta_0 X_i) = 0 \right),
$$

when the empirical version of $E(Y_i - \beta X_i) = E[E((Y_i - \beta X_i) \mid X_i)] = 0, i = 1, ..., n$, is taken into account. However, we also have

$$
E(X_i(Y_i - \beta X_i)) = E[E(X_i(Y_i - \beta X_i) \mid X_i)] = E[X_i E((Y_i - \beta X_i) \mid X_i)] = 0, i = 1, ..., n.
$$

Then, one can propose the H_0 – empirical likelihood in the form

$$
\max_{0 < p_1, ..., p_n < 1} \left(\prod_{i=1}^{n} p_i : \sum_{i=1}^{n} p_i = 1, \sum_{i=1}^{n} p_i (Y_i - \beta_0 X_i) = 0, \sum_{i=1}^{n} p_i X_i (Y_i - \beta_0 X_i) = 0 \right).
$$

Moreover, it is clear that $E(X_i^k (Y_i - \beta X_i)) = 0, i = 1, ..., n, k = 0, 1, 2, 3...$ Therefore, in general, we can define that the H_0 – empirical likelihood is

$$
L_k(\beta_0) = \max_{0 < p_1, ..., p_n < 1} \left(\prod_{i=1}^{n} p_i : \sum_{i=1}^{n} p_i = 1, \sum_{i=1}^{n} p_i (Y_i - \beta_0 X_i) = 0, \right.
$$

$$
\left. \sum_{i=1}^{n} p_i X_i (Y_i - \beta_0 X_i) = 0, ..., \sum_{i=1}^{n} p_i X_i^k (Y_i - \beta_0 X_i) = 0 \right).
$$

In this case, the nonparametric version of Wilks' theorem regarding the empirical likelihood ratio test statistic $n^{-n}/L_k(\beta_0)$ can provide the result that $2 \log(n^{-n}/L_k(\beta_0))$ has an asymptotic chi-square distribution with $k + 1$ degrees of freedom under the null hypothesis. It can be anticipated that, for a fixed sample size n, relatively small values of k provide a "good" Type I error rate control via Wilks' theorem, since k defines the number of constraints to be in effect when the empirical likelihood is derived. However, relatively large values of k will increase the power of the test. The question to be evaluated in this study is the following: What are the optimal values of k that, depending on n, lead to an appropriate Type I error rate control and maximize the power of the empirical likelihood ratio test? Theoretically, this issue corresponds to higher order approximations to the Type I error rate and the power of the test.

14.6 Penalized Empirical Likelihood Estimation

The *penalized* parametric likelihood methodology is well addressed in the modern statistical literature. In parallel with the penalized parametric likelihood techniques, this research proposes and examines their nonparametric counterparts, using the material of Chapters 5, 10, Section 10.5, and methods shown in Qin and Lawless (1994).

14.7 An Improvement of the AUC-Based Interference

In Section 7.3.1, it is shown that, for the diseased population $X \sim N(\mu_1, \sigma_1^2)$ and for the non-diseased population $Y \sim N(\mu_2, \sigma_2^2)$, a closed form of the AUC

is $A = \Phi\left(\dfrac{\mu_1 - \mu_2}{\sqrt{\sigma_1^2 + \sigma_2^2}}\right)$. Then, in the case with $\mu_1 = \mu_2$, the AUC cannot assist in

detecting differences between the distributions of X and Y when $\sigma_1^2 \neq \sigma_2^2$. Towards this end, we propose considering the AUC based on the random variables $Z(X, X^2)$ and $Z(Y, Y^2)$, where X^2, Y^2 are chi-square distributed and the function Z is chosen to maximize the AUC, $\Pr\{Z(X, X^2) > Z(Y, Y^2)\}$ (see Section 7.5 in this context). As a first stage in this statement of the problem, we can consider $Z(u, v) = u + av$, where $a = \arg\max_\lambda \Pr\left(X + \lambda X^2 > Y + \lambda Y^2\right)$.

14.8 Composite Estimation of the Mean based on Log-Normally Distributed Observations

Let iid data points $X_1, ..., X_n$ be observed. Assume that X_1 is distributed as the random variable e^ξ, where $\xi \sim N(\mu, \sigma^2)$ with unknown parameters μ, σ^2. The problem is to estimate $\theta = EX_1$. Since $\theta = \exp(\mu + \sigma^2 / 2)$, the maximum likelihood estimation can provide the estimator $\hat{\theta} = \exp(\hat{\mu} + \hat{\sigma}^2 / 2)$ of θ, where

$\hat{\mu}, \hat{\sigma}^2$ are the maximum likelihood estimators of μ, σ^2. However, it can be anticipated that the simple estimator $\bar{\theta} = \sum_{i=1}^{n} X_i / n$ of $\theta = EX_1$ can outperform $\hat{\theta}$ for relatively small values of n. The research issue in this project is related to how to combine $\hat{\theta}$ and $\bar{\theta}$ to optimize the confidence interval estimation of θ, depending on n.

References

Ahmad, I. A. (1996). A class of Mann-Whitney-Willcoxon type statistics. *American Statistician*, **50**, 324–327.

Armitage, P. (1975). *Sequential Medical Trials*. New York, NY: John Wiley & Sons.

Armitage, P. (1981). Importance of prognostic factors in the analysis of data from clinical trials. *Controlled Clinical Trials*, **1**(4), 347–353.

Armitage, P. (1991). Interim analysis in clinical trials. *Statistics in Medicine*, **10**(6), 925–937.

Armstrong, D. (2015). *Advanced Protocols in Oxidative Stress III*. New York, NY: Springer.

Balakrishnan, N., Johnson, N. L. and Kotz, S. (1994). *Continuous Univariate Distributions*. New York, NY: Wiley Series in Probability and Statistics.

Balakrishnan, N. and Lai, C.-D. (2009). *Continuous Bivariate Distributions*. New York, NY: Springer.

Bamber, D. (1975). The area above the ordinal dominance graph and the area below the receiver operating characteristic graph. *Journal of Mathematical Psychology*, **12**(4), 387–415.

Barnard, G. A. (1946). Sequential tests in industrial statistics. *Supplement to the Journal of the Royal Statistical Society*, **8**(1), 1–26.

Bartky, W. (1943). Multiple sampling with constant probability. *Annals of Mathematical Statistics*, **14**(4), 363–377.

Bauer, P. and Kohne, K. (1994). Evaluation of experiments with adaptive interim analyses. *Biometrics*, **50**(4), 1029–1041.

Bayarri, M. J. and Berger, J. O. (2000). P values for composite null models. *Journal of the American Statistical Association*, **95**, 1127–1142.

Belomestnyi, D. V. (2005). Reconstruction of the general distribution by the distribution of some statistics. *Theory of Probability & Its Applications*, **49**, 1–15.

Berger, J. O. (1980). *Statistical Decision Theory: Foundations, Concepts, and Methods*. New York, NY: Springer-Verlag.

Berger, J. O. (1985). *Statistical Decision Theory and Bayesian Analysis*. New York, NY: Springer-Verlag.

Berger, J. O. (2000). Could Fisher, Jeffreys and Neyman have agreed on testing? *Statistical Science*, **18**. 1–12.

Berger, J. O. and Sellke, T. (1987). Testing a point null hypothesis: The irreconcilability of P values and evidence. *Journal of the American Statistical Association*, **82**(397), 112–122.

Berger, J. O., Wolpert, R. L., Bayarri, M. J., DeGroot, M. H., Hill, B. M., Lane, D. A. and LeCam, L. (1988). The likelihood principle. *Lecture Notes—Monograph Series*, **6**, iii–v, vii–xii, 1–199.

Berger, R. L. and Boss, D. D. (1994). P values maximized over a confidence set for the nuisance parameter. *Journal of the American Statistical Association*, **89**, 1012–1016.

Bernardo, J. M. and Smith, A. F. M. (1994). *Bayesian Theory*. Toronto: Wiley.

Bickel, P. J. and Doksum, K. A. (2007). *Mathematical Statistics: Basic Ideas and Selected Topics*. 2nd ed., Vol. I, Updated Printing. Upper Saddle River, NJ: Pearson Prentice Hall.

Bleistein, N. and Handelsman, R. A. (1975). *Asymptotic Expansions of Integrals*. New York, NY: Courier Corporation.

Booth, J. G. and Sarkar, S. (1998). Monte Carlo approximation of bootstrap variances. *American Statistician*, **52**(4), 354–357.

Borovkov, A. A. (1998). *Mathematical Statistics*. The Netherlands: Gordon & Breach Science Publishers.

Box, G. E. (1980). Sampling and Bayes' inference in scientific modelling and robustness. *Journal of the Royal Statistical Society. Series A (General)*, **143**(4), 383–430.

Box, G. E. and Cox, D. R. (1964). An analysis of transformations. *Journal of the Royal Statistical Society. Series B (Methodological)*, **26**(2), 211–252.

Bressoud, D. M. (2008). *A Radical Approach to Lebesgue's Theory of Integration*. New York, NY: Cambridge University Press.

Broemeling, L. D. (2007). *Bayesian Biostatistics and Diagnostic Medicine*. New York, NY: Chapman & Hall.

Brostrom, G. (1997). A martingale approach to the changepoint problem. *Journal of the American Statistical Association*, **92**, 1177–1183.

Bross, I. D., Gunter, B., Snee, R. D., Berger, R. L., et al. (1994). Letters to the editor. *American Statistician*, 48, 174–177.

Browne, R. H. (2010). The t-test p value and its relationship to the effect size and $P(X>Y)$. *American Statistician*, **64**(1), 30–33.

Campbell, G. (1994). Advances in statistical methodology for the evaluation of diagnostic and laboratory tests. *Statistics in Medicine*, 13(5–7), 499–508.

Carlin, B. P. and Louis, T. A. (2011). *Bayesian Methods for Data Analysis*. Boca Raton, FL: CRC Press.

Chen, M. H. and Shao, Q. M. (1999). Monte Carlo estimation of Bayesian credible and HPD intervals. *Journal of Computational and Graphic Statistics*, **8**, 69–92.

Chen, X., Vexler, A. and Markatou, M. (2015). Empirical likelihood ratio confidence interval estimation of best linear combinations of biomarkers. *Computational Statistics & Data Analysis*, **82**, 186–198.

Chow, Y. S., Robbins, H. and Siegmund, D. (1971). *Great Expectations: The Theory of Optimal Stopping*. Boston, MA: Houghton Mifflin.

Chuang, C.-S. and Lai, T. L. (2000). Hybrid resampling methods for confidence intervals. *Statistica Sinica*, **10**(1), 1–32.

Chung, K. L. (1974). *A Course in Probability Theory*. San Diego, CA: Academic Press.

Chung, K. L. (2000). *A Course in Probability Theory*. 2nd ed. London: Academic Press.

Claeskens, G. and Hjort, N. L. (2004). Goodness of fit via non-parametric likelihood ratios. *Scandinavian Journal of Statistics*, **31**(4), 487–513.

Copas, J. and Corbett, P. (2002). Overestimation of the receiver operating characteristic curve for logistic regression. *Biometrika*, **89**(2), 315–331.

Cornish, E. A. and Fisher, R. A. (1937). Moments and cumulants in the specification of distributions. *Review of the International Statistical Institute*, **5**, 307–322.

Cox, R. (1962). *Renewal Theory*. New York, NY: Methuen & Company.

Crawley, M. J. (2012). *The R Book*. United Kingdom: John Wiley & Sons.

Csörgö, M. and Horváth, L. (1997). *Limit Theorems in Change-Point Analysis*. New York, NY: Wiley.

Cutler, S., Greenhouse, S., Cornfield, J. and Schneiderman, M. (1966). The role of hypothesis testing in clinical trials: Biometrics seminar. *Journal of Chronic Diseases*, **19**(8), 857–882.

Daniels, M. and Hogan, J. (2008). *Missing Data in Longitudinal Studies: Strategies for Bayesian Modeling and Sensitivity Analysis*. New York, NY: Chapman & Hall.

Davis, C. S. (1993). The computer generation of multinomial random variates. *Computational Statistics & Data Analysis*, **16**(2), 205–217.

Davison, A. C. and Hinkley, D. V. (1997). *Bootstrap Methods and Their Application*. Cambridge: Cambridge University Press.

De Bruijn, N. G. (1970). *Asymptotic Methods in Analysis*. Amsterdam: Dover Publications.

DeGroot, M. H. (2005). *Optimal Statistical Decisions*. Hoboken, NJ: John Wiley & Sons.

Delwiche, L. D. and Slaughter, S. J. (2012). *The Little SAS Book: A Primer: A Programming Approach*. Cary, NC: SAS Institute.

Dempster, A. P. and Schatzoff, M. (1965). Expected significance level as a sensitivity index for test statistics. *Journal of the American Statistical Association*, 60, 420–436.

Desquilbet, L. and Mariotti, F. (2010). Dose-response analyses using restricted cubic spline functions in public health research. *Statistics in Medicine*, **29**(9), 1037–1057.

DiCiccio, T. J., Kass, R. E., Raftery, A. and Wasserman, L. (1997). Computing Bayes factors by combining simulation and asymptotic approximations. *Journal of the American Statistical Association*, **92**(439), 903–915.

Dmitrienko, A., Molenberghs, G., Chuang-Stein, C. and Offen, W. (2005). *Analysis of Clinical Trials Using SAS: A Practical Guide*. Cary, NC: SAS Institute.

Dmitrienko, A., Tamhane, A. C. and Bretz, F. (2010). *Multiple Testing Problems in Pharmaceutical Statistics*. New York, NY: CRC Press.

Dodge, H. F. and Romig, H. (1929). A method of sampling inspection. *Bell System Technical Journal*, **8**(4), 613–631.

Dragalin, V. P. (1997). The sequential change point problem. *Economic Quality Control*, **12**, 95–122.

Edgar, G. A. and Sucheston, L. (2010). *Stopping Times and Directed Processes (Encyclopedia of Mathematics and Its Applications)*. New York, NY: Cambridge University Press.

Efron, B. (1979). Bootstrap methods: Another look at the jackknife. *Annals of Statistics*, **7**(1), 1–26.

Efron, B. (1981). Nonparametric standard errors and confidence intervals. *The Canadian Journal of Statistics/La Revue Canadienne de Statistique*, **9**(2), 139–158.

Efron, B. (1986). How biased is the apparent error rate of a prediction rule? *Journal of the American Statistical Association*, **81**(394), 461–470.

Efron, B. and Morris, C. (1972). Limiting risk of Bayes and empirical Bayes estimators. *Journal of the American Statistical Association*, **67**, 130–139.

Efron, B. and Tibshirani, R. J. (1994). *An Introduction to the Bootstrap*. Boca Raton, FL: CRC Press.

Eng, J. (2005). Receiver operating characteristic analysis: A primer. *Academic Radiology*, **12**(7), 909–916.

Evans, M. and Swartz, T. (1995). Methods for approximating integrals in statistics with special emphasis on Bayesian integration problems. *Statistical Science*, **10**(3), 254–272.

Everitt, B. S. and Palmer, C. (2010). *Encyclopaedic Companion to Medical Statistics*. Hoboken, NJ: John Wiley & Sons.

Fan, J., Farmen, M. and Gijbels, I. (1998). Local maximum likelihood estimation and inference. *Journal of the Royal Statistical Society: Series B (Statistical Methodology)*, **60**(3), 591–608.

Fan, J., Zhang, C. and Zhang, J. (2001). Generalized likelihood ratio statistics and Wilks phenomenon. *Annals of Statistics*, **29**(1), 153–193.

Fawcett, T. (2006). An introduction to ROC analysis. *Pattern Recognition Letters*, **27**(8), 861–874.

Feuerverger, A. and Mureika, R. (1977). The empirical characteristic function and its applications. *Annals of Statistics*, **5**, 88–97.

Finkelestein, M., Tucker, H. G. and Veeh, J. A. (1997). Extinguishing the distinguished logarithm problems. *Proceedings of the American Mathematical Society*, **127**, 2773–2777.

Firth, D. (1993). Bias reduction of maximum likelihood estimates. *Biometrika*, **80**, 27–38.

Fisher, R. (1925). *Statistical Methods for Research Workers*. Edinburgh: Oliver & Boyd.

Fisher, R. A. (1921). On the "probable error" of a coefficient of correlation deduced from a small sample. *Metron*, **1**, 3–32.

Fisher, R. A. (1922). On the mathematical foundations of theoretical statistics. *Philosophical Transactions of the Royal Society A*, **222**, 309–368.

Fluss, R., Faraggi, D. and Reiser, B. (2005). Estimation of the Youden index and its associated cutoff point. *Biometrical Journal*, **47**, 458–472.

Food and Drug Administration. (1988). *Guideline for the Format and Content of the Clinical and Statistical Sections of New Drug Applications*. FDA, U.S. Department of Health and Human Services, Rockville, MD.

Freeman, H. A., Friedman, M., Mosteller, F. and Wallis, W. A. (1948). *Sampling Inspection*. New York, NY: McGraw-Hill.

Freiman, J. A., Chalmers, T. C., Smith, H. Jr. and Kuebler, R. R. (1978). The importance of beta, the type II error and sample size in the design and interpretation of the randomized control trial. Survey of 71 "negative" trials. *New England Journal of Medicine*, **299**(13), 690–694.

Gardener, M. (2012). *Beginning R: The Statistical Programming Language*. Canada: John Wiley & Sons.

Gavit, P., Baddour, Y. and Tholmer, R. (2009). Use of change-point analysis for process monitoring and control. *BioPharm International*, **22**(8), 46–55.

Gelman, A., Carlin, J. B., Stern, H. S. and Rubin, D. B. (2003). *Bayesian Data Analysis*. Boca Raton, FL: CRC Press.

Gelman, A., Carlin, J. B., Stern, H. S., Dunson, D. B., Vehtari, A. and Rubin, D. B. (2013). *Bayesian Data Analysis*. Boca Raton, FL: CRC Press.

Genz, A. and Kass, R. E. (1997). Subregion-adaptive integration of functions having a dominant peak. *Journal of Computational and Graphical Statistics*, **6**(1), 92–111.

Geweke, J. (1989). Bayesian inference in econometric models using Monte Carlo integration. *Econometrica: Journal of the Econometric Society*, **57**(6), 1317–1339.

Ghosh, M. (1995). Inconsistent maximum likelihood estimators for the Rasch model. *Statistics & Probability Letters*, **23**(2), 165–170.

Gönen, M., Johnson, W. O., Lu, Y. and Westfall, P. H. (2005). The Bayesian two-sample t-test. *American Statistician*, **59**(3), 252–257.

Good, I. (1992). The Bayes/non-Bayes compromise: A brief review. *Journal of the American Statistical Association*, **87**(419), 597–606.

Gordon, L. and Pollak, M. (1995). A robust surveillance scheme for stochastically ordered alternatives. *Annals of Statistics*, **23**, 1350–1375.

Green, D. M. and Swets, J. A. (1966). *Signal Detection Theory and Psychophysics*. New York, NY: Wiley.

Grimmett, G. and Stirzaker, D. (1992). *Probability and Random Processes*. Oxford: Oxford University Press.

Gurevich, G. and Vexler, A. (2005). Change point problems in the model of logistic regression. *Journal of Statistical Planning and Inference*, **131**(2), 313–331.

Gurevich, G. and Vexler, A. (2010). Retrospective change point detection: From parametric to distribution free policies. *Communications in Statistics—Simulation and Computation*, **39**(5), 899–920.

Hall, P. (1992). *The Bootstrap and Edgeworth Expansions*. New York, NY: Springer.

Hammersley, J. M. and Handscomb, D. C. (1964). *Monte Carlo Methods*. New York, NY: Springer.

Han, C. and Carlin, B. P. (2001). Markov chain Monte Carlo methods for computing Bayes factors. *Journal of the American Statistical Association*, **96**(455), 1122–1132.

Hartigan, J. (1971). Error analysis by replaced samples. *Journal of the Royal Statistical Society. Series B (Methodological)*, **33**(2), 98–110.

Hartigan, J. A. (1969). Using subsample values as typical values. *Journal of the American Statistical Association*, **64**(328), 1303–1317.

Hartigan, J. A. (1975). Necessary and sufficient conditions for asymptotic joint normality of a statistic and its subsample values. *Annals of Statistics*, **3**(3), 573–580.

Hosmer, D. W. Jr. and Lemeshow, S. (2004). *Applied Logistic Regression*. Hoboken, NJ: John Wiley & Sons.

Hsieh, F. and Turnbull, B. W. (1996). Nonparametric and semiparametric estimation of the receiver operating characteristic curve. *Annals of Statistics*, **24**(1), 25–40.

Hwang, J. T. G. and Yang, M-c. (2001). An optimality theory for MID p-values in 2×2 contingency tables. *Statistica Sinica*, **11**, 807–826.

James, W. and Stein, C. (1961). Estimation with quadratic loss. *Proceedings of the Fourth Berkeley Symposium on Mathematical Statistics and Probability*, **1**, 361–379.

Janzen, F. J., Tucker, J. K. and Paukstis, G. L. (2000). Experimental analysis of an early life-history stage: Selection on size of hatchling turtles. *Ecology*, **81**(8), 2290–2304.

Jeffreys, H. (1935). Some tests of significance, treated by the theory of probability. *Mathematical Proceedings of the Cambridge Philosophical Society*, **31**(2), 203–222.

Jeffreys, H. (1961). *Theory of Probability*. Oxford: Oxford University Press.

Jennison, C. and Turnbull, B. W. (2000). *Group Sequential Methods with Applications to Clinical Trials*. New York, NY: CRC Press.

Johnson, M. E. (1987). *Multivariate Statistical Simulations*. New York, NY: John Wiley & Sons.

Julious, S. A. (2005). Why do we use pooled variance analysis of variance? *Pharmaceutical Statistics*, **4**, 3–5.

Kass, R. E. (1993). Bayes factors in practice. *Statistician*, **42**(5), 551–560.

Kass, R. E. and Raftery, A. E. (1995). Bayes factors. *Journal of the American Statistical Association*, **90**(430), 773–795.

Kass, R. E. and Vaidyanathan, S. K. (1992). Approximate Bayes factors and orthogonal parameters, with application to testing equality of two binomial proportions. *Journal of the Royal Statistical Society. Series B (Methodological)*, **54**(1), 129–144.

Kass, R. E. and Wasserman, L. (1995). A reference Bayesian test for nested hypotheses and its relationship to the Schwarz criterion. *Journal of the American Statistical Association*, **90**(431), 928–934.

Kass, R. E. and Wasserman, L. (1996). The selection of prior distributions by formal rules. *Journal of the American Statistical Association*, **91**(435), 1343–1370.

Kass, R. E., Tierney, L. and Kadane, J. B. (1990). The validity of posterior asymptotic expansions based on Laplace's method. *Bayesian and Likelihood Methods in Statistics and Econometrics: Essays in Honor of George A. Barnard*. Geisser, S., Hodges, J. S., Press, S. J. and ZeUner, A. (Eds.), New York, NY: North-Holland.

Kepner, J. L. and Chang, M. N. (2003). On the maximum total sample size of a group sequential test about binomial proportions. *Statistics & Probability Letters*, **62**(1), 87–92.

Koch, A. L. (1966). The logarithm in biology 1. Mechanisms generating the log-normal distribution exactly. *Journal of Theoretical Biology*, **12**(2), 276–290.

Konish, S. (1978). An approximation to the distribution of the sample correlation coefficient. *Biometrika*, **65**, 654–656.

Korevaar, J. (2004). *Tauberian Theory*. New York, NY: Springer.

Kotz, S., Balakrishnan, N. and Johnson, N. L. (2000). *Continuous Multivariate Distributions, Models and Applications*. New York, NY: John Wiley & Sons.

Kotz, S., Lumelskii, Y. and Pensky, M. (2003). *The Stress-Strength Model and Its Generalizations: Theory and Applications*. Singapore: World Scientific Publishing Company.

Krieger, A. M., Pollak, M. and Yakir, B. (2003). Surveillance of a simple linear regression. *Journal of the American Statistical Association*, **98**, 456–469.

Lai, T. L. (1995). Sequential changepoint detection in quality control and dynamical systems. *Journal of the Royal Statistical Society. Series B (Methodological)*, **57**(4), 613–658.

Lai, T. L. (1996). On uniform integrability and asymptotically risk-efficient sequential estimation. *Sequential Analisis*, **15**, 237–251.

Lai, T. L. (2001). Sequential analysis: Some classical problems and new challenges. *Statistica Sinica*, **11**, 303–408.

Lane-Claypon, J. E. (1926). *A Further Report on Cancer of the Breast with Special Reference to Its Associated Antecedent Conditions*. Ministry of Health. Reports on Public Health and Medical Subjects (32), London.

Lasko, T. A., Bhagwat, J. G., Zou, K. H. and Ohno-Machado, L. (2005). The use of receiver operating characteristic curves in biomedical informatics. *Journal of Biomedical Informatics*, **38**(5), 404–415.

Lazar, N. A. (2003). Bayesian empirical likelihood. *Biometrika*, **90**(2), 319–326.

Lazar, N. A. and Mykland, P. A. (1999). Empirical likelihood in the presence of nuisance parameters. *Biometrika*, **86**(1), 203–211.

Lazzeroni, L. C., Lu, Y. and Belitskaya-Levy, I. (2014). P-values in genomics: Apparent precision masks high uncertainty. *Molecular Psychiatry*, **19**, 1336–1340.

Le Cam, L. (1953). On some asymptotic properties of maximum likelihood estimates and related Bayes' estimates. *University of California Publications in Statistics*, **1**, 277–330.

Le Cam, L. (1986). *Asymptotic Methods in Statistical Decision Theory*. New York, NY: Springer-Verlag.

Lee, E. T. and Wang, J. W. (2013). *Statistical Methods for Survival Data Analysis*. Hoboken, NJ: John Wiley & Sons.

Lehmann, E. L. and Casella, G. (1998). *Theory of Point Estimation*. New York, NY: Springer-Verlag.

Lehmann, E. L. and Romano, J. P. (2006). *Testing Statistical Hypotheses*. New York, NY: Springer-Verlag.

Limpert, E., Stahel, W. A. and Abbt, M. (2001). Log-normal distributions across the sciences: Keys and clues on the charms of statistics, and how mechanical models resembling gambling machines offer a link to a handy way to characterize log-normal distributions, which can provide deeper insight into variability and probability—Normal or log-normal: That is the question. *BioScience*, **51**(5), 341–352.

Lin, C.-C. and Mudholkar, G. S. (1980). A simple test for normality against asymmetric alternatives. *Biometrika*, **67**(2), 455–461.

Lin, Y. and Shih, W. J. (2004). Adaptive two-stage designs for single-arm phase IIA cancer clinical trials. *Biometrics*, **60**(2), 482–490.

Lindsey, J. (1996). *Parametric Statistical Inference*. Oxford: Oxford University Press.

Liptser, R. Sh. and Shiryayev, A. N. (1989). *Theory of Martingales*. London: Kluwer Academic Publishers.

Liu, A. and Hall, W. (1999). Unbiased estimation following a group sequential test. *Biometrika*, **86**(1), 71–78.

Liu, C., Liu, A. and Halabi, S. (2011). A min–max combination of biomarkers to improve diagnostic accuracy. *Statistics in Medicine*, **30**(16), 2005–2014.

Lloyd, C. J. (1998). Using smoothed receiver operating characteristic curves to summarize and compare diagnostic systems. *Journal of the American Statistical Association*, **93**(444), 1356–1364.

Lorden, G. and Pollak, M. (2005). Nonanticipating estimation applied to sequential analysis and changepoint detection. *The Annals of Statistics*, **33**, 1422–1454.

Lucito, R., West, J., Reiner, A., Alexander, J., Esposito, D., Mishra, B., Powers, S., Norton, L. and Wigler, M. (2000). Detecting gene copy number fluctuations in tumor cells by microarray analysis of genomic representations. *Genome Research*, **10**(11), 1726–1736.

Lukacs, E. (1970). *Characteristic Functions*. London: Charles Griffin & Company.

Lusted, L. B. (1971). Signal detectability and medical decision-making. *Science*, **171**(3977), 1217–1219.

Mallows, C. L. (1972). A note on asymptotic joint normality. *Annals of Mathematical Statistics*, **39**, 755–771.

Marden, J. I. (2000). Hypothesis testing: From p values to Bayes factors. *Journal of the American Statistical Association*, **95**, 1316–1320.

Martinsek, A. T. (1981). A note on the variance and higher central moments of the stopping time of an SPRT. *Journal of the American Statistical Association*, **76**(375), 701–703.

McCulloch, R. and Rossi, P. E. (1991). A Bayesian approach to testing the arbitrage pricing theory. *Journal of Econometrics*, **49**(1), 141–168.

McIntosh, M. W. and Pepe, M. S. (2002). Combining several screening tests: Optimality of the risk score. *Biometrics*, **58**(3), 657–664.

Meng, X.-L. and Wong, W. H. (1996). Simulating ratios of normalizing constants via a simple identity: A theoretical exploration. *Statistica Sinica*, **6**(4), 831–860.

Metz, C. E., Herman, B. A. and Shen, J. H. (1998). Maximum likelihood estimation of receiver operating characteristic (ROC) curves from continuously-distributed data. *Statistics in Medicine*, **17**(9), 1033–1053.

Mikusinski, P. and Taylor, M. D. (2002). *An Introduction to Multivariable Analysis from Vector to Manifold*. Boston, MA: Birkhäuser.

Montgomery, D. C. (1991). *Introduction to Statistical Quality Control*. New York, NY: Wiley.

Nakas, C. T. and Yiannoutsos, C. T. (2004). Ordered multiple-class ROC analysis with continuous measurements. *Statistics in Medicine*, **23**(22), 3437–3449.

Newton, M. A. and Raftery, A. E. (1994). Approximate Bayesian inference with the weighted likelihood bootstrap. *Journal of the Royal Statistical Society. Series B (Methodological)*, **56**(1), 3–48.

Neyman, J. and Pearson, E. S. (1928). On the use and interpretation of certain test criteria for purposes of statistical inference: Part II. *Biometrika*, **20A**(3/4), 263–294.

Neyman, J. and Pearson, E. S. (1933). The testing of statistical hypotheses in relation to probabilities a priori. *Mathematical Proceedings of the Cambridge Philosophical Society*, **29**(4), 492–510.

Neyman, J. and Pearson, E. S. (1938). Contributions to the theory of testing statistical hypotheses. *Journal Statistical Research Memoirs (University of London)*, **2**, 25–58.

Obuchowski, N. A. (2003). Receiver operating characteristic curves and their use in radiology 1. *Radiology*, **229**(1), 3–8.

Owen, A. B. (1988). Empirical likelihood ratio confidence intervals for a single functional. *Biometrika*, **75**(2), 237–249.

Owen, A. B. (1990). Empirical likelihood ratio confidence regions. *The Annals of Statistics*, **18**(1), 90–120.

Owen, A. B. (1991). Empirical likelihood for linear models. *The Annals of Statistics*, **19**(4), 1725–1747.

Owen, A. B. (2001). *Empirical Likelihood*. Boca Raton, FL: CRC Press.

Pepe, M. S. (1997). A regression modelling framework for receiver operating characteristic curves in medical diagnostic testing. *Biometrika*, **84**(3), 595–608.

Pepe, M. S. (2000). Receiver operating characteristic methodology. *Journal of the American Statistical Association*, **95**(449), 308–311.

Pepe, M. S. (2003). *The Statistical Evaluation of Medical Tests for Classification and Prediction*. Oxford: Oxford University Press.

Pepe, M. S. and Thompson, M. L. (2000). Combining diagnostic test results to increase accuracy. *Biostatistics*, **1**(2), 123–140.

Petrone, S., Rousseau, J. and Scricciolo, C. (2014). Bayes and empirical Bayes: Do they merge? *Biometrika*, **101**(2), 285–302.

Petrov, V. V. (1975). *Sums of Independent Random Variables*. New York, NY: Springer.

Piantadosi, S. (2005). *Clinical Trials: A Methodologic Perspective*. Hoboken, NJ: John Wiley & Sons.

Pocock, S. J. (1977). Group sequential methods in the design and analysis of clinical trials. *Biometrika*, **64**(2), 191–199.

Pollak, M. (1985). Optimal detection of a change in distribution. *The Annals of Statistics*, **13**, 206–227.

Pollak, M. (1987). Average run lengths of an optimal method of detecting a change in distribution. *The Annals of Statistics*, **5**(2), 749–779.

Powers, L. (1936). The nature of the interaction of genes affecting four quantitative characters in a cross between Hordeum deficiens and Hordeum vulgare. *Genetics*, **21**(4), 398.

Proschan, M. A. and Shaw, P. A. (2016). *Essentials of Probability Theory for Statisticians*. New York, NY: Chapman & Hall/CRC.

Provost, F. J. and Fawcett, T. (1997). Analysis and visualization of classifier performance: Comparison under imprecise class and cost distributions. In *Proceedings of the Third International Conference on Knowledge Discovery and Data Mining*, AAAI Press, 43–48.

Qin, J. (2000). Combining parametric and empirical likelihoods. *Biometrika*, **87**(2), 484–490.

Qin, J. and Lawless, J. (1994). Empirical likelihood and general estimating equations. *The Annals of Statistics*, **22**(1), 300–325.

Qin, J. and Leung, D. H. (2005). A semiparametric two-component "compound" mixture model and its application to estimating malaria attributable fractions. *Biometrics*, **61**(2), 456–464.

Qin, J. and Zhang, B. (2005). Marginal likelihood, conditional likelihood and empirical likelihood: Connections and applications. *Biometrika*, **92**(2), 251–270.

Quenouille, M. H. (1949). Problems in plane sampling. *The Annals of Mathematical Statistics*, **20**(3), 355–375.

Quenouille, M. H. (1956). Notes on bias in estimation. *Biometrika*, **43**(3–4), 353–360.

R Development Core Team. (2014). *R: A Language and Environment for Statistical Computing*. R Foundation for Statistical Computing, Vienna, Austria.

Reid, N. (2000). Likelihood. *Journal of the American Statistical Association*, **95**, 1335–1340.

Reiser, B. and Faraggi, D. (1997). Confidence intervals for the generalized ROC criterion. *Biometrics*, **53**(2), 644–652.

Richards, R. J., Hammitt, J. K. and Tsevat, J. (1996). Finding the optimal multiple-test strategy using a method analogous to logistic regression the diagnosis of hepatolenticular degeneration (Wilson's disease). *Medical Decision Making*, **16**(4), 367–375.

Ritov, Y. (1990). Decision theoretic optimality of the CUSUM procedure. *The Annals of Statistics*, **18**, 1464–1469.

Robbins, H. (1959). Sequential estimation of the mean of a normal population. *Probability and Statistics (Harold Cramér Volume)*. Stockholm: *Almquist and Wiksell*, pp. 235–245.

Robbins, H. (1970). Statistical methods related to the law of the iterated logarithm. *The Annals of Mathematical Statistics*, **41**, 1397–1409.

Robbins, H. and Siegmund, D. (1970). Boundary crossing probabilities for the Wiener process and sample sums. *The Annals of Mathematical Statistics*, 41, 1410–1429.

Robbins, H. and Siegmund, D. (1973). A class of stopping rules for testing parametric hypotheses. In *Proceedings of Sixth Berkeley Symposium of Mathematical Statistics and Probability*, University of California Press, 37–41.

Robert, C. P. and Casella, G. (2004). *Monte Carlo Statistical Methods*. 2nd ed., New York, NY: *Springer*.

Sackrowitz, H. and Samuel-Cahn, E. (1999). P values as random variables-expected p values. *The American Statistician*, **53**, 326–331.

SAS Institute Inc. (2011). *SAS® 9.3 Macro Language: Reference*. Cary, NC: SAS Institute.

Schiller, F. (2013). Die Verschwörung des Fiesco zu Genua. Berliner: CreateSpace Independent Publishing Platform.

Schisterman, E. F., Faraggi, D., Browne, R., Freudenheim, J., Dorn, J., Muti, P., Armstrong, D., Reiser, B. and Trevisan, M. (2001a). Tbars and cardiovascular disease in a population-based sample. *Journal of Cardiovascular Risk*, **8**(4), 219–225.

Schisterman, E. F., Faraggi, D., Browne, R., Freudenheim, J., Dorn, J., Muti, P., Armstrong, D., Reiser, B. and Trevisan, M. (2002). Minimal and best linear combination of oxidative stress and antioxidant biomarkers to discriminate cardiovascular disease. *Nutrition, Metabolism, and Cardiovascular Disease*, **12**, 259–266.

Schisterman, E. F., Faraggi, D., Reiser, B. and Trevisan, M. (2001b). Statistical inference for the area under the receiver operating characteristic curve in the presence of random measurement error. *American Journal of Epidemiology*, **154**, 174–179.

Schisterman, E. F., Perkins, N. J., Liu, A. and Bondell, H. (2005). Optimal cut-point and its corresponding Youden index to discriminate individuals using pooled blood samples. *Epidemiology*, **16**, 73–81.

Schisterman, E. F., Vexler, A., Ye, A. and Perkins, N. J. (2011). A combined efficient design for biomarker data subject to a limit of detection due to measuring instrument sensitivity. *The Annals of Applied Statistics*, **5**, 2651–2667.

Schwarz, G. (1978). Estimating the dimension of a model. *The Annals of Statistics*, **6**(2), 461–464.

Schweder, T. and Hjort, N. L. (2002). Confidence and likelihood. *Scandinavian Journal of Statistics*, **29**(2), 309–332.

Serfling, R. J. (2002). *Approximation Theorems of Mathematical Statistics*. Canada: John Wiley & Sons.

Shao, J. and Tu, D. (1995). *The Jackknife and Bootstrap*. New York, NY: Springer Science & Business Media.

Shao, J. and Wu, C. F. J. (1989). A general theory for jackknife variance estimation. *The Annals of Statistics*, **17**, 1176–1197.

Shapiro, D. E. (1999). The interpretation of diagnostic tests. *Statistical Methods in Medical Research*, **8**(2), 113–134.

Siegmund, D. (1968). On the asymptotic normality of one-sided stopping rules. *The Annals of Mathematical Statistics*, **39**(5), 1493–1497.

Simon, R. (1989). Optimal two-stage designs for phase II clinical trials. *Controlled Clinical Trials*, **10**(1), 1–10.

Singh, K., Xie, M. and Strawderman, W. E. (2005). Combining information from independent sources through confidence distributions. *The Annals of Statistics*, **33**(1), 159–183.

Sinharay, S. and Stern, H. S. (2002). On the sensitivity of Bayes factors to the prior distributions. *The American Statistician*, **56**(3), 196–201.

Sinnott, E. W. (1937). The relation of gene to character in quantitative inheritance. *Proceedings of the National Academy of Sciences of the United States of America*, **23**(4), 224.

Sleasman, J. W., Nelson, R. P., Goodenow, M. M., Wilfret, D., Hutson, A., Baseler, M., Zuckerman, J., Pizzo, P. A. and Mueller, B. U. (1999). Immunoreconstitution after ritonavir therapy in children with human immunodeficiency virus infection involves multiple lymphocyte lineages. *The Journal of Pediatrics*, **134**, 597–606.

Smith, A. F. and Roberts, G. O. (1993). Bayesian computation via the Gibbs sampler and related Markov chain Monte Carlo methods. *Journal of the Royal Statistical Society. Series B (Methodological)*, **55**(1), 3–23.

Smith, R. L. (1985). Maximum likelihood estimation in a class of nonregular cases. *Biometrika*, **72**(1), 67–90.

Snapinn, S., Chen, M. G., Jiang, Q. and Koutsoukos, T. (2006). Assessment of futility in clinical trials. *Pharmaceutical Statistics*, **5**(4), 273–281.

Stein, C. (1956). Inadmissibility of the usual estimator for the mean of a multivariate normal distribution. *Proceedings of the Third Berkeley Symposium on Mathematical Statistics and Probability*, **1**, 197–206.

Stigler, S. M. (1986). *The History of Statistics: The Measurement of Uncertainty before 1900*. Cambridge, MA: Belknap Press of Harvard University Press.

Stigler, S. M. (2007). The epic story of maximum likelihood. *Statistical Science*, **22**, 598–620.

Subkhankulov, M. A. (1976). *Tauberian Theorems with Remainder Terms*. Moscow: Nauka.

Su, J. Q. and Liu, J. S. (1993). Linear combinations of multiple diagnostic markers. *Journal of the American Statistical Association*, **88**(424), 1350–1355.

Suissa, S. and Shuster, J. J. (1984). Are Uniformly Most Powerful Unbiased Tests Really Best? *The American Statistician*, **38**, 204–206.

Tierney, L. and Kadane, J. B. (1986). Accurate approximations for posterior moments and marginal densities. *Journal of the American Statistical Association*, **81**(393), 82–86.

Tierney, L., Kass, R. E. and Kadane, J. B. (1989). Fully exponential Laplace approxima-tions to expectations and variances of nonpositive functions. *Journal of the Amer-ican Statistical Association*, **84**(407), 710–716.

Titchmarsh, E. C. (1976). *The Theory of Functions*. New York, NY: Oxford University Press.

Trafimow, D. and Marks, M. (2015). Editorial in basic and applied social psychology. *Basic and Applied Social Pschology*, **37**, 1–2.

Tukey, J. W. (1958). Bias and confidence in not quite large samples. *Annals of Mathe-matical Statistics*, **29**, 614–623.

Vexler, A. (2006). Guaranteed testing for epidemic changes of a linear regression model. *Journal of Statistical Planning and Inference*, **136**(9), 3101–3120.

Vexler, A. (2008). Martingale type statistics applied to change points detection. *Com-munications in Statistics—Theory and Methods*, **37**(8), 1207–1224.

Vexler, A. A. and Dtmirenko, A. A. (1999). Approximations to expected stopping times with applications to sequential estimation. *Sequential Analysis*, **18**, 165–187.

Vexler, A. and Gurevich, G. (2009). Average most powerful tests for a segmented regression. *Communications in Statistics—Theory and Methods*, **38**(13), 2214–2231.

Vexler, A. and Gurevich, G. (2010). Density-based empirical likelihood ratio change point detection policies. *Communications in Statistics—Simulation and Computa-tion*, **39**(9), 1709–1725.

Vexler, A. and Gurevich, G. (2011). A note on optimality of hypothesis testing. *Journal MESA*, **2**(3), 243–250.

Vexler, A., Hutson, A. D. and Chen, X. (2016a). *Statistical Testing Strategies in the Health Sciences*. New York, NY: Chapman & Hall/CRC.

Vexler, A., Liu, A., Eliseeva, E. and Schisterman, E. F. (2008a). Maximum likelihood ratio tests for comparing the discriminatory ability of biomarkers subject to limit of detection. *Biometrics*, **64**(3), 895–903.

Vexler, A., Liu, A. and Schisterman, E. F. (2010a). Nonparametric deconvolution of density estimation based on observed sums. *Journal of Nonparametric Statistics*, **22**, 23–39.

Vexler, A., Liu, A., Schisterman, E. F. and Wu, C. (2006). Note on distribution-free estimation of maximum linear separation of two multivariate distributions. *Nonparametric Statistics*, **18**(2), 145–158.

Vexler, A., Liu, S., Kang, L. and Hutson, A. D. (2009a). Modifications of the empirical likelihood interval estimation with improved coverage probabilities. *Communi-cations in Statistics—Simulation and Computation*, **38**(10), 2171–2183.

Vexler, A., Schisterman, E. F. and Liu, A. (2008b). Estimation of ROC based on stably distributed biomarkers subject to measurement error and pooling mixtures. *Sta-tistics in Medicine*, **27**, 280–296.

Vexler, A., Tao, G. and Hutson, A. (2014). Posterior expectation based on empirical likelihoods. *Biometrika*, **101**(3), 711–718.

Vexler, A. and Wu, C. (2009). An optimal retrospective change point detection policy. *Scandinavian Journal of Statistics*, **36**(3), 542–558.

Vexler, A., Wu, C., Liu, A., Whitcomb, B. W. and Schisterman, E. F. (2009b). An exten-sion of a change point problem. *Statistics*, **43**(3), 213–225.

Vexler, A., Wu, C. and Yu, K. F. (2010b). Optimal hypothesis testing: From semi to fully Bayes factors. *Metrika*, **71**(2), 125–138.

Vexler, A., Yu, J. and Hutson, A. D. (2011). Likelihood testing populations modeled by autoregressive process subject to the limit of detection in applications to longi-tudinal biomedical data. *Journal of Applied Statistics*, **38**(7), 1333–1346.

Vexler, A., Yu, J., Tian, L. and Liu, S. (2010c). Two-sample nonparametric likelihood inference based on incomplete data with an application to a pneumonia study. *Biometrical Journal*, **52**(3), 348–361.

Vexler, A., Yu, J., Zhao, Y., Hutson, A. D. and Gurevich, G. (2017). Expected P-values in light of an ROC curve analysis applied to optimal multiple testing procedures. *Statistical Methods in Medical Research*. doi:10.1177/0962280217704451. In Press.

Vexler, A., Zou, L. and Hutson, A. D. (2016b). Data-driven confidence interval estimation incorporating prior information with an adjustment for skewed data. *American Statistician*, **70**, 243–249.

Ville, J. (1939). *Étude critique de la notion de collectif. Monographies des Probabilités (in French)*. 3. Paris: Gauthier-Villars.

Wald, A. (1947). *Sequential Analysis*. New York, NY: Wiley.

Wald, A. and Wolfowitz, J. (1948). Optimum character of the sequential probability ratio test. *Annals of Mathematical Statistics*, **19**(3), 326–339.

Wasserstein, R. L. and Lazar, N. (2016). The ASA's statement on p-values: Context, process, and purpose. *American Statistician*, **70**, 129–133.

Wedderburn, R. W. (1974). Quasi-likelihood functions, generalized linear models, and the Gauss–Newton method. *Biometrika*, **61**(3), 439–447.

Whitehead, J. (1986). On the bias of maximum likelihood estimation following a sequential test. *Biometrika*, **73**(3), 573–581.

Wieand, S., Gail, M. H., James, B. R. and James, K. L. (1989). A family of nonparametric statistics for comparing diagnostic markers with paired or unpaired data. *Biometrika*, **76**(3), 585–592.

Wilks, S. S. (1938). The large-sample distribution of the likelihood ratio for testing composite hypotheses. *Annals of Mathematical Statistics*, **9**(1), 60–62.

Williams, D. (1991). *Probability with Martingales*. New York, NY: Cambridge University Press.

Yakimiv, A. L. (2005). *Probabilistic Applications of Tauberian Theorems*. Boston, MA: Martinus Nijhoff Publishers and VSP.

Yakir, B. (1995). A note on the run length to false alarm of a change-point detection policy. *Annals of Statistics*, **23**, 272–281.

Yu, J., Vexler, A. and Tian, L. (2010). Analyzing incomplete data subject to a threshold using empirical likelihood methods: An application to a pneumonia risk study in an ICU setting. *Biometrics*, **66**(1), 123–130.

Zellner, A. (1996). *An Introduction to Bayesian Inference in Econometrics*. New York, NY: Wiley.

Zhou, X. and Reiter, J. P. (2010). A note on Bayesian inference after multiple imputation. *American Statistician*, **64**, 159–163.

Zhou, X.-H. and Mcclish, D. K. (2002). *Statistical Methods in Diagnestie Medicine*. New York, NY: Wiley.

Zhou, X.-H., Obuchowski, N. A. and McClish, D. K. (2011). *Statistical Methods in Diagnostic Medicine*. Hoboken, NJ: John Wiley & Sons.

Zimmerman, D. W. and Zumbo, B. D. (2009). Hazards in choosing between pooled and separate-variance t tests. *Psiologica*, **30**, 371–390.

Zou, K. H., Hall, W. and Shapiro, D. E. (1997). Smooth non-parametric receiver operating characteristic (ROC) curves for continuous diagnostic tests. *Statistics in Medicine*, **16**(19), 2143–2156.

Author Index

Subject Index

Printed in the United States
by Baker & Taylor Publisher Services